Essentials for Health Protection

T0177674

Essentials for Health Protection
Four key components

Emily Ying Yang Chan
Assistant Dean and Professor,
Faculty of Medicine,
The Chinese University of Hong Kong
Visiting Professor,
Nuffield Department of Health,
The University of Oxford

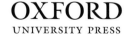

OXFORD
UNIVERSITY PRESS

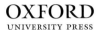

Great Clarendon Street, Oxford, OX2 6DP,
United Kingdom

Oxford University Press is a department of the University of Oxford.
It furthers the University's objective of excellence in research, scholarship,
and education by publishing worldwide. Oxford is a registered trade mark of
Oxford University Press in the UK and in certain other countries

Published in the United States of America by Oxford University Press
198 Madison Avenue, New York, NY 10016, United States of America

British Library Cataloguing in Publication Data
Data available

Library of Congress Control Number: 2019947974

ISBN 978–0–19–883547–9

Printed in Great Britain by
Bell & Bain Ltd., Glasgow

To my family, Eric, Ellie, Ernest, and Einstein, for their love and support

Contents

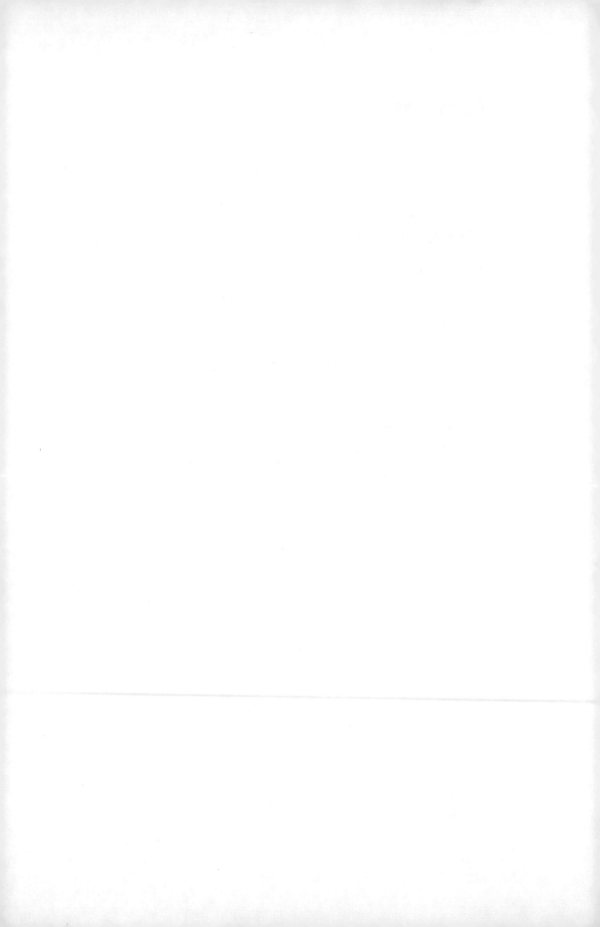

Foreword

Health protection is one of the three key domains of public health, together with health improvement and health services. It covers a long-established set of functions to protect individuals, groups, and populations from various hazards. In Hong Kong, the Centre for Health Protection was established under the Department of Health of the Government of the Hong Kong Special Administrative Region in 2004 to strengthen the capacity of Hong Kong's public health system to deal with various public health challenges. In addition to infectious disease control tracing back to John Snow's classic cholera outbreak study and environmental health exemplified in the UK Clean Air Acts of the 1950s, health protection has increasingly expanded into new grounds, covering new hazards. One of the new attempts to delineate the health protection practice is the document 'Health Protection Policy Toolkit: Health System Strengthening for Health Security', compiled by the Commonwealth Secretariat and Public Health Wales in 2016 for the Commonwealth Health Ministers Meeting, which was later updated as the 'Health Protection Policy Toolkit: Health as an Essential Component of Global Security' in 2017. Based on the Systems Framework for Healthy Policy as a suggested way for 53 Commonwealth member countries to coordinate and organize their health protection services, the toolkit aims to provide a comprehensive and practical resource for policy-makers to strengthen regional, national, and global health protection as part of an overall health system. It defines health protection as encompassing activities that ensure robust health security at local, national, and global levels, which cover four major components: communicable disease control, emergency preparedness and response, environmental health, and climate change and sustainability. The document argues that health protection services can prevent and manage disease outbreaks associated with pathogens and environmental hazard exposures, as well as increase resilience in coping with other emergencies and extreme climate change events.

Based on this framework and her expertise and experience in global health and humanitarian medicine and with the full support of The Chinese University of Hong Kong (CUHK) Jockey Club School of Public Health and Primary Care (JCSPHPC), Professor Emily Chan has addressed the key aspects in the four essential health protection components in this book. This is a very welcome effort. I believe that this book will help bring health protection practice and research up to date by revisiting classical and re-emerging infectious disease and environmental hazards and presenting new and emerging health hazards from climate change and more frequent natural and human-caused disasters and emergencies that are receiving increased attention from the Centre for Health Protection here in Hong Kong to the World Health Organization globally. Recent repeated outbreaks and extreme events in various parts of the world have reminded us the inadequacies of national as well as international health systems. As part of the effort to strengthen the wider health system, a comprehensive discipline of health protection will facilitate the provision of high-quality health services to populations from the local to the global.

I congratulate Professor Chan on her academic persistence in making this valuable reference work a reality and I recommend this book to students, practitioners, researchers, and policy-makers who share the vision of protecting human health from the major hazards of the globalizing world.

Eng-kiong Yeoh
Professor of Public Health,
Director JC School of Public Health and Primary Care,
The Chinese University of Hong Kong

Foreword

As a clinician, teacher, and researcher in infectious disease, tropical medicine, and global health, I fully support Professor Emily Chan's emphasis on the importance of health protection in the field of public health, as well as medicine in general. Professor Chan's new book, *Essentials for Health Protection: Four Key Components*, builds on her expertise and that of her team at the Collaborating Centre for Oxford University and Chinese University of Hong Kong (CUHK) for Disaster and Medical Humanitarian Response (CCOUC). Established as a joint research centre of the two universities and of the Nuffield Department of Medicine and CUHK Faculty of Medicine in 2011, CCOUC has excelled in research, education, and community knowledge transfer in emergency preparedness and response, as well as climate change and sustainability. These areas form two of the four key components of health protection as identified in the Commonwealth Secretariat policy document 'Health Protection Policy Toolkit: Health System Strengthening for Health Security' prepared for the Commonwealth Health Ministers Meeting in 2016. Defining health protection as encompassing activities that ensure robust health security at local, national, and global levels, and covering four major components—communicable disease control, emergency preparedness and response, environmental health, and climate change and sustainability—this document provides a useful framework for a comprehensive overview.

Using her expertise and experience in global health and humanitarian medicine, and supported by her CCOUC team and the newly established Division of Global Health and Humanitarian Medicine at CUHK Jockey Club School of Public Health and Primary Care (JCSPHPC), Professor Chan has examined the four key health protection domains in this globally oriented resource for students, researchers, practitioners, and policy-makers in health protection, as well as the four sub-fields from a global health perspective. As one of her academic collaborators, I am impressed by Professor Chan's energy. She has significant responsibilities in classroom and field teaching, research, knowledge transfer, and policy consultancy activities, ranging from school and university to regional and global levels. This new book is a timely and valuable contribution to the evolving field of global health. Professor Chan introduces the basic concepts and principles not only in the fields of emergency preparedness and climate change, where she is well recognized, but also in the traditional public health areas of communicable disease control and the developing global health subject of environmental and planetary health.

Addressing the four essential components of health protection beyond a particular nation in a single volume, this book will help readers develop a comprehensive view of the commonalities and differences across various domains of health protection. This will enable the reader to develop insights into understanding, mitigating, and reducing related health risks tailored to issues unique to their own countries and regions. I recommend this book as a very useful resource for students, practitioners, and policy-makers from health and non-health background alike, and essential for anyone seeking to understand health protection through the prism of global health and humanitarian medicine.

Christopher P. Conlon, MD, FRCP
Professor of Infectious Diseases,
Head of Department
Nuffield Department of Medicine,
University of Oxford

Acknowledgements

This content of this book originates from the teaching and research of public health, global health, and Health Emergency and Disaster Risk Management (Health-EDRM) conducted at the JC School of Public Health and Primary Care (JCSPHPC), The Chinese University of Hong Kong and Nuffield Department of Medicine, the University of Oxford. Case studies were developed based on activities and fieldwork of the Collaborating Centre for Oxford University and CUHK for Disaster and Medical Humanitarian Response (CCOUC) and Centre for Global Health in China and Asia. Through the academic research, consultancies, and the policy advisory role I have undertaken during the past decade, I realize that there is an urgent need for a textbook/reference document to describe the trans-national, interdisciplinary, and integrated approach to health protection that applies in the global context.

The author gratefully acknowledges the copyediting assistance and friendship of Mr Chi-shing Wong of CCOUC. The patience and professional facilitation from Ms Nicola Wilson, Ms Hillevi Sellen, their colleagues, and the supporting team at Oxford University Press are also deeply appreciated. My sincere gratitude goes to the generous support, trust, and encouragement from the two universities behind CCOUC, The Chinese University of Hong Kong (CUHK) and the University of Oxford, specifically to their former and incumbent Vice-Chancellors, Professor Andrew Hamilton, Professor Louise Richardson, Professor Joseph Sung, and Professor Rocky S. Tuan; the former and incumbent Deans of CUHK Faculty of Medicine, Professor Tai-fai Fok and Professor Francis Ka-leung Chan; the former and incumbent Directors of JCSPHPC, Professor Sian M. Griffiths and Professor Eng-kiong Yeoh; Interim Head of Department, Oxford University Nuffield Department of Medicine (NDM), Professor Chris Conlon, and last but not least, Mr Darren Nash, Associate Head of NDM.

My special thanks also goes to Professor Shui-shan Lee (Head of the Division of Infectious Diseases and Deputy Director of Stanley Ho Centre for Emerging Infectious Diseases, JCSPHPC) and Professor Shelly Lap-ya Tse (Head of the Division of Occupational and Environmental Health and Director of the Centre for Occupational and Environmental Health Studies, JCSPHPC) for their support for this book project, as well as to Professor William B. Goggins III and the Climate Change and Health Study group at JCSPHPC, Professor Samuel Yeung-shan Wong, Professor Henry Lik-yuen Chan, Professor Colin A. Graham, Professor Kin-fai Ho, Professor David Shu-cheong Hui, Professor Kevin K. C. Hung, Professor Jean H. Kim, Professor Kin-on Kwok, Professor Xiang-qian Lao, Professor Vincent C. T. Mok, Professor Virginia Murray, Professor Rajib Shaw, Professor Martin C. S. Wong, Professor Tze Wai Wong, Professor Justin C. Y. Wu, Professor May Pui-shan Yeung, Professor Ignatius Tak-sun Yu, Professor Benny C. Y. Zee, Ms Gloria Kwong-wei

Chan, Dr Peter Ka-hung Chan, Ms Carol Sin-yee Chiu, Mr Cheuk-pong Chiu, Ms Janet Yiu-wai Chow, Ms Sharon Chow, Ms Caroline Dubois, Ms Janice Ying-en Ho, Mr Keith Yun-chau Hon, Mr Zhe Huang, Ms Heidi Hung, Dr Ryoma Kayano, Ms Christine Pui-yan Ko, Dr Holly Ching-yu Lam, Ms May Hang-mei Lee, Mr Kevin Sida Liu, Mr Eugene Siu-kai Lo, Ms Hermione Hin-man Lo, Ms Asta Yi-tao Man, Ms Kaffee Ka-ki Mok, Ms Rosanna Tse-ying So, Dr Greta Chun-huen Tam, Ms Sophine Nok-sze Tsang, Mr Zhe Wang, Ms Carol Ka-po Wong, Dr Tony K. C. Yung, all students helpers at CCOUC, and staff members of the Division of Global Health and Humanitarian Medicine at JCSPHPC. Finally, my sincere appreciation is offered to my JCSPHPC colleagues, Professor Chok-wan Chan, Mr and Mrs Robert and Irene Che-yun Lee Yau, Professor and Mrs NK and Olivia Leung, and all friends who have assisted in the publication of this book for their encouragement, inspiration, support, assistance, and friendship. As always, special appreciation must go to Mr Eric S. K. Yau and our children, Ellie and Ernest.

Emily Ying Yang Chan
Hong Kong, April 2019

Case Contributors

Gloria Kwong Wai Chan, BSSc (CUHK), MSSc (CUHK) is a professional journalist by training. After spending years in political news reporting in Hong Kong, she joined the international medical humanitarian organization, Médecins Sans Frontières, as the Director of Communications for the organization's communication effort in Hong Kong, China, and South-East Asia. Her expertise was employed in the frontline of a number of emergencies over the world. Before joining the Collaborating Centre for Oxford University and CUHK for Disaster and Medical Humanitarian Response (CCOUC) in 2014, she was the Chief Executive of the Hong Kong Medical Association. Ms Chan currently serves as Deputy Director of CCOUC and is undertaking her doctoral degree study on co-production of health with reinforcement of social network on community level.

Peter Ka-hung Chan, BSc (CUHK), MSc (Oxon), DPhil (Oxon), AFHEA (UK), was initially trained in public health in the JC School of Public Health and Primary Care of The Chinese University of Hong Kong, University of Copenhagen, and Johns Hopkins Bloomberg School of Public Health. Subsequently, he obtained his MSc in Global Health Science and DPhil in Population Health from the University of Oxford. He is now a postdoctoral environmental epidemiologist working in Oxford. His research interests include household and ambient air pollution, climate change, non-communicable disease, and the application of multi-omics analysis in understanding environmental risk exposures.

Sharon Chow, BSSc (CUHK), MSc (HKU), was the CEO of Wu Zhi Qiao (Bridge to China) Charitable Foundation (2007–18). Since the inception of the Foundation in 2007, Ms Chow has been instrumental in shaping the mission, strategic development, and overall operation of the Foundation. Dedicated to blending modern green technology with traditional wisdom supported by in-depth research, the Foundation has supported comprehensive research and demonstrative sustainable building projects in rural China with regional significance and environmental and social impacts. Ms Chow served on the International Scientific Review Panel at the World Sustainable Building Environment Conference (2017) and on the Advisory Committee of Humanitarian Initiative in School of Public Health in CUHK (2009). She started her doctoral study in early 2019 with a focus on sustainability, housing, and health.

Caroline Dubois, BSc (UCL), MSc (UCL), was a research assistant at the Collaborating Centre for Oxford University and CUHK for Disaster and Medical Humanitarian Response in Hong Kong. She obtained her postgraduate degree in Global Health and Development and was previously a Project Officer at Gavi, the Vaccine Alliance, working on partner engagement for the immunization programme's technical assistance, with a focus on Francophone Africa.

Janice Ying-en Ho, BSc (U. Michigan), PhD Candidate (CUHK), is a third-year PhD candidate in Public Health at The Chinese University of Hong Kong. Previously, she has worked for the Collaborating Centre for Oxford University and CUHK for Disaster and Medical Humanitarian Response (CCOUC), World Resources Institute, and the World Green Organisation. She obtained her Bachelor's degree from the University of Michigan with a double major in environmental science and psychology. Her research interests include vulnerable populations and health impacts of climate change.

Zhe Huang, BMS (Guangzhou Medical University), MPH (CUHK), is a project officer at CCOUC with a particular focus on climate change and data analysis. He received his Master of Public Health from The Chinese University of Hong Kong, majoring in epidemiology and biostatistics, and he obtained a Bachelor's degree in public affairs management from Guangzhou Medical University in China. He has participated in field-based assessments and interventions in rural China. He started his doctoral study in 2018 with a focus on biostatistics and climate change and health.

Heidi H. Y. Hung, BSocSc & LLB (University of Hong Kong), MSt (Oxon), was trained as a policy-maker in the Hong Kong SAR Government after her study in international law as a Rhodes Scholar in Oxford. She has experience in global anti-poverty campaign as a Senior Manager in Oxfam Hong Kong. She is currently a PhD candidate in public health focusing on chronic diseases among the working poor, including their emergency preparedness.

Jean H. Kim, MSc, ScD, is Head and Associate Professor of the Division of Epidemiology, the Jockey Club School of Public Health and Primary Care at The Chinese University of Hong Kong (CUHK). Professor Kim is a social epidemiologist who has conducted extensive research in sociobehavioural topics related to globalization and health including addiction behaviours, reproductive and adolescent health. She was the former co-Director of the Master of Public Health programme at CUHK. Kim is currently active in regional alcohol policy research.

Kin-on Kwok, BSc, MPhil, PhD, is an Assistant Professor at the Jockey Club School of Public Health and Primary Care at The Chinese University of Hong Kong. Dr Kwok is an infectious disease epidemiologist and mathematical modeller with a focus on infectious disease epidemiology, surveillance, and infection control policy. His research interest is in understanding the transmission dynamics, epidemiology, and evolution of infectious diseases. His previous work has contributed to the understanding and control of SARS and influenza. He is currently active on multiple projects on antimicrobial resistance epidemiology and surveillance.

Holly Ching-yu Lam, BEng (CUHK), MSc (CUHK), PhD (CUHK), obtained her Master's degree in Department of Statistics at The Chinese University of Hong Kong and her PhD degree in the JC School of Public Health and Primary Care (JCSPHPC, CUHK). Her research interests are climate-related health issues and environmental epidemiology. She joined JCSPHPC in 2010. She worked on cancer epidemiological research projects and then switched to the environmental epidemiology team at the same school. Dr Lam completed her 3-year postdoctoral fellowship at the Collaborating Centre for Oxford University and CUHK for Disaster and Medical Humanitarian Response and mainly works on weather-, climate change-, and disaster risk-related health studies.

May Hang-mei Lee, BSc (CUHK), MPhil (CUHK), is currently a part-time doctoral student at the JC School of Public Health and Primary Care of CUHK with an interest in research related to nutrition, breast cancer, and cancer screening. She has conducted several research projects related to the nutrition for primary and secondary school students, as well as cancer patients, before joining the Hong Kong Breast Cancer Foundation (HKBCF). Currently at the HKBCF, she is responsible for managing the Hong Kong Breast Cancer Registry and conducts research on other breast cancer-related topics.

Hermione Hin-man Lo, BNurs (HKU), MScNurs (PolyU), PRCC (Intensive Care), completed her Master of Public Health student at The Chinese University of Hong Kong. She is a registered nurse who practised at Queen Mary Hospital before joining the Residential Care Home for Elderly at the Tanner Hill under the Hong Kong Housing Society. She is currently a Lecturer at the Nethersole School of Nursing at The Chinese University of Hong Kong. Her research interests include global public health policies in the ageing population and dementia care strategies.

Xiang Qian Lo, MB (Sun Yat-sen), MM (PUMC), PhD (HKU), works at the JC School of Public Health and Primary Care of The Chinese University of Hong Kong. His research focuses on air pollution and health. Professor Lao's research work has been widely reported in the media, greatly increasing public awareness of air pollution, and inspiring people to pursue better air quality. He was invited by the Hong Kong Government to join a working group responsible for reviewing Hong Kong's air quality standards and exploring possibilities for tightening these.

Asta Yi-tao Man, BA (Sarah Lawrence College), MPH (ISMMS), was a research assistant at CCOUC with an interest in mental health and communicable diseases in disaster settings. She received her Bachelor's degree in liberal arts and sciences, concentrating on microbiology and creative writing. She then went on to receive a Masters in Public Health in the United States, majoring in global health. At CCOUC, she conducted research on natural hazards and risk communication in Hong Kong as well as assisted international engagements pertaining to disaster risk reduction.

Shelly Lap-ah Tse, BMed (Fudan), PgD Dip. Occ. Hyg. (CUHK), PhD (CUHK), ICOH (member), FHKIOEH (fellow), is Head and Associate Professor of the Division of Occupational and Environmental Health and Director of the Centre for Occupational and Environmental Health Studies, the JC School of Public Health and Primary Care, The Chinese University of Hong Kong. She obtained her Bachelor of Medicine in Fudan

University and PhD degree at The Chinese University of Hong Kong. Professor Tse received further training in cancer epidemiology at the NCI/NIH in the United States and in occupational hygiene. She now serves as the Chairman of Advisory Committee/Environmental Hygiene (CUHK) and Vice-President of Hong Kong Institute of Occupational and Environmental Hygiene. Tse is the CUHK PI leader of tripartite collaboration with Utrecht University and University of Toronto on the exposome and public health, in particular shift work and circadian disruption. She enjoys close collaboration with NCI/NIH on breast cancer study and IARC/WHO regarding the SYNERGY Project on lung cancer. She received the Second Class Award of State Scientific and Technological Progress Award in 2014/2015 on silicosis, mechanisms, and prevention (4th), and has more than 170 research publications. Her main research interests are in occupational and environmental health and epidemiology.

Zhe Wang, MPH (Chinese Center for Disease Control and Prevention), is an Associate Professor in Public Health Emergency Center at the Chinese Center for Disease Control and Prevention. His research interest includes emergency preparedness and response for natural disaster. He has participated in many field relief operations in natural disasters at home and abroad including the Yushu earthquake in 2011, the Ludian earthquake in 2014, and the Nepal earthquake in 2015.

Carol Ka-Po Wong, BSSc (CUHK), MIPA (HKU), MPH (CUHK), is the Head of Training and Development at CCOUC with an interest in the care of older people in disaster settings. She has years of project management experience in NGOs in Asia, with a focus on slum health, and disaster risk reduction and response.

Chi Shing Wong, BSSc (CUHK), MSc (LSE), has a background in Journalism and Communication. Having worked as a journalist in a local English newspaper, he received his Master in Comparative Politics at the London School of Economics and Political Science, focusing on democratization, ethnic politics and nationalism with regional foci in China and Southeast Asia, and researched on political identity at the University of Oxford afterwards. Upon his return to Hong Kong, Mr Wong has worked in various teaching, research, and administrative positions at local academic institutions. Mr Wong is currently working as Publications Manager at the Collaborating Centre for Oxford University and CUHK for Disaster and Medical Humanitarian Response.

About the Author

Emily Ying Yang Chan, MBBS (HKU), BS (Johns Hopkins), SM PIH (Harvard), MD (CUHK), DFM (HKCFP), FFPH, FHKAM (Community Medicine), FHKCCM, serves as Professor and Assistant Dean (External Affairs) at the Faculty of Medicine, and Head of Division of Global Health and Humanitarian Medicine and Associate Director (External Affairs and Collaboration) at the JC School of Public Health and Primary Care, The Chinese University of Hong Kong (CUHK). She is Director of the Collaborating Centre for Oxford University and CUHK for Disaster and Medical Humanitarian Response (CCOUC), the Centre for Global Health (CGH), the Centre of Excellence (ICoE-CCOUC) of Integrated Research on Disaster Risk (IRDR), and Deputy Director of the CUHK Jockey Club Multi-Cancer Prevention Programme. Professor Chan is also Co-chairperson of the WHO Thematic Platform for Health Emergency & Disaster Risk Management (H-EDRM) Research Network, a member of the Asia Science Technology and Academia Advisory Group (ASTAAG) of the United Nations Office for Disaster Risk Reduction (UNISDR), and a member of the Third China Committee for Integrated Research on Disaster Risk (IRDR China). She serves as Visiting Professor (Public Health) at Oxford University Nuffield Department of Medicine, Honorary Professor at Li Ka Shing Faculty of Medicine, University of Hong Kong, and Fellow at FXB Center, Harvard University.

Her research interests include disaster and humanitarian medicine, climate change and health, global and planetary health, Human Health Security and Health Emergency and Disaster Risk Management (Health-EDRM), remote rural health, implementation and translational science, ethnic minority health, injury and violence epidemiology, and primary care. Awarded the 2007 Nobuo Maeda International Research Award of the American Public Health Association, Professor Chan has published more than 300 international peer-reviewed academic/technical/conference articles. She also had extensive experience as a frontline emergency relief practitioner in the mid-1990s, which spanned across twenty countries. Professor Chan was also awarded Caring Physicians of the World Award in 2005, Ten Outstanding Young Persons of the World Award in 2005, *National Geographic* Chinese Explorer Award in 2016, National Teaching Achievement Award of People's Republic of China in 2018, and nominee of the biennial United Nations Sasakawa Award for Disaster Risk Reduction in 2019. She is author/editor of numerous book titles and articles, including *Public Health Humanitarian Responses to Natural Disasters* (Routledge, 2017), *Building Bottom-up Health and Disaster Risk Reduction Programme* (Oxford University Press, 2018), *Climate Change and Urban Health* (Routledge, 2019), and *Disaster Public Health and Older People* (Routledge, 2019).

Chapter 1

Introduction

Health protection is one of the major knowledge themes in the field of public health. Its actions and approaches aim to prevent, protect, and manage health risks as well as diseases and environmental hazards (i.e. communicable and non-communicable diseases and injuries arising from environmental hazard exposures). Effective health protective measures may enhance well-being as well as improve individual and community resilience during health and emergency crises that cost substantial human life and provoke adverse health outcomes. Protection of health and well-being of individuals often constitutes the core commitments of national governments to their citizens and is central to the claims to individual liberty and rights in the argument of the betterment of the society (e.g. quarantine during disease outbreak or the ban on cigarette smoking). In global governance systems, International Health Regulations (IHR) (i.e. the existing international framework of health protection), the United Nations 2030 Agenda for Sustainable Development (i.e. Goal 3 of the Sustainable Development Goals), and the Sendai Framework for Disaster Risk Reduction are all examples of global policy commitments and agreements in health protection at the global level (Commonwealth Secretariat, 2017; United Nations, 2015; World Health Organization, 2016). Global consensus in health protection measures and policies often leads to effective actions in disease prevention (e.g. the global smallpox eradication campaign) and health improvement. Such international collaboration attempts also demonstrate common shared values and objectives of protecting people from potential preventable risks and harm.

To protect human health and well-being effectively, practitioners and policy-makers need to understand the causes and patterns of health risks, their related manifestations in disease outcomes, and the impact of them on human well-being. Similarly, the ability to analyse disease trends and patterns as well as the capacity to identify, plan, and implement appropriate measures provide important knowledge bases for devising solutions and approaches to protect the health and well-being of a population. Meanwhile, health protection requires multidisciplinary collaboration and action. With ever-changing human living contexts and health risks associated with modern living ecosystems, policies, and actions within the health sector alone will be insufficient to maximize prevention and responses for minimizing potential adverse impact on at-risk populations. Health protection in modern world calls on various sectors to work together and to identify the best way to minimize harm in a population.

Essentials for Health Protection: Four Key Components is a textbook for undergraduate and postgraduate students in medicine and public health who are interested in obtaining

Essentials for Health Protection. Emily Ying Yang Chan, Oxford University Press (2020).
© Oxford University Press
DOI: 10.1093/oso/9780198835479.001.0001

an overview of the key concepts, principles, and building blocks of health protection in public health practice. This book has four major objectives. First and foremost, it intends to provide an overview of the key public health concepts and principles that are essential to the examination of trends, issues, and approaches in health protection for the well-being of people in the twenty-first century. There is currently no relevant textbook that allows students of the subject to approach health protection systematically; existing publications tend to focus on the specialized and professional level that may deter learners from approaching the subject early in their career.

Second, this book also attempts to fill the current gap in the availability of relevant textbooks and reference materials that discuss health protection in a globalized human living environment. Most existing textbooks in this subject area either focus only on theories and concepts or use national policy and practice examples from a single country or region alone. Health protection, as discussed here, is based on an increasingly globalized reality that renders a single-country response/management approach ineffective in protecting people from potential preventable risks and harm.

Third, as illustrated in the book's contents, the determinants of health risks and factors that affect the efficacy of health protection are often inter- and multidisciplinary. Current education and knowledge systems are structured in a discrete and compartmentalized manner. Any cross-disciplinary learning and techniques may be hampered by the lack of relevant textbooks and reference materials that seek to enable interdisciplinary education efforts. Thus, in addition to its intended readers who might be students in health-related subjects and medical professionals who are interested in community health protection, this book also caters for the non-health professional and policy-maker who may be actively involved and engaged in health protection efforts. In addition, the discussion of how health protection practices might be linked to non-health sectors and the frontiers of health risks as consequences of socio-economic developments and technological advancements will be beneficial to a wider audience.

Finally, this book's discussion of new frontiers of health protection aims to tackle the latest challenges that might affect health protection. In addition to the discussion of the four main areas of public health protection including communicable disease control, emergency preparedness and disaster response, environmental health, and the impact of climate change on health, this book will also explore a number of dynamics and new health protection frontiers. Various text boxes and case examples are included throughout to illustrate the current status of health protection globally and impart the latest controversies and dynamics that might change the landscape and reality of health protection practices and development.

This book comprises nine chapters. Chapter 1 provides the background, objectives, and an overall description of the book's structure. Chapter 2 explains the main concepts and principles of public health relevant to understanding the topic of health protection and an analysis of the issues involved and approaches taken. Chapter 3 describes one of the five main topics of this book, namely the impact of climate change on human health. Climate change is arguably one of the most important global environmental changes that affects health protection in our living ecosphere (Chan, 2019). It is a complex topic that involves many academic disciplines. For students to appreciate how climate change might affect human health, it requires the understanding of a range of basic knowledge across a number of disciplines (such as physical, behavioural, political, and management sciences). The current education and knowledge system is structured in a discrete and compartmentalized manner that hampers cross-disciplinary learning and techniques. This chapter aims to describe how human health may influence and be affected by various impacts involved in climate change.

Chapter 4 describes the issues and approaches in emergency preparedness and responses in healthcare. When a disaster strikes, not only does it bring about direct human health consequences such as death and injury but it may also compromise health systems and health-maintaining lifeline infrastructures sufficiently enough to render affected communities vulnerable to secondary health risks and impact (Chan, 2017). Public health efforts, such as emergency preparedness and disaster responses, are often the key determinants to ensure survival and protection. This chapter explains how health protection efforts might be prepared, planned, and executed throughout the emergency cycle and might be mounted up to save lives. Chapter 5 discusses another important health protection topic, the control of infectious diseases. Communicable diseases, commonly known as infectious diseases, have repeatedly led to catastrophic consequences in human history (e.g. the Black Death in the thirteenth and fourteenth centuries and the Spanish flu in the twentieth century). Whilst a single chapter might be too superficial an attempt to explain the range of issues and frontiers of infectious diseases and their control, this chapter outlines the key principles, characteristics, and approaches in infectious disease control that matter in health protection. People and their environment are interlinked and the combination of health risks and human behavioural and environmental contexts poses potential harm to human health. These interfaces need constant monitoring through surveillance and evaluation to achieve the objectives of health protection. Chapter 6 reviews the key knowledge areas in environmental science and discusses how potential environmental factors might affect human health and well-being.

Chapter 7 explores the latest developments in concepts and theories in health protection. It explores the ideas of sustainability and planetary health. Although major scientific and technological advancement might provide more opportunities for improving quality of life, the sustainability of current patterns of consumption is being questioned. Specific emphasis is placed on how intergenerational justice in resources and decision-making might be associated with human health. Chapter 8 explicates and discusses the challenges of health protection that are likely to compromise the effectiveness of our ability to protect our well-being and ecosphere in the twenty-first century. Specifically, human population has been experiencing a mosaic of health transitions due to various changes of specific determinants such as demography, epidemiology, nutrition, urbanization, and energy (Caldwell, Findley, Caldwell, Santow, Crawford, et al., 1990). Not only have such changes affected human well-being but other living systems and the natural environments have been intimately affected too. Consequences of the changes will be likely to affect future generations. A new range of health protection challenges might result and new approaches in risk management such as Health Emergency and Disaster Risk Management (Health-EDRM, World Health Organization, 2019) require attention. Chapter 9 offers a conclusion.

This book is written to be an easily accessible reference to update healthcare professionals, non-health actors, and policy-makers on how an integrated public health approach may be used to conceptualize matters related to health protection. A better understanding of public health concepts may enable better appreciation and comprehension of the complexities that are associated with health risks, needs, and approaches to address the health protection challenges ahead.

References

Caldwell, J., Findley, S., Caldwell. P., Santow, G., Crawford, W., Brand, J., … Broers-Freeman, D. (1990). *What We Know About Health Transition: The Cultural, Social and Behavioral Determinants of Health*. Canberra: Australia National University Printing Services.

Chan, E. Y. Y. (2017). *Public Health Response in Emergency and Humanitarian Crisis*. London: Routledge.

Chan, E. Y. Y. (2019). *Climate Change and Urban Health: The Case of Hong Kong as a Subtropical City*. London: Routledge.

Commonwealth Secretariat (2017). Health protection policy toolkit: Health as essential component of global security. Available at: https://www.thecommonwealth-healthhub.net/wp-content/uploads/2017/05/HPToolkitwordversionEd2-CHMM-2017.pdf.

United Nations (2015). Transforming our world: The 2030 Agenda for Sustainable Development. Available at: <https://sustainabledevelopment.un.org/content/documents/21252030%20Agenda%20for%20Sustainable%20Development%20web.pdf>.

World Health Organization (2016). International Health Regulations (2005). Available at: <https://www.who.int/ihr/publications/9789241580496/en/>.

World Health Organization (2019). Health emergency and disaster risk management framework. World Health Organization.

Chapter 2

Core Principles of Public Health in Health Protection Practices

Health protection is a core technical competency in the public health discipline and for its practitioners. It encompasses activities and programmes that maintain health security at local, national, and global levels, protect the public from avoidable health risks, and minimize health impact of these risks. A number of chapters in this book highlight important health protection issues such as climate change and sustainability, emergency preparedness, communicable disease control, and environmental and planetary health. This chapter describes the key public health concepts that may be fundamental to understanding of health protection.

Public health

Definition of health and public health

As defined by the World Health Organization (WHO, 1946), 'health' is a state of complete physical, social, and mental well-being, and not merely the absence of disease or infirmity. Public health is a multidisciplinary subject that integrates various disciplines and practices. It encompasses three levels: individual, community, and global health. Public health involves research and practice in the prevention of diseases and the promotion of health in the general population. Public health differs from clinical medicine which focuses on disease management of individual patients. Nevertheless, both public health and clinical medicine share the emphasis on application of evidence-based medicine approach to conduct research and holding to the standard of patient-centred value in order to achieve the goal of good health.

Three domains of public health

Within the discipline of public health, there are three major domains of public health practices. **Health protection** involves prevention and control of diseases. Disease prevention can be classified into three levels: (i) primary prevention refers to preventing diseases from developing, which includes most health promotion and protection activities; (ii) secondary prevention involves taking measures to identify diseases early and prevent diseases from exacerbating once early symptoms have emerged; and (iii) tertiary prevention concerns curing or mitigating the symptoms of diseases and reducing clinical complication development, such as controlling and monitoring infectious diseases,

Essentials for Health Protection. Emily Ying Yang Chan, Oxford University Press (2020).
© Oxford University Press
DOI: 10.1093/oso/9780198835479.001.0001

environmental health, occupational health, and vaccination. **Health improvement** refers to processes that enable people to enhance their current health status, as well as controlling health risks and improving their own well-being. Its activities include health education, which encourages the public to healthy lifestyles. Examples include the promotion of a balanced diet, health education, and sex education. **Health services and management** covers how a healthcare system and its services are being organized. A majority of the population's health needs are fulfilled by primary care, which is the first point of contact for patients and their families in the healthcare system, provides patients with disease treatment and preventive care, as well as coordinating and integrating inter-professional healthcare services.

Measuring health and indicators for diseases

Health-impact pyramid

An agent or event may cause different impacts on an individual's health. For any situation, the most severe health impact is death. However, for most health-affecting events, although people develop symptoms, discomfort, and other health effects, a majority of these adverse health impacts may be resolved and relieved without specific care needs. Meanwhile, a proportion of the population may need to seek help or healthcare like over-the-counter medicine to relieve the discomfort. Some may seek primary medical help and the vulnerable (people with underlying health issues) may require professional healthcare or even hospitalization due to exacerbation of the underlying conditions (see Figure 6.8).

Frequently, Objective indicators such as hospital admission rates and mortality rate may reflect health impact. Conversely, data collection related to individual behavioural, self-help, and informal health support may be more difficult. For instance, patients with severe illness may not seek healthcare services provided by the government and they are not required to report their use of self-medication to any authority.

Determinants of health

Health outcomes are determined by multiple factors. Among the existing theories which explain factors affecting health, Dahlgren and Whitehead's 'determinants of health' (or 'rainbow diagram') is one most often applied. This framework highlights that health is the result of multiple factors. The innermost layer, also known as the non-modifiable risk factors, described biological traits such as age, gender, and genes that are unchangeable and might affect disease development of an individual or a target subgroup.

The subsequent outer layers of the framework are modifiable risk factors. Individual behavioural and lifestyle factors such as diet, physical exercise, and sleeping patterns might affect the well-being of an individual. These behavioural habits may be modified by psychological factors, education, information access, policies which can alter health risk, and disease manifestation. Social context and supporting networks may affect health outcomes because these social environments (e.g. family, peers, and neighbours) may influence environmental and behavioural context. **Social epidemiology** is the study of social determinants of the distribution of diseases within a population. Analysis of the various levels (micro: individual; meso: household; and macro: a large area) of characteristics will facilitate the better understanding of how outcomes might be associated with factors that might be modifiable. Social factors such as early life influences, food, stress, social status, exclusion, and support, work, unemployment, whether an individual is addicted to toxic substances, and access to transport are found to be directly associated with health (Wilkinson and Marmot, 2003). **Deprivation** might be in the form of material (e.g. income, which affects material access) and social (manifested in the employment and suboptimal living environment, e.g. social exclusion). People living in deprivation are found to be associated with poorer health outcomes, lower life expectancy, a high risk of addiction (tobacco, alcohol, drug), and a higher risk of contracting noncommunicable diseases. **Social capital** describes the social networks that support and strengthen health resilience and outcomes. It bonds and bridges members within and beyond community groups and may be considered at the micro, meso, and macro levels. Social capital, at all levels, is found to be associated with economic affluence, low crime levels, educational attainment, and good health (Lewis, Sheringam, Bernal, and Crayford, 2015). **Macro-determinants of health** such as globalization, economy, culture, religion, and environmental conditions are all important factors that affect health. Cultural factors might influence beliefs of disease aetiology and treatment options. The main theme of the 'rainbow diagram' is that except the innermost layer, all health determinants could be modified. Due to their interconnected nature, various layers of health determinants, including their risk factors and specific solutions, should be considered simultaneously when exploring a health issue (see Fig. 2.3, Chan, 2018).

Indicators for the burden of disease

There are a number of approaches in measuring health and the description of the disease burden. **Mortality rate** is one of the most common indicator for measuring population health. It refers to the proportion of people dying of a disease or a given incident in a particular population and reflects the peril deriving from a particular cause of death. It may also serve to reveal the level of healthcare vis-à-vis preventable death in a particular region. **Morbidity rate** refers to the proportion of people who are in an unhealthy state, physically or psychologically, in a given population. Three morbidity indicators are commonly used to describe the disease burden. **Prevalence** refers to the proportion of people in a given population who suffer from a particular disease. It is mainly used to measure the extent and state of distribution of a particular disease in a given population at a certain point of time. **Incidence** refers to the occurrence of new cases of disease or injury in a population over a specified period of time. Incidence is mainly used to measure the risk and trend of a certain disease in a particular population. **Disability-adjusted life years (DALYs)** is the indicator quantifies the years of healthy lifespan lost (YLLs) and the years lived with disability (YLDs) of an individual. It is calculated based on data including morbidity rate, mortality rate, average age of onset, and duration of a disease, assuming that the disease brings dire peril to health by way of shortening lifespan in terms of both early death and disability in terms of normal activities or work. It is one of the ways to measure and calculate the economic burden of a disease to a population. Another important concept related to the burden of disease is the concept of risk. **Risk** is the likelihood of event occurrence. It might be calculated as the proportion of individuals who are free of the disease at the time of the investigation, who might later develop the diseases. **Population attributable risk** (PAR) is the excess rate of disease attributable to the exposure to the risk or condition in a target population (including both exposed and non-exposed members).

Epidemiology and demography

When compared with previous decades, people live a longer and healthier life. With longer life expectancy, advances in medical technology, and scientific discoveries in medicine, health risk and disease patterns also evolve with demographic and socio-economic changes. **Demography** is the study of population structure and its trends. A population's characteristics (e.g. age, gender, and occupation choices) change with **births, deaths, migration**, and **ageing**, and these demographic drivers will in turn affect health, medical, and social needs. **Epidemiology** is the study of disease distribution in a population and risk factors determining the disease distribution and progression. In public health, epidemiology is a vital tool for describing and monitoring health risks factors and disease occurrence. Epidemiological studies may examine and reveal current and future public health threats and patterns.

Disease burden

Diseases might be categorized in different ways (e.g. by anatomical site or origin of diseases). Among these categorizations, 'communicability', namely being communicable and non-communicable, is the most frequently disease description used. **Communicable diseases**, also known as infectious diseases, are the major causes for morbidity and mortality in human history. These diseases transmit 'specific infectious agent (or its toxic products) from an infected person, animal … to a susceptible host, either directly or indirectly' (Guest, Ricciardi, Kawachi, and Lang, 2013, p. 166). Diseases may be transmitted among persons/animals. Disease occurrence is associated with by behavioural, social, environmental, and biological determinants of the susceptible community. Social and environmental changes from urbanized lifestyles, deforestation, and increased living density may also influence the infectious diseases burden at global level. A suboptimal health-enabling environment and health risk-associated behavioural patterns have rendered communicable diseases the largest public health threats for preventable child and adolescent mortality. Meanwhile, antibiotics overuse has created new, emerging communicable diseases, such as multidrug-resistant tuberculosis (TB) and vancomycin-resistant *Staphylococcus aureus* that affect individuals in developing and developing contexts alike. Increased international movements of people and expansion of international trade have also increased the risk of communicable diseases in developed communities.

Non-communicable diseases (NCDs) are diseases that do not pass among living entities or humans hence are not communicable in nature. Although non-communicable diseases represent a wide range of conditions, some common NCD characteristics exist. NCDs do not transmit from person to person. They tend to progress slowly and may lead to chronic or permanent illness. Their occurrence may be influenced by multiple risk factors and treatment for NCDs might require continuous and/or permanent, life-sustaining medical treatment, such as daily medication or kidney dialysis. Many of the NCDs have life-threatening acute complications such as brain haemorrhage from uncontrolled high blood pressure. Due to their cumulative and continuous medical cost, NCDs increase household economic burden (e.g. loss of employment/income) and health expenditure. Although NCDs can be both acute (e.g. stroke and accidents/violence) and chronic (e.g. hypertensions and diabetes), many common NCDs are chronic in nature. Medical services for NCDs require a range of health services and support, such as prevention, treatment, rehabilitation, and palliative care.

Globally, NCDs accounted for 71% (41 million) of total global deaths annually. Common chronic NCDs include cardiovascular diseases (e.g. coronary heart disease or stroke), hypertension, cancers, chronic respiratory diseases (e.g. chronic obstructed pulmonary disease), diabetes, mental health disorders, injuries, renal diseases, and chronic neurologic disorders (e.g. Alzheimer's, dementias, and epilepsy). Over 80% of all NCD deaths were caused by one of four NCDs: cardiovascular diseases (17.9 million); cancers (9.0 million); respiratory diseases (3.9 million); and diabetes (1.6 million). More than 75% of NCD deaths (32 million) occurred in low- and middle-income countries (WHO, 2018). In many developing countries, both communicable and non-communicable diseases remain as the double burden of healthcare needs.

Mental health problems are mostly non-communicable in nature and are prevalent worldwide and constitute more than 10% of the global burden of disease measured in disability-adjusted life years (DALY). Common mental disorders include depression, anxiety disorders, bipolar affective disorder, schizophrenia and other psychoses, dementia, and intellectual disabilities and developmental disorders including autism. Globally, reports indicate that an increasing number of people are reported to be affected by adverse mental health outcomes and there is a general increase in demand for public health intervention to address mental health needs. Meanwhile, unlike other non-communicable diseases, such as cardiovascular diseases or diabetes, there are many barriers to addressing mental health patterns and need adequately. Physical invisibility, lack of expertise, prejudice against, and stigma of people with mental illness have often buried the impact of mental health problems, resulting in their impact is often underestimated and individuals affected are neglected.

Injuries are important non-communicable diseases in the twenty-first century. They are commonly classified based on 'intentionality', divided into **intentional** (e.g. suicide, homicide, assault, and self-harm) and **unintentional** (e.g. traffic accidents, drowning, and falls) injuries. Intentional injury, which is often associated with violence, might be further classified into self-directed violence (suicide), or collective violence (war). Violence can result in injury, death, psychological harm, mal-development, or deprivation. Evidence suggests that there are demographic patterns associated with higher risks of injury sub-types. For example, injuries tend to be more prevalent among adolescent boys than girls. Furthermore, poisoning, drowning, burns, and maltreatment by caregivers affect pri-marily small children, while road traffic accidents, interpersonal violence, and sports injuries tend to affect older children and adolescents. Older people are more likely to experience household falls. Understanding the nature of diseases, injuries, and their asso-ciated risk factors is thus crucial for public health decision-making for health protection in planning and programme implementation. Furthermore, with limited resources, the understanding of national and global disease burden and trends can help prioritize the most needed interventions for the target population.

Development and health risk transition

As defined by the World Health Organization (WHO, 2009), health risk might be de-scribed as those factors which might raise the probability of adverse health outcomes and physical, mental, and social well-being of an individual or community. It should be noted that health risks changes with age (as described earlier as physiological changes occur throughout the life course) as well as environmental and circumstantial changes occur in living context through time. Major health risks changes with socio-economic develop-ment. For instances, traditional health risks might be associated with suboptimal hygiene and nutrition status and expose individual and community to unsafe water, infections, and nutritional deficiencies. With industrialization, economic, and social development as well as urbanization, health risks may evolve into risks that may evolve to associate with lifestyle, economic disparities, occupational hazards, and access to healthcare and services. The WHO has proposed public health interventions (e.g. vaccination), improved infra-structure (e.g. water, sanitation, electricity), scientific advancement and improvement in medical care, and population ageing might affect the type and extent of health risks (WHO, 2009; McCracken and Philips, 2017). Thus, with the diversity of population structure and stages of socio-economic development across the global communities, health risks should be viewed as combinations of specific risk factors in the context being studied.

Globalization and health

Globalization alters biological, environmental, and social factors that affect health and well-being of human population. For example, global population movements (e.g. travel) change the transmission risks of communicable and non-communicable diseases (e.g. cardiovas-cular diseases) and accidents. Case Box 2.1 describes the outbreaks of communicable dis-eases and the challenge they posed towards global public health security in this century.

Case Box 2.1 Globalization, Health Risks, and Protection

The following three cases described how globalization might affect major diseases transmission in populations around the world.

Case 1 Severe Acute Respiratory Syndrome (SARS)

In February 2003, an infected doctor from Guangdong Province, China visited Hong Kong Special Administrative Region for an academic conference and stayed in a hotel in the city. Since he came into contact with the hotel guests from all over the world (e.g. taking the same lift), it was hypothesized that infected contacts transmitted the viruses to other countries. Within four months, almost 4,000 diagnosed cases could be traced back to have contacted this Guangdong Province doctor (Fleck, 2003).

Case 2 Middle East Respiratory Syndrome (MERS)

In May 2015, South Korea reported its first case of Middle East Respiratory Syndrome (MERS). The patient was a Korean national who had visited four countries in the Middle East before the onset of the disease (Hui, Perlman, & Zumla, 2015). The condition was then spread across hospitals in Seoul and other districts in South Korea. By July, diagnosed cases was reported to be 186, with a death toll of 38 (Cho, Kang, Ha, Park, Lee, Ko, et al., 2016). Many countries issued travel warning subsequently and it costed major economic and tourism losses.

Case 3 Ebola virus disease

In March 2014, Ebola virus disease cases were reported in West Africa. The disease first appeared in Guinea, a West African country, and spread rapidly to Sierra Leone and Liberia, Guinea's two neighbours (World Health Organization Ebola Response Team, Aylward, Barboza, et al., 2014). Meanwhile, some infected people brought the virus to other West African countries including Senegal and Mali. An infected Liberian on vacation in the United States later received treatment and eventually died (Parmet and Sinha, 2015). Along with the confirmed case in the United States, there were also healthcare workers infected in Spain (World Health Organization, 2014a, 2014b, 2014c). The epidemic continued to spread till the end of 2014. The mortality rate of human infected cases in this major outbreak was about 50% (World Health Organization, 2019).

Public health approaches

Life-course approach

The life-course approach recognizes that human experience throughout the life course may contribute to well-being and health outcomes. It argues that functional (physical) capacity increases in childhood, peaks in early adulthood, and eventually declines with the ageing process. The WHO (2000) has proposed two main perspectives of how life course affect health. The first model assumes that there are critical periods in one's life and certain exposure and behavioural factors during specific periods might imply a lasting or lifelong impact on one's health and well-being. An example of such influences is detrimental exposure in the intrauterine foetal period, which might be the origin and lead to the development of diseases in later life. The second model describes the impact of an accumulation of risks. It suggests factors that might increase disease risks accumulate gradually over the life course. The cumulative impact or damage will increase with intensity and exposure duration in biological systems through the lifespan. Regardless of the models, the concept recognizes that health is influenced by contextual and dynamic experiences early in life and thus supports a health and social policy that enriches maternal and child health. The concept of 'life-course health development' (LCHD) has underlined some health policy and system developments (Halfon, Larson, Lu, Tullis, and Russ, 2014) and ageing health outcomes (Dannefer and Daub, 2009).

Pathway of care

This is a concept that illustrates how health needs may be addressed at various points of an individual's health journey. Activities/interventions might target 'health protection', 'disease prevention', and 'health promotion' in health risks to keep an individual free from disease. If the individual is affected by a condition, his/her healthcare experiences will progress through diagnosis, treatment, and rehabilitation, and finally, palliative care if he/she is in the terminal stage of a disease. Thus, attempts of health protection may target and implement a spectrum of services that ranges from disease prevention/protection to health promotion, diagnosis, treatment, rehabilitation ('tertiary prevention'), and palliative care (Chan, 2017).

Hierarchy of prevention

Hierarchy of prevention is the disease-prevention framework proposed by Leavell and Clark (1958). The concept may be applied to all aspects of health protection and disease prevention and classifies disease prevention into three broad levels: primary, secondary, and tertiary. **Primary prevention** typically targets both general and at-risk populations, aiming to prevent occurrence of disease through health protection and health improvement strategies. Health protection strategies include health screening, vaccination programmes, and enforcing regulations, legislation, and policies. Health improvement strategies encompass various population-based health promotion activities, such as health education to promote physical exercise and healthy diet. **Secondary prevention** generally targets high-risk population groups and aims to detect early, slow down, or stop existing disease progression or development of disability with prompt interventions, such as early screening, diagnosis, and treatment. **Tertiary prevention** targets those who have already been affected by a disease and aims to cure the disease or to reduce the risk of disability with therapeutic and rehabilitative measures. Services in this category include treatment, rehabilitation, and palliative care. In addition to the three prevention levels, **primordial** or **pre-primary prevention** has also become increasingly important for the conceptualization of health prevention practice, particularly in environmental health protection. Primordial prevention activities focus on reducing health threats and risks in general. For instance, environmental control measures seek to improve air quality and reduce potential environmental hazards, such as biological or chemical hazards (Davidson, 2013).

Principles of health promotion

Health promotion, as adopted at the Ottawa conference of the WHO in 1986, is defined as the process of enabling people to increase control over, and to improve, their health (WHO, 1986). It emphasizes that in order to reach a state of complete physical, mental, and social well-being, an individual or group must be able to identify and to realize aspirations, to satisfy needs, and to change or cope with the environment. The Charter specified ways in which actions could be taken to achieve 'health for all' around the world. Some basic prerequisites for health protection include creating supportive environments, enabling community participation, developing personal skills for health, reorienting healthcare services towards prevention and health promotion, and building wide-ranging public policies that protect the environment and promote health. Many theories have been developed to conceptualize health promotion approaches. Tannahill (1985) described three overlapping spheres of activity in health promotion, namely disease prevention, health education, and health protection.

Health promotion initiatives tend to promote universal interventions that reduce risks for the whole population versus target interventions in health protection efforts. Notably, **prevention paradox** describes the fact that although certain actions that might be taken to reduce disease risks across a population might be successful to reduce overall population risks, individuals might reap only minimum benefit from the population-based actions (Rose, 1981). It is thus important to publicize health promotion efforts carefully in order to understand its implication on different subgroups in a community (Hunt and Emslie, 2001). Failure to acknowledge the potential prevention paradox impact of interventions might lead to community mistrust or rejection of health promotion efforts.

Health education is one of the many approaches to achieve health promotion. Individuals and community groups receive their information and education not only from official planned channels (e.g. government, school systems) but also from informal communication such as friends, family, newspaper, the Internet, and the media. In addition to targeting people's beliefs, attitudes, and behaviour, health education should aim to enable individual to make informed decisions about lifestyle choices that may affect health and well-being. Appropriate settings for health promotion might improve effectiveness of health protection and well-being improvement. Some common settings for health promotion include school, workplaces, institutions (e.g. prisons), and healthcare settings. These settings can provide resources, structured information, and access to the target population for relevant health promotion goals.

There are a number of health promotion models (e.g. health-belief models, stages of changes, and theory of planned behaviour) which facilitate the understanding of behavioural patterns and identify appropriate approaches to address the promotion needs. These models, regardless of target of interventions at the intrapersonal, interpersonal, or community levels, aim to define the scope and aims of health promotion, improve understanding of the motivation behind individuals' behaviour, and facilitate the development of relevant health promotion programmes that address behaviours that are causing health concern. In addition to targeting behavioural changes through health education, health promotion might also apply levers at the community and national levels to create a supportive environment that alters the level of risk or enhances health promoting behavioural. *Banning* the availability of harmful products (e.g. alcohol or cigarettes), *restriction* of usage (e.g. smoke-free environments), sales (of illicit drugs), advertising, and information (legislation of tobacco advertisement, enforcing warning and labelling in products) all target availability and access to harmful products. At the national level, fiscal measures such as taxation and subsidies (for health-enhancing products such as fresh food and vegetables) may help address unfavourable externalities and creating the context in which health protection efforts may be implemented effectively.

Health system

To understand how public health may be protected and supported by a given system, it is necessary to understand what constitutes a 'health system'. According to the WHO (n.d.), a '**health system**' includes all units, individuals, and behaviours that aim to improve, resume, protect, and maintain health of the population. Conceptually, there are six main components in a health system. **Leadership and governance** concerns with the oversight, coalition, regulation, and policy of a country or region's health system. It describes how health system might be organized. As its structures vary across countries and regional context, governance and leadership may vary widely across countries. The second essential component in a healthcare system is the **healthcare financing structure**. The collection, allocation, and utilization of resources as well as risk management are important to a well-functioning health system. Potentially, financing mechanisms affect health outcomes and access to services. The third essential element is the **health workforce**. For a healthcare system to function efficiently, workers' competence in a range of skill specialization is required. Doctors, nurses, pharmacists, physiotherapists, and nutritionists all fulfil important roles and complement each other to address the healthcare needs of the community. The fourth core component includes **medical products and technology**, which include medical products, vaccines, medical technologies, and safety protocols and guidelines that ensure medical care of high quality, highly effective, and safe. Globally, the availability of medical products and technologies might be associated with economic capacity, education, and policies of a system. The fifth area is related to **information and research**. In the era of technology and innovation, the exchange and management of information, as well as the application of new findings in medical science, can improve people's health. A smoothly run health system can disseminate, reliably, timely, and effectively, any information and re- sults of scientific research relevant to determinants of health, health impacts, and the health system, thus enhancing good health in the community. Last but not least, the sixth element of a health system is **service delivery**. A high-quality health system can provide appropriate and comprehensive healthcare services, ranging from primary care and specialist treatment to recovery. In conclusion, the objectives of a health system are to address health needs and improve well-being in society, respond to the needs of society in terms of healthcare, en- sure that healthcare does not become a huge financial burden to patients, and increase the efficacy of services. The ultimate target is to achieve full coverage of healthcare and medical services, and maximize health and well-being of the entire population.

Levels of care

A well-organized health system can offer appropriate and comprehensive healthcare services along the pathway of care to prevent risks, protect well-being, and address needs. The ultimate aims of any health systems are to achieve full coverage of healthcare and medical services and to enhance the health of the entire population in society. To achieve these objectives, the healthcare needs of society needs to be addressed and service efficacy be enhanced without bankrupting the service system and household financial capacity. Health services include all service provision along the pathway of care, for example dealing with the diagnosis and treatment of disease, or the promotion, maintenance, and restoration of good health. Service provision re- quires inputs such as money, staff, equipment, and drugs; and good service delivery concerns quality, access, safety, and coverage. Effective and equitable service provision is possible when all the six building components are combined to allow the efficient delivery of high-quality, timely health interventions (see also the earlier discussion about 'health system'). Health service delivery may be categorized into three levels of health service provision. **Primary healthcare** (PHC), which comprises the main health and medical services in most developing countries, typically serves as the entry point to the health system and aims to provide basic packages of preventive and cura- tive health services to the population. These services might include health and nutri- tion education, health-maintaining habits (e.g. boiling water before drinking, washing hands after using the latrine); disease prevention (immunization, elimination of stag- nant water for vector-borne disease prevention); diagnosis and treatment of common diseases (injury, diarrhoea). Primary care providers may be healthcare workers such as general practitioners, nurse practitioners, or physician assistants. **Secondary healthcare** is usually provided in service facilities (outpatient or inpatient such as in hospital) that offer specialist medical care (e.g. surgery) and involves more elaborate and complex services (laboratory diagnosis) and treatment support. **Tertiary-level care** is highly specialized care on referral from primary and secondary healthcare for advanced medical investigation and treatment, such as organ transplant units, burns care units, etc. In many developing countries, these services are usually very limited and often only available in national-level hospitals.

Meanwhile, care for patents or the needy may be provided by informal healthcare procedures. In many communities and health systems, complementary and alternative treatments are considered **informal health practices**. Whilst these therapies might be different from conventional Western medicine and health models, they might constitute main health and service providers of the general population to address health needs and well-being maintenance. For example, in the United Kingdom, 31% of people took vitamin, minerals, and dietary supplements but more than 50% of these individuals never reviewed information or received advice about the underlying risks and benefits of consuming such supplements (Mchugh and Moon, 2008). Another important source of informal health-related help and care in a community is family care. **Family care** might be the most crucial care provider but frequently not accounted for or formally included at the level of care planning. **Self-help group(s)** are potential sources of medical information, social capital, and health assistant that may be organized by patient/stakeholder groups. These community groups typically aim to bridge the knowledge and information gap between professional availability and the desire to obtain information and experiences related to disease and care support. In addition, the **lay referral system** might also be used for social support and care provision, symptoms interpretation, and seeking advices for choice of care and providers (Friedson, 1959). Thus, an individual may experience a long time lag between becoming unwell and seeking professional help. With the rise of the Internet and electronic communication platforms (e.g. email systems), self-help groups for medical conditions appear to become more virtual and globalized (Lewis et al., 2015). Meanwhile, the dynamics of how these informal care systems might facilitate or hamper health protection and communication are yet to be examined.

Health protection

Ghebrehewet and colleagues (2016) suggest that health protection practices include three interrelated areas, namely **emergency preparedness, resilience, and response (EPPR); communicable disease control;** and **environmental public health** (Ghebrehewet, Stewart, Baxter, Shears, Conrad, et al., 2016). Emergency preparedness, resilience and response (EPPR) covers the prevention, investigation, control, and management of incidents and events that might have serious consequences to human well-being. Incidents might include but are not limited to natural disaster response, communicable diseases control, human-caused incidents, and complex emergencies (war/conflict) responses. The discussion of emergency preparedness is often multidisciplinary and requires a continuous effort throughout the normal, impact, and recovery period (see Chapter 4). Communicable diseases control (see Chapter 5) concerns the prevention, investigation, control, and management of communicable diseases. In the globalized context, communicable disease control requires functional local and national systems as well as international cooperation and agreements. Environmental public health (see Chapter 6) includes prevention and addresses health risks or threats resulting from natural and human-made environment. Environmental issues are often complex and dynamic in nature. They may lack specific definition or solutions and present as physical, psychological, and social health impact of a potential environmental hazard (e.g. water source pollution, power lines construction, etc.). In recent years, one of the most prominent environmental health concerns is the development of health protection practices and discussion relates to **climate change**, **sustainability**, and **health**.

Conceptually, the management of health risks and hazards may have similar principles. An 'all-hazard approach', is advocated by the WHO (World Health Organization Regional Office for Europe, n.d.) to address health protection in a community. Activities and policies related to public health risk and hazard management might be implemented in four major areas, namely planning and preparedness, prevention and early detection, investigation and control, and overall public health management and leadership (Ghebrehewet et al., 2016).

Planning and preparedness

Strategies and plans may be developed to prevent and mitigate health risks and threats from communicable disease, pollution, and environmental risks. Moreover, susceptibility and impact on individuals varies with age, underlying health status (e.g. immunocompromised individuals), and socio-demographic factors. To plan for health protection, various conceptual pathways might be used. For communicable diseases, the agent (e.g. infectious agent) host (people) environment (e.g. displacement camp and urban area) pathway can be a key framework that can underlie planning. For environmental health concerns, source (e.g. pollution) pathway (e.g. biological involvement-ingesting, inhalation) receptor (human) framework may help facilitate discussion and preparedness. For EPPR and climate related-health concerns, both these conceptual pathways may be useful. In addition to identifying a planning framework, partnership and platforms for communications and action planning would need to be established and maintained. Risk registries, surveillance systems, community education and promotion, and the multidisciplinary learning platform could enable coordination and implementation. Contingency plans and community drills/exercise for evacuation may also be important approaches to address various extreme event risks related to EPPR (Chan, 2017).

Prevention and early detection

In public health practices, there are a number of approaches to facilitate prevention and early detection of public health risks. Vaccination campaigns, clean water provision, sewage, and waste disposal management, as well as health education and hygiene promotion are some examples of prevention activities aiming to confine health hazards to achieve health protection for communities. Surveillance report review, fire alarms, and air-quality monitoring are some examples of early hazard detection mechanisms to minimize the health impact of a health threat to communities.

Investigation and control

Investigation and control are common practices in communicable disease control and health risk management arising from emergencies and environmental health concerns. Control measures may range from isolation to quarantine and banning of products that might cause health threats. Other initiatives include the provision of prophylaxis, public health advices, basic essential services, and material support to maintain health and well-being (including water and sanitation, food and nutrition, shelter and non-food items, health services, and information) (Bolton and Burkle, 2013; Chan, 2017).

Management and leadership

Whilst various actions are implemented by multi-disciplinary actors in an attempt to address health protection, leadership, terms of references, and clear management structure are important elements to ensure health protection actions and policies are effective.

Science and hierarchy of evidence in health protection

The paradigm of evidence-based policy and programme has underlined public health practice in the twenty-first century. However, whilst research efforts are being promoted to generate evidence to support health protection programmes, many of such research outcomes may not be directly translatable to actual policy and practice. The public health relevance of research should be clearly mapped out during research planning and design stage. Well-developed research planning and findings might inform intervention programme options, approaches, strategies, development, programme implementation, and monitoring. Research findings might also serve to refine existing knowledge and develop new theories to address evolutionary needs associated with health protection in modern life (see Chapter 9).

Hierarchy of evidence may guide evidence implementation to support health protection in the community. Systematic review and meta-analysis, randomized control trials (RCTs), cohort studies, case control, cross-sectional surveys, case series, and case reports are the most common research designs that generate scientific evidence to support health protection efforts. Among these study designs, meta-analysis design, which combines multiple related study trials with similar quality studies to examine exposure and outcomes, represents research evidence of the highest quality available for understanding the problem/issue of concern. Nevertheless, only limited topics in specific study areas have enough available published studies to synthesize evidence for meta-analysis studies. For new emerging medical and health risks as well as contexts, there may be no existing studies or experiences available to inform public health protection decisions.

Depending on research questions and available information/data, specific study designs may have to be used to answer a research question. When a topic of interest is to be examined by different research designs, the adoption of an evidence ranking system to assess quality and evidence robustness might be instrumental in differentiating the quality of evidence for policy/programme choices (OCEBM Levels of Evidence Working Group, 2016). Regardless of topics, another important research objective related to health protection and assessment of risks are related to causation and association. A statistical association does not necessary mean causation; to ascertain the causal link between two variables/concerns, temporality (sequence of events, the events must precede effect), strength, consistency, specificity, biological gradient, plausibility, coherence, experimental, and analogy are the nine major criteria to be fulfilled (Hill, 1965). Thus, although statistical association might reflect relationship between exposure and outcome, such relationship might arise from bias, chance, and confounding factors, and the direction of relationship (e.g. reverse causality) cannot be determined.

Regardless of research design, the interpretation and implication of study findings must also take into account the issue of **ecological fallacy** because results indicated by aggregate population data may not applied to individuals. When trying to understand the impact of health in a small, local area, the prevalence and risks of a particular disease may be vastly different from the prevalence in regional/national level. Thus, even though extrapolating national-level health survey data may offer insights on local context, extra efforts (e.g. commissioned research of local study) might be important. In addition, although it is beyond the scope of this book to discuss research quality, health protection practitioners should at least be aware of and learn about the latest ongoing research findings and how these findings may be implemented in practice.

Conclusion

Health protection is a core competency in public health practice. Although this chapter highlights only some of the core principles in public health, these concepts are useful ideas and frameworks for understanding the health risks and challenges related to health protection discussed in the next chapters of the book.

References

Bolton, P., and Burkle, F. M. (2013). Emergency response. In C. Guest, W. Ricciardi, I. Kawachi, and I. Lang (eds), *Oxford Handbook of Public Health Practice* (3rd edn). Oxford University Press, pp. 210–21.

Chan, E. Y. Y. (2017). *Public Health Humanitarian Responses to Natural Disasters*. London: Routledge.

Chan, E. Y. Y., (2018). *Building Bottom-Up Health and Disaster Risk Reduction Programmes*. London: Oxford University Press.

Cho, S. Y., Kang, J. M., Ha, Y. E., Park, G. E., Lee, J. Y., et al. (2016). MERS-CoV outbreak following a single patient exposure in an emergency room in South Korea: an epidemiological outbreak study. *Lancet 388*(10048) 3–9.

Dannefer, D. and Daub, A. (2009). Extending the interrogation: Life span, life course, and the constitution of human aging. *Advances in Life Course Research 14*(1) 15–27.

Davidson, W. (2013). Principles of prevention: The four stages theory of prevention. Available at: https://www.academia.edu/10916848/Principles_of_Prevention_The_Four_Stages_Theory_of_Prevention_PDF_File?auto=download.

Fleck, F. (2003). How SARS changed the world in less than six months. *Bull World Health Organ 81*(8) 625–6.

Friedson, E. (1959). Specialties without roots: The utilization of new services. *Hum Organ 18*(3) 112–16.

Ghebrehewet, S., Stewart, A. G., Baxter, D., Shears, P., Conrad, D., et al. (2016). *Health Protection Principles and Practice*. Oxford: Oxford University Press.

Guest, C., Ricciardi, W., Kawachi, I., and Lang I. (eds) (2013). *Oxford Handbook of Public Health Practice* (3rd edn). Oxford: Oxford University Press.

Halfon, N., Larson, K., Lu, M., Tullis, E., and Russ, S. (2014). Lifecourse health development: Past, present and future. *Matern Child Health J 18*(2) 344–65.

Hill, A. B. (1965). The environment and disease: Association or causation? *J R Soc Med 58* 296–300.

Hunt, K. and **Emslie, C.** (2001). Commentary: The prevention paradox in lay epidemiology-Rose revisited. *Int J Epidem 30*(3) 442–6.

Hui, D. S., **Perlman, S.**, and **Zumla, A.** (2015). Spread of MERS to South Korea and China. *Lancet Respiratory Medicine 3*(7) 509–10.

Leavell, H. R. and **Clark, E. G.** (1958). *Preventive Medicine for the Doctor in his Community: An Epidemiologic Approach* (2nd edn). New York, NY: McGraw-Hill.

Lewis, G., **Sheringam, J.**, **Bernal, J. L.**, and **Crayford, T.** (2015). *Mastering Public Health: A Postgraduate Guide to Examinations and Revalidation* (2nd edn). Boca Raton, LA: CRC Press.

McCracken, L. and **Phillips, D. R.** (2017). *Global Health: An Introduction to Current and Future Trends* (2nd edn). London: Routledge.

McHugh, S. and **Moon, N.** (2008). *Consumer Consumption of Vitamin and Mineral Food: Consumer of Vitamin and Mineral Food Agency*. London: Centre Office of Information.

Oxford Centre of Evidence-Based Medicine Levels of Evidence Working Group (2016). The Oxford 2011 Levels of Evidence. Available at: http://www.cebm.net/index.aspx?o=5653.

Parmet, W. E. and **Sinha, M. S.** (2015). A panic foretold: Ebola in the United States. *Critcal Public Health 27*(1) 148–55.

Rose, G. (1981). Strategy of prevention: Lessons from cardiovascular disease. *Br Med J 282*(6279) 1847–51.

Tannahill, A. (1985). What is health promotion? *Health Ed J 44*(4) 167–8.

Wilkinson, R. and **Marmot, M.** (eds). (2003). *Social Determinants of Health: The Solid Facts* (2nd edn). Copenhagen: WHO. Available at: http://www.euro.who.int/__data/assets/pdf_file/0005/98438/e81384.pdf.

World Health Organization (n.d.). Health systems strengthening: Glossary. Available at: http://www.who.int/healthsystems/hss_glossary/en/index5.html.

World Health Organization (1946). Constitution of the World Health Organization. Available at: http://apps.who.int/gb/bd/PDF/bd48/basic-documents-48th-edition-en.pdf#page=7.

World Health Organization. (1986). The Ottawa Charter for Health Promotion. Available at: https://www.who.int/healthpromotion/conferences/previous/ottawa/en/.

World Health Organization (2000). The implications for training of embracing: A life course approach to health. Available at: http://www.who.int/ageing/publications/lifecourse/alc_lifecourse_training_en.pdf.

World Health Organization (2009). Global health risks: Mortality and burden of disease attributable to selected major risks. Available at: https://www.who.int/healthinfo/global_burden_disease/GlobalHealthRisks_report_full.pdf.

World Health Organization. (2014a). Ebola situation in Senegal remains stable. Available at: https://www.who.int/mediacentre/news/ebola/12-september-2014/en/.

World Health Organization. (2014b). Ebola virus disease—Spain. Available at: https://www.who.int/csr/don/09-october-2014-ebola/en/

World Health Organization (2014c). Mali confirms its first case of Ebola. Available at: https://www.who.int/mediacentre/news/ebola/24-october-2014/en/.

World Health Organization (2018). Noncommunicable diseases. Available at: http://www.who.int/news-room/fact-sheets/detail/noncommunicable-diseases.

World Health Organization. (2019). Ebola virus disease. Available at: https://www.who.int/en/news-room/fact-sheets/detail/ebola-virus-disease.

World Health Organization Ebola Response Team, Aylward, B., Barboza, P., et al. (2014). Ebola virus disease in West Africa—the first 9 months of the epidemic and forward projections. *N Engl J Med 371*(16) 1481–95.

World Health Organization Regional Office for Europe (n.d.). Disaster preparedness and response: Policy. Available at: http://www.euro.who.int/en/health-topics/emergencies/disaster-preparedness-and-response/policy.

Chapter 3

Climate Change and Health

Climate change poses one of the biggest public health threats in the twenty-first century. According to estimates by World Health Organization, climate change will lead to excess annual deaths of 250,000 between 2030 and 2050. Direct health impact of climate change includes changing patterns of respiratory and cardiovascular diseases and morbidity and mortality as a result of more frequent and severe extreme temperatures. Climate change also have indirect health impact by facilitating the breeding of mosquitoes as vectors of diseases such as malaria and dengue fever and reduce access to clean water and food supply. Adaptation and mitigation are the two main approaches to alleviate and manage the health risks of climate change to achieve climate-resilient pathways for sustainable development.

Overview of climate change

Weather and climate

Weather is how the atmosphere behaves at a specific time and location, and it has variations such as snow, rain, typhoons, and the temperature. **Climate** is the synthesis of weather conditions in a given area, defined by the collation of long-term statistics of the meteorological elements in that area (World Meteorological Organization, 1992a).

Climate change and global warming

The United Nations Framework Convention on Climate Change (UNFCCC) defines climate change as a change of climate that is attributed directly or indirectly to human activity that alters the composition of the global atmosphere and that is in addition to natural climate variability observed over comparable time periods (United Nations, 1992). According to the Intergovernmental Panel on Climate Change (IPCC), climate change refers to a change in the state of the climate that can be identified (e.g. using statistical tests) by changes in the mean and/or the variability of its properties, and persists for an extended period, typically decades or longer (IPCC, 2007a).

The level of carbon dioxide in the atmosphere has increased 40% since the Industrial Revolution. The major cause is the extensive burning of fossil fuels closely followed by deforestation (IPCC, 2013). **The greenhouse effect** is a natural process that maintains the energy balance of the Earth's climate system. About one-third of the solar energy that reaches the top of the Earth's atmosphere is reflected back into space and dispersed. The remaining two-thirds is absorbed by the Earth's surface. The Earth radiates the energy

Essentials for Health Protection. Emily Ying Yang Chan, Oxford University Press (2020).
© Oxford University Press
DOI: 10.1093/oso/9780198835479.001.0001

Table 3.1 The Major Anthropogenic Greenhouse Gases that Increase the Greenhouse Effect

Greenhouse gases	Sources
Carbon dioxide, CO_2	Industries that burn fossil fuels, including energy industry, commercial industries, the transportation industry, and domestic use.
Methane, CH_4	Mining, energy industry, agricultural and farming, waste landfill and disposal, etc.
Nitrous oxide, N_2O	Agricultural (especially the use of fertilizer containing nitrogen), energy industry, waste disposal, etc.
Hydrofluorocarbons, HFCs	Domestic and commercial refrigerators, etc.
Tropospheric ozone, O_3	Vehicles, commercial industries, energy industry, etc.

back into space after the planet's surface gets warm. Much of the solar energy is absorbed by the greenhouse gases in the atmosphere, which increase the air temperature to keep the Earth surface temperature at around 14 °C. If there were no greenhouse gases the surface temperature would drop to –19 °C which is not suitable for human life.

Global warming is the common term used for climate change. Specifically, it refers to the increase of the Earth's average surface temperature caused by human activity which releases greenhouse gases. The Earth's surface is wrapped in a layer of gases that make up the atmosphere. Among all the components, carbon dioxide, methane, and nitrous oxide have increased due to human activities and the increase will boost the greenhouse effect and worsen global warming (see Table 3.1). **Global warming** occurs when the atmospheric greenhouse gases concentration increases sharply and more of the energy emitted from Earth surface is reflected back to the surface by the atmosphere. This phenomenon exacerbates the greenhouse effect and increases the surface average temperature (Elder, n.d.). Two main factors are assumed to have caused climate change. These include natural and anthropogenic factors. Natural factors include changes in Earth's orbit around the Sun, changes in oceanic circulation, and the El Niño and La Niña phenomena. Anthropogenic factors that based on human activities, such as burning fossil fuels which affects the proportion of gases in the atmosphere, have also changed elements in the climate system and can result in change of global climate patterns.

Important phenomena of climate change

Through direct surveys and Radar Satellite Remote Sensing Technology, scientists have observed that the Earth's current climate differs from that of previous centuries and becomes increasingly erratic. Four important phenomena of climate change include changes in ambient temperature, rainfall pattern, sea-level rise, and frequencies of extreme weather events.

Average temperature changes and the increase in extreme temperature events

Since the start of twentieth century, most regions globally have been affected by the rise in average temperatures. The average surface temperature has risen 0.85 °C (IPCC,

2013) over the past 100 years. Although there is an overall global temperature increase, cold air from the North Pole also invades the low-latitude districts, leading to severe cold spells. Overall, global human communities are experiencing more hot days, but also unexpected extreme temperature events.

Change of precipitation patterns

Global warming has a direct impact on precipitation. When the temperature increases by 1 °C, the air can contain approximately 7% more water vapour. As the total content of water vapour in the atmosphere increases, the global average precipitation changes. The change in annual average precipitation from 1951 to 2010 is more significant marked than the change from 1901 to 2010. The frequency and intensity of heavy rain has also increased. Heavy rain may present intense precipitation in a particular region which is far higher than the annual average for that region at that time. However, as heavy rain is usually a single event, it is not equal to the increase of total precipitation in a certain region (IPCC, 2014). For drought-prone areas, one episode of heavy precipitation may not be able to relieve scarcity and perennial water insecurity.

Sea-level rise

Coastal and low-lying areas may be flooded by the rising level of sea water, which also leads to general destruction of infrastructure (seawater intrusion), contamination of freshwater sources, and soil salinization (IPCC, 2013). Since the start of the twentieth century, the global average sea level has risen by 1.7 mm each year (IPCC, 2007b). Sea levels have been rising faster over the past 160 years than the average increase in levels over the previous 2,000 years. This phenomenon poses a huge threat to the economic, social, and environmental context in coastal areas (IPCC, 2007b). There are three main reasons that cause the rise in sea levels, namely ocean warming, glacier and ice-sheet melting, and increased depletion of underground water stores. **Ocean warming** (thermal expansion) occurs as the globe gets warmer, seawater is heated and expands. It was estimated that 50% of sea-level rise happens because of this effect. **Glaciers** form when there is year-round snow which gathers and turns into ice and they can melt in the summer. Global warming speeds up the snow melt rate and diminishes snow which upsets the balance of glacier accumulation and melting. Glaciers melting causes more fresh water to flow to the ocean. **Increasing depletion of underground water supplies** due to the increasing amount of underground water extracted for agricultural, industrial, and domestic water usage allows this water to finds its way into rivers and ends up flowing into the sea, leading to a rise in sea levels.

Extreme climate-related events and disasters

Climate change phenomena, such as temperature increases, sea-level rise, and extreme precipitation cause more large-scale natural hazards (such as storm, flooding, and drought, refer to Chapter 4) that tend to affect extensive geographic areas and human population.

Drought

Drought refers to either a prolonged absence or marked deficiency of precipitation, or a period of abnormally dry weather sufficiently prolonged for the lack of precipitation to cause a serious hydrological imbalance (World Meteorological Organization, 1992b). In general, drought may happen when there is no rainfall for a long period of time, the demand of water exceeds its supply, or usable water resources are polluted.

Flooding

Flooding concerns the impact of flood waters on humans and the environment and is defined as (i) the overflowing by water of the normal confines of a watercourse or other body of water; or (ii) the accumulation of drainage water over areas which are not normally submerged (World Meteorological Organization, 2012). Apart from consistent heavy rain, anthropogenic, topographic, and other climatic factors also cause flooding.

Relationship between globalization and climate change

The problems brought about by climate change have become more frequent and their impacts are affecting multiple countries. Climate change has thus become the most important global issue this century. **Intergenerational environmental justice**, population movement, economic impact, sustainable development, insecurity in water resources and food production crises, and the increase in the risk of infectious diseases are some key globalized climate change impacts that affect human well-being.

Environmental justice is one of the main challenges to **sustainability** since the Industrial Revolution. Humans have been generating a huge volume of greenhouse gases in their economic activities. Developed countries have been contributed to the largest amount of greenhouse gases, while developing countries have to suffer a higher risk of disaster due to their geographical location and lack of resources. **Climate change-related events** can have a severe impact on human health. For example, in 2015, São Paulo in Brazil was affected by severe drought and local citizens conserved water in various containers (e.g. buckets, swimming pools), but without a cover these containers were ideal breeding grounds for mosquitoes and increased the risk of dengue fever. A total of 563 confirmed cases and 17 death cases from dengue fever were recorded during that urban drought period in Brazil (Jelmayer and Chao, 2015). Climate change also provokes natural disasters which lead to people losing their homes and livelihood and becoming environmental refugees. The United Nations Environment Programme describes environmental refugees as people 'who have been forced to leave their traditional habitat, temporarily or permanently, because of a marked environmental disruption (natural and/or triggered by people) that jeopardised their existence and/or seriously affected the quality of their life' (El-Hinnawi, 1985). According to data released by the United Nations Office for Disaster Risk Reduction (UNISDR) in 2015, the global economy lost US$1.4 trillion between 2005 and 2014 due to natural disasters (see Figure 3.1 and Case Box 3.1), a majority of which were climate-related.

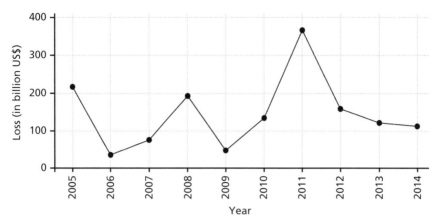

Figure 3.1 The economic impact of disasters from 2005 to 2014

Source: Data from United Nations Office for Disaster Risk Reduction. (2015). The economic and human impact of disasters in the last 10 years. Available at: <http://www.unisdr.org/files/42862_economichumanimpact20052014uni sdr.pdf>

The impact of climate change on public health and determinants of health

Although climate change may bring some health benefits—for example, a decrease in the mortality rate in winter in cold regions—its global health impact is largely negative. Apart from the casualties and related diseases directly caused by extreme weather, climate change also poses a threat to human health by altering various health determinants. Food production, the quality and quantity of the water supply, air quality, and the resilience of medical and public health infrastructure all are indirectly affected by climate and will influence health outcomes (see Tables 3.2 and 3.3).

Case Box 3.1 Climate Change Refugee: The Movement of Tuvalu

The Western Pacific island nation of Tuvalu was the first country to announce the nationwide relocation of its population due to rising sea levels. Tuvalu, located in Oceania, is only 4 metres above sea level which has been rising 5 mm per year since 1993 according to satellite images. It is estimated that the sea level will cover more than half the land by 2050. Since 2002, Tuvaluans have been moving to New Zealand due to climate change and the New Zealand Government has considered accepting some in the name of 'climate change refugees'.

Sources: Bedford and Bedford (2010); Australian Bureau of Meteorology and Commonwealth Scientific and Industrial Research Organisation (2011); Australian Government (August 2012).

Table 3.2 Climate Change and the Determinants of Health

The determinants of health	Expected changes	Health risks
Environmental conditions	◆ Overall global average ambient temperature rise and increase in frequency and intensity of extreme temperature ◆ Changes in the distribution and transmission of infectious diseases due to extreme temperature, humidity, and rainfall	◆ Extreme hot and cold weather events leading to an increase in the incidence rate of disease and mortality ◆ The increased risk of infectious disease outbreaks. World Health Organization (WHO) estimates there will be 2 billion people at risk of dengue fever by 2080
Water resources	◆ The increase in the number of people who lack access to safe drinking water due to decrease in rainfall, faster water evaporation, urbanization pressure for limited safe water supply to address needs, and population growth ◆ Water quality affected by contamination (e.g. due to flooding)	◆ The increased risk of diarrhoea with the lack of clean drinking water ◆ Human security events such as conflicts and wars due to disputes over water sources, along with potential increase in human casualties and health risks
Food	◆ Potential decrease in crop and food production due to hot weather and abnormal precipitation	◆ Increase in risks of food shortage and insecurity, and nutritional crises
Living places	◆ The increased risk of coastal areas being flooded due to sea-level rise	◆ Increased risks of infectious diseases, injuries, and mental health consequences

Source: World Health Organization (2008).

Vulnerability

The frequency and intensity of climate-related events are vital in determining the extent of the impact and damage. Meanwhile, there are other factors affecting people and their social vulnerability. A clear definition of *risk* and *vulnerability* can help people comprehend the reasons why different populations are affected differently by climate change. **Risk** is defined as 'the probability of harmful consequences, or expected losses (deaths, injuries, property, livelihoods, economic activity disrupted or environment damaged) resulting from interactions between natural or human-induced hazards and vulnerable conditions' (UNISDR, 2009). Climate change may affect the factors that alter risks. These factors include hazard, exposure, and vulnerability. **Hazard** refers to dangerous phenomena which may cause a negative impact; **exposure** refers to people, property, systems, or other elements present in hazard zones that are thereby subject to potential losses; **vulnerability** refers to the characteristics and circumstances of a community, system, or asset that make it susceptible to the damaging effects of a hazard.

Table 3.3 Examples of Adaption Approaches, Policy Framework, and Adaptation Policies to Reduce Adverse Impact by Health and Non-Health Sectors

	Adaptation approach	Policies framework	Adaptation policies
Health aspect	Strengthening health infrastructure and contingency services	◆ Planning health response measures and emergency medical service for extreme temperature and weather events ◆ Monitoring the climate sensitive disease patterns ◆ Checking drinking water safety	◆ Formulating public health policies that raise the awareness of climate change risk, enhancing self-care possibilities, and strengthening the health service and regional and international cooperation
Non-health aspect	Enhancing water resources utilization efficiency	◆ Improving utilization efficiency of water resources ◆ Enabling recycling of water resources ◆ Adopting desalination technology to produce water for drinking or irrigation ◆ Improving rainwater collection, storage, and preservation	◆ Formulating national policies to manage water resources and water-related hazards
	Capacity improvement of agricultural industry for food production	◆ Adjusting the planting time and diversifying types of crops to reduce the chance of crop failure ◆ Protecting and improving land use, e.g. controlling soil erosion by planting trees	◆ Reforming land-use rights ◆ Providing incentives such as training, finance, subsidies, and tax credits ◆ Formulating research policies that can support farmers and relevant stakeholders to adapt to climate challenges in agricultural industries
	Strengthening and diversifying energy source	◆ Strengthening the distribution infrastructure; use underground cables for utilities ◆ Reducing dependence on a single source ◆ Utilization of renewable energy sources	◆ Formulating national energy policies and introduce financial incentives to encourage the use of alternative sources ◆ Incorporating climate change into design standards and architecture
	Consolidating infrastructure resilience	◆ Consolidating the dunes, and building up seawalls and storm barriers ◆ Cultivating marsh or wetlands to act as buffers against rising sea levels and flooding ◆ Refraining from building and urban development within coastal flood plains	◆ Setting up land-use regulations ◆ Incorporating climate change into design standards and architecture

(continued)

Table 3.3 Continued

Adaptation approach	Policies framework	Adaptation policies
Facilitating transport adaptation	◆ Designing and planning roads, rail, and other infrastructure to cope with warming and drainage	◆ Optimizing transport routes to increase movement efficiency and reduce unnecessary travel and traffic ◆ Integrating climate change considerations into national transport policy
Facilitating tourism industry and livelihood adaptation	◆ Diversifying and expanding tourist highlights ◆ Adapting contexts with climate change: moving the ski slopes to higher altitudes and glaciers; using artificial snow; developing summer activity options in traditional ski resorts	◆ Integrated planning (e.g. carrying capacity), and links with other sectors ◆ Financial incentives such as subsidies and tax credits

Source: IPCC (2007a).

Although both developed and developing countries must face the threat of climate change, developing countries are at a higher risk. As developing countries lack the necessary infrastructure facilities, response system, and resources that are found in developed nations, they are more vulnerable when facing climate change. A community's vulnerability depends on factors such as facility access, service availability, and socioeconomic and environmental conditions. People who are more vulnerable tend to suffer from a higher health risk. Population expansion, ageing, and population movement change an area's social structure and require relevant adjustment and public health planning to address health risks and medical needs (World Health Organization and World Meteorological Organization, 2012).

Risk factors for vulnerability

Key risk factors leading to human vulnerability include **lack of facilities and access to services**, **reliance on monotonous economic activities** (e.g. an agriculture-based economy), **vulnerable populations** (e.g. minority groups and indigenous people), and **at-risk environment/geography**. People who live in an area without a sufficient health infrastructure have a limited capacity for preparedness and response to climate change. Poor populations inhabiting in areas with insufficient facilities tend to be at a higher risk. Agriculture-based economy communities with populations living and relying entirely on natural environment also have higher risk of losing their livelihood because of climate change. For example, farmers may face a higher risk of crop failure due to a long cold period or heavy rain. The morbidity and mortality rates of women and children are known to be higher than adult men in disasters. In developing countries, 90% of the post-disaster cases of malaria, diarrhoea, and malnutrition-related diseases affect children below the age of five. Older people and chronically ill patients need persistent and special care after disasters, otherwise their health suffers severely (Chan, 2019b). The impact of climate change is closely related to geographic susceptibility to drought, flooding, and regular water security. Residents in these communities are likely to suffer serious water and food insecurity and experience the lack of access to clean drinking water and poor crop yield. With the frequent population movement after disasters and the lack of social support, victims from ethnic minorities may suffer poorer physical and mental health. Indigenous inhabitants who live in their original environment may be forced to give up their traditional style of living (United Nations Department for Economic and Social Affairs, 2009).

The major health impacts of extreme weather

Extreme weather affects human health and public health protection at different levels. Extreme temperature, such as heatwaves and cold spells, may increase the incidence and risks of infectious diseases, non-infectious diseases, and injuries. As a result, human health may suffer and service burden will increase in medical, social, and welfare systems (Chan, 2019a; see Case Box 3.2 and Figure 3.2).

Case Box 3.2 The Relationship between Temperature and Public Health

The Collaborating Centre for Oxford and CUHK for Disaster and Medical Humanitarian Response (CCOUC) published two studies on temperature and public health in 2012 and 2013 respectively. The first study analyses the relationship between hot weather in Hong Kong and the death toll. It shows that the death toll increases 1.8% for every 1 °C above 28.2 °C. The second study reveals the relationship between the temperature in Hong Kong and the number of inpatients from 1998 to 2009. It shows that during the period June to September, the number of inpatients increased 4.5% for every 1 °C above 29 °C; during November to March, when the temperature was between 8.2 °C and 26.9 °C, the number of inpatients increased 1.4% for every 1 °C drop. The major reason for the rise in both the number of inpatients and the death toll was the increase in the number of people suffering from respiratory tract diseases and infectious diseases. Another study from the CCOUC focuses on health-seeking behaviours and shows that when the temperature reaches 30 °C to 32 °C, the frequency of health-related calls started to increase. About 49% of calls were made for explicit health-related reasons including dizziness, shortness of breath, and general pain. These research findings provide important data for the government departments and NGOs to formulate relevant policies and contingency plans to secure citizens' health. Overall, when the maximum temperature of that day is higher than the threshold, the frequency of health-related calls rises significantly.

Sources: Chan (2019a); Chan, Goggins, Kim, and Griffiths (2010); Chan, Goggins, Kim, Griffiths, and Ma (2011); Chan, Goggins, Yue, and Lee (2013).

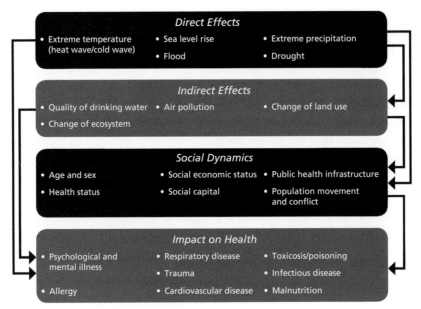

Figure 3.2 The impact of climate change on health
Source: Watts, Adger, Agnolucci, Blackstock, Byass, et al. (2015).

Health impact of heatwaves

According to the definition given by the World Meteorological Organization (WMO), a heatwave is a period of abnormally hot weather. It occurs in an area when the area is invaded by hot air or when its temperature persistently and significantly increases for days or even weeks. With global climate change, it is expected that heatwaves will become more frequent and episodes will be stronger and last a longer period than in earlier years. Such events will pose threats to public health and individual well-being (IPCC, 2012; see Case Box 3.3 and Figure 3.3). With more people using air-conditioning equipment in hot weather and increased air particulates, outdoor and indoor air pollutions (coupled with poor ventilation) are likely to increase the incidence rate of **respiratory tract diseases**. Strong sunshine also increases the intensity of ozone at ground level and may potentially

Case Box 3.3 A 2015 Heatwave in India

In May 2015, persistent fatal heatwaves affected India. Some Indian cities reported ambient temperature of 48 °C and the heatwave was reported to have caused 2,500 deaths. In Andhra Pradesh, a city in south-eastern India, more than 1,700 people died. The medical institutions were so overcrowded that they launched a public appeal to minimize outdoor activities and movement.

Sources: Burton (2015); Associated Press (31 May 2015).

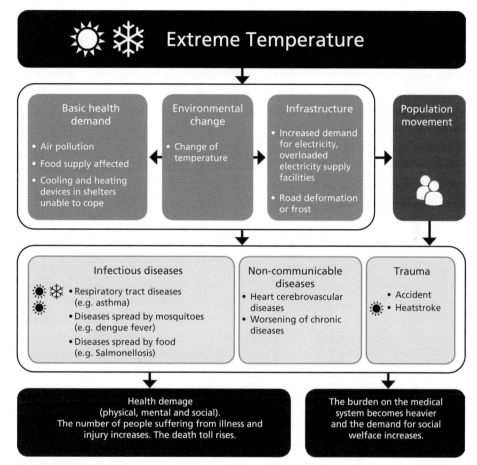

Figure 3.3 Pathways linking extreme temperature and human health

affect the respiratory system and people with underlying health risks such as asthma and chronic obstructive pulmonary disease. In addition, as the temperature increases, some comparatively cold regions become warm and the habitat range of mosquitoes expands towards high-latitude areas. Increases in the risk of **communicable diseases** such as intestinal pathogenic bacteria infection (which is spread via drinking water), salmonella (which is spread through eating contaminated food), and dengue fever, malaria, and West Nile virus (which are spread by mosquitoes) are also reported in scientific literature. High temperatures may hasten open water evaporation, decrease fresh water available and lead to drought in susceptible areas. Inappropriate water storage may encourage mosquito breeding and increase the risk of vector-borne infectious diseases. Increased ambient temperature may also increase human physiological vulnerability to exacerbation of health risks in people with chronic condition in cardiovascular and cerebrovascular disease, and deteriorate the functions of other organs that may be sensitive to overheating.

Health impact of cold spells

A cold spell (or cold wave) is a sudden and significant drop of temperature over a large geographic area. Due to global warming, there are likely to be fewer cold days than in former years but sporadic cold waves will remain a major extreme temperature event that affects communities in northern latitudes (IPCC, 2007c). During a cold wave, apart from the abnormal outdoor temperature, poor housing design and inability to maintain indoor thermal comfort may affect human health. High-risk groups of people, such as the elderly and those suffering from long-term diseases, who lack indoor heating will face an increased risk of illness and death. Morbidity rate of those with respiratory diseases is likely to rise. Periods of cold weather may lead to surge in incidences of **respiratory diseases** because it increases the activity of influenza viruses and boosts their transmission in enclosed indoor environment with poor ventilation. Besides, cold and dry air may directly stimulate the narrowing of respiratory tract, which may lead to exacerbating of chronic diseases such as asthma and COPD. Cold temperature may constrict weather can narrow the capillaries near skin surface and cause an increase in blood pressure. It can also cause dilated cardiomyopathy, an increase in the number of blood platelets, and an increase in blood viscosity. These may lead to **cardiovascular and cerebrovascular diseases**. In cold weather, the constriction of human blood vessels may affect blood circulation and lead to muscle stiffness. Clumsiness of clothing and muscle stiffness may predispose to injuries (e.g. those resulting from falls among older people and young children). Sporadic cold spells may affect unprepared communities that are not typically affected by cold spells (see Case Box 3.4).

Major health impacts of rainfall increase

A rise in the total annual rainfall or sporadic periods of heavy rain will both affect the environmental and ecological system and increase the risk of water-related diseases. Heavy rain may lead to secondary natural disasters, including flooding and landslips (see Case

---

Case Box 3.4 Cold Wave in a Subtropical City: Hong Kong

On 22 January 2016, an extremely cold weather phenomenon occurred in Hong Kong. Hong Kong Observatory (2015) recorded an ambient temperature of 3.1 °C in the city on 24 January, the lowest temperature reached in 59 years. The temperature on Tai Mo Shan, the highest peak, dropped to −6 °C. More than 100 people became trapped in mountains and required emergency rescue by fire services and police force.

The Education Bureau responded by announcing school suspension for all kindergartens, special schools for children with physical disabilities, intellectual disabilities, and primary schools on the subsequent day. The Home Affairs Department had opened 17 temporary cold shelters in different districts and provided resources (such as blankets) for the needy.

Source: Chan, Huang, Mark, and Guo (2017).

Case Box 3.5 2014 Heavy Rain in Hong Kong

On 30 March 2014, Hong Kong, a subtropical city in southern China, was affected by heavy rain and reported hail storm in some areas. During the heavy rain, the Drainage Services Department received 29 flooding reports. The Hong Kong Observatory was prompted to issue Yellow, Red, and Black Rainstorm Warnings and a Landslip Warning within a short period of time. The downpour led to major flight delays and traffic congestion. Flooding was reported in major underground railway stations and urban shopping malls were drenched as the heavy rain poured through their ceilings like a waterfall. Catastrophic economic loss was reported by the agricultural community.

Sources: Kao (31 March 2014); Hong Kong Observatory (23 March 2015).

Box 3.5). Heavy rain and associated flooding may pollute clean drinking water sources and cause intestinal diseases. Water-and food-borne diseases, such as dysentery, giardiasis, cryptosporidiosis, hepatitis A, cholera, and typhoid fever, may be spread through the consumption of food and water and affect a large group of population (refer also to Chapter 5). Stagnant water may serve as a breeding ground for mosquitoes, bacteria, and fungi which may lead to an increase in transition of diseases such as Japanese encephalitis, malaria, and dengue fever (see Case Box 3.6). Figure 3.4 describes how increased rainfall might affect health outcomes.

Major health impacts of sea-level rise

As the speed at which sea levels are rising is comparatively slow, the potential impact is usually neglected. Nevertheless, rising sea levels will seriously affect human life, property, livelihood, and access to safe drinking water and food, especially in some coastal areas in lowland or delta regions. Figure 3.5 highlights the impact of sea-level rise on human health outcomes.

An increase in the rate of infectious diseases might result from suboptimal urban drainage system, flooded with seawater intrusion. Fresh water is polluted which can lead to a water shortage or the outbreak of diseases which are spread by water, such as intestinal diseases. Populations might be forced to move when their homes are destroyed by flood water. Floods can also cause casualties, and people's mental health can be damaged. Sea-level rise might also lead to **malnutrition due to food insecurity**. When seawater seeps into the soil it causes salinization. Wetlands are polluted and fish, birds, and plants lose their habitats which leads to ecological imbalance. It can also cause human food shortages and, ultimately, malnutrition, or lead to conflicts over scarce resources.

Major health impacts of flooding

Flooding can affect human lives. Drowning, pollution of the sources of fresh water, interruption of the health system, and water scarcity leading to forced mass migration are

Case Box 3.6 Malaria

Malaria is the leading cause of mortality and morbidity in developing countries. In 2015, it caused 214 million cases and 438,000 deaths. About 3.2 billion people are at risk worldwide. Around 90% of all malaria deaths occurred in sub-Saharan Africa and 70% among children under five. Malaria is caused by the *Plasmodium* parasite, transmitted via the bites of infected vectors, the female Anopheles mosquitoes. In the human body, the parasites multiply initially in the liver, then in the blood (inside the red blood cells), causing fever, headache, and vomiting between 10 and 15 days after the bite. Some forms of malaria can develop into severe cases that, if left untreated, may result in death. Key interventions for malaria management include treatment with artemisinin-based combination therapies (ACTs), insecticidal net use, and indoor insecticide spraying. Meanwhile, the breeding of mosquitoes is highly dependent on weather variables (i.e. **temperature, rainfall**, and **humidity**). Its survival is limited to areas with ambient temperatures between 16 °C and 40 °C. Optimal transmission temperature is around 28°C to 30 °C. Higher temperatures increase the vector's metabolic rate, hence the demand for more frequent blood meals. Higher temperatures also speed up parasite growth in the body of the mosquito, which make vectors more infective. Furthermore, the early onset of the rainy season has been associated with increased malaria incidence (Thomson, Doblas-Reyes, Mason, Hagedorn, Connor, et al., 2006). Humidity also determines the lifespan of mosquitoes (Chaves and Koenraadt, 2010) and hence transmission capacity. Although active interventions since 2000 have decreased global malaria incidence and mortality rates by 37% and 60%, respectively (WHO, 2016), malaria still contributes to significant burden of preventable death in an at-risk developing context.

common ways how flooding may be associated with health and well-being. Figure 3.6 describes how flooding events might affect human health and well-being.

Most casualties caused by flooding are due to **traumatic injury**. Drowning, electrical shock, and trauma, and the speed, height, and volume of flood water cause significant mortality worldwide. For example, flash floods are more fatal than other kinds of flooding. In general, people at the highest risk of home drowning are mostly older people. Flooding-related trauma includes contusions and laceration. In addition, if hospitals and clinics are damaged by flooding, patients may not be able to visit doctors and receive timely treatment. The victims of flooding may also suffer from **mental health** consequences like anxiety, depression, and sleep disorders brought on by the damage floods cause such as witnessing houses collapsing, suffering the loss of property and livelihood, and being forced to move away from one's home.

Indirect health impacts are also common and might be long-lasting. The incidence of these diseases after disasters is more common in developing settings. Water treatment and public health facilities in developed countries are comparatively well-maintained and

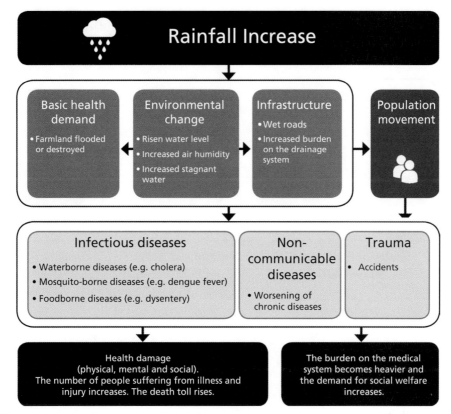

Figure 3.4 The health outcomes of rainfall increase

therefore less likely to host outbreaks of infectious diseases. Drinking water can be polluted easily by flood water after disasters, thus increasing the risk of diseases spread by water like cholera, leptospirosis, and hepatitis A. In addition, although the initial deluge washes away mosquito eggs, the stagnant water left after flooding becomes a hotbed of breeding mosquitoes and the incidence rate of diseases spread by the insects such as dengue fever and malaria increases accordingly. There are also data that show that respiratory tract, skin, and eye infection cases also increase after flooding. Shortage of food and subsequence malnutrition might also result from flooding. Crops may be submerged and the food supply is affected (see Case Box 3.7).

Major health impacts of drought

Water is essential to maintaining life, but from 1994 to 2013, there were more than 1 billion people throughout the world adversely affected by drought and water insecurity. It causes crops failure, a shortage of drinking water, and large-scale outbreaks of infectious diseases. It can also have a long-term effect on the environment, the social economy, and health (Centre for Research on the Epidemiology of Disasters, 2015). Figure 3.7 describes potential health impacts of drought events.

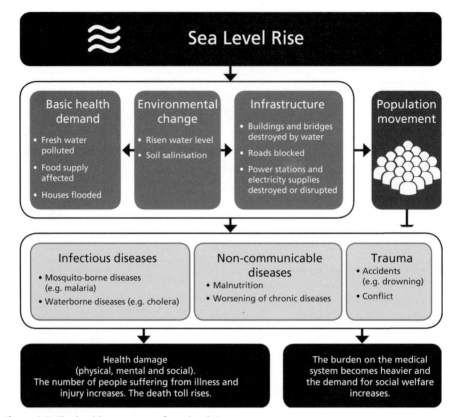

Figure 3.5 The health outcomes of sea-level rise

Drought may lead to a shortage of water resources and can affect local hygiene practices. For example, citizens may lack clean water to wash themselves and their food.
Microorganisms may thrive due to dried-up rivers and lakes and they could pollute the
remaining water sources. When there is a water stress and shortage, more people tend to
share the same water source which, in turn, increases the risk of water pollution and the
incidence rate of diseases spread by water, such as cholera, typhoid fever, and diarrhoea
increases. Besides, dry soil can lead to dust which may increase the incidence rate of
respiratory tract infection, cardiovascular disease, and cardiopulmonary diseases. After
drought, some vectors, like worms, reproduce rapidly as their natural enemies sharply decrease. This leads to a greater risk of outbreak of diseases like dengue fever, malaria, and
Japanese encephalitis. Food production sharply decreases during dry weather, resulting
in a shortage of food and a rise in cases of malnutrition (Stanke, Kerac, Prudhomme,
Medlock, and Murray, 2013). Communities whose livelihood depends of agriculture are
severely affected by persistent dry weather as it affects their livelihood and they may be
forced to move; the negative feelings that follow are detrimental to mental health (see
Case Box 3.8).

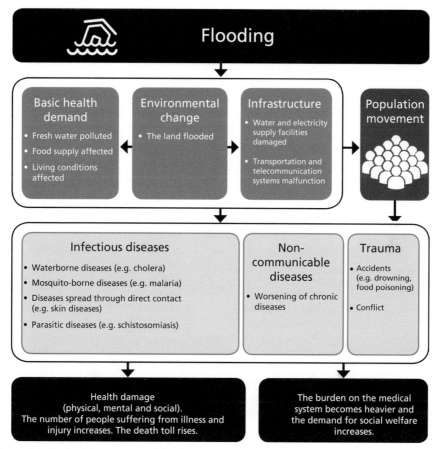

Figure 3.6 The health outcomes of flooding

Case Box 3.7 2015 Flooding in Myanmar

In August 2015, persistent heavy rain caused flooding in Myanmar. More than 100 people died and over 1 million people were affected. The western regions were inundated and suffered from the heaviest damage with some areas covered by several metres of stagnant water. Roads, bridges, and houses in the disaster areas were severely damaged, more than 500,000 hectares of crops were destroyed, and there was serious threat to the safety of food and drinking water.

Source: FloodList (22 October 2015).

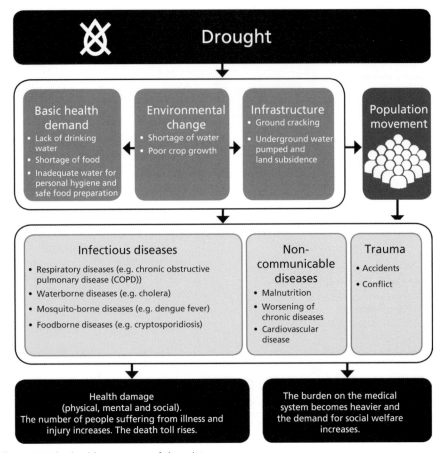

Figure 3.7 The health outcomes of drought

Case Box 3.8 Drought in Vietnam

Since late 2015, the middle and southern regions of Vietnam have been suffering from persistent and severe drought. Affected by the strong El Niño, 39 out of 63 provinces in Vietnam suffered from a shortage of water and the storage of fresh water in lakes decreased. Communities around the Mekong Delta was most severely affected and most damaged. The water level of the Mekong Delta reached its lowest point since 1926 with residents nearby facing a shortage of both domestic and agricultural water. Farmers living there have lost their livelihood. The Mekong Delta also suffered from the intrusion of seawater as the sea level rose. The soil was seriously salinized and crop production decreased sharply with more than 1.75 million residents affected.

Sources: ReliefWeb (14 April 2016); Daiss (25 May 2016).

Major health impacts of complex emergencies

Climate change increases living and environmental stress and thus the occurrence of complex emergencies, such as conflicts and wars. According to the World Health Organization (WHO), complex emergencies are 'situations of disrupted livelihoods and threats to life produced by warfare, civil disturbance and large-scale movements of people in which any emergency response has to be conducted in a difficult political and security environment'. Many developing countries face the threat of a complex emergency. These usually follow on from destabilizing situations including **political instability** (e.g. internal war, civil unrest, and violence); **economic instability** (e.g. national poverty and disparity between the rich and the poor); **environmental instability** (e.g. the effect brought about by persistent drought); and **population instability** (e.g. rapid growth in urban cities and large-scale migration) (see Case Box 3.9).

Complex emergency-based events may lead to excess trauma and injury (including physical violence and sexual violence); infectious diseases (as the surveillance and health system is damaged); a lack of health service facilities; malnutrition (as an unstable food supply means that people may lack sufficient nutrition and suffer from mild or severe malnutrition); and mental health risks (as populations forced to move away are separated from their family and friends). The lack of social support and suffering from different trauma will also lead to mental health problems.

Case Box 3.9 Complex Emergencies in Niger

Niger, a landlocked country in West Africa, is fragile in the face of climate change. Although more than 80% of its population work in the agricultural and farming industry, nearly 60% of people live under the poverty line. Due to the high dependence on the agricultural and farming industry, when a drought occurs, the country will face food insecurity. With the absence of self-sufficient internal food supply, its population will rely on food import and foreign food assistance. Domestic food shortages usually lead to high food prices which result in complex emergencies that lead to large-scale population movement, illness, and death.

In 2015, a serious food crisis occurred in Niger. Severe drought and locust plague had curtailed food production in many parts of Niger and caused severely restricted food supply. Food prices tripled in rural areas and doubled in urban areas. Most people could barely afford to feed themselves and 15,000 children suffered from malnutrition. The Government tried to sell food at subsidised prices but a large number of people still could not afford it. Some citizens marched through the streets of the capital, Niamey, calling on the Government to distribute free food while many others crossed over into neighbouring Nigeria to escape this disaster.

Climate change and diseases

The environmental impact of climate change may impose great social burdens on the protection of public health of the affected community. Apart from changes in the living environment and incidence of climate-related extreme events and disasters, climate change may alter disease patterns and their manifestation.

Communicable diseases

Risks of communicable disease are likely to alter with changes in distribution of pathogens and vectors, as well as improper hygiene practices. Warmer air or sea temperatures, increased precipitation, plus human factors such as urban crowding and deforestation create more favourable conditions for pathogens and vectors, leading to the prevalence of water-, food-, and vector-borne diseases.

Water-borne diseases

Access to clean water is essential for health. The quality and quantity of water available to a given population depends on complex interactions in climate systems. About one-third of the world's population is facing moderate to high water stress. Climate change-related events, such as floods, droughts, excessive precipitation, increased temperature, and rising sea levels influence the interactions, resulting in changes in water availability, quality, and access. Water shortage may increase water-borne disease risks. **Water-borne diseases** are infections caused by pathogens that can be spread by contaminated water via various faecal–oral routes such as drinking contaminated water, recreational use of suboptimal water sources, or eating contaminated food (Centers for Disease Control and Prevention, n.d.). Whilst diarrhoea and vomiting are the most common clinical symptoms, water-borne diseases also cause other symptoms such as malnutrition, skin infections, and organ damage.

Scientific evidence indicates that climate change has led to an increase in water-borne diseases due to changes in weather patterns. **Excessive precipitation** increases water run-off, which potentially overwhelms water and sewage treatment facilities and contaminates fresh water sources. Excessive precipitation may also cause river/urban floods and spread contaminated floodwaters. Cholera outbreaks are associated with flooding combined with population displacement when access to fresh water is compromised. **Rising air temperature** may encourage growth of planktonic species in water sources, which may increase the incidence of pathogens in human consumption. **Droughts** reduce water availability, which may limit dilution effects and decrease the water quality by increasing concentrations of effluent pathogens, sediments, and minerals. Water highly concentrated in pollutants may also overwhelm ageing water-treatment plants and increase the chances of spreading contaminated water. **Changes in ocean and coastal ecosystems** might alter water pH value, nutrient, salinity, and seawater currents can affect water availability and quality. Exposure to contaminated seawater increases the risk of fungal skin diseases, eye infections, and respiratory illnesses (National Institute of Environmental Health Sciences,

2010). **Rise in sea temperature** may contribute to the emergence of marine bacterial water-borne infectious diseases such as **Vibrio infections** in Northern Europe (Baker-Austin, Trinanes, Taylor, Hartnell, Siitonen, et al., 2012). Health risks increase for people with restricted access to treated water or who depend on untreated surface water from rivers and streams for daily activities. Furthermore, reduced water availability could affect local sewage systems. Even for developed countries with established water-treatment in-frastructures, urban floods compounded by aged sewage infrastructure may increase the water-borne disease risk.

Food-borne diseases

Along with water, food is another basic component to maintain health. A warmer climate may increase the incidence of food-borne diseases. These may be caused by ingesting food contaminated with infectious agents (such as bacteria, viruses, parasites in uncooked meat or vegetables) and by ingesting chemical or toxic substances, persistent organic pol-lutants, such as dioxins, and heavy metals (WHO, 2015). Food may become contaminated at any point in production and distribution. The most common clinical symptoms are gastrointestinal, such as nausea, vomiting, and diarrhoea. Nevertheless, food-borne dis-eases can cause long-lasting disability and death.

Changes in climate and weather patterns may increase food-borne disease risks by altering pathogen growth, survival, habitable ranges, transmission patterns, and the environmental context that the pathogen may thrive. The incidence of disease is associated with **ambient temperature**, which may increase as warmer temperatures create more favourable breeding conditions for pathogens. Furthermore, human factors, such as eating raw food like sushi in hot weather and eating outdoors increases the risk of pathogen exposure. Activities of pathogen-bearing pests (e.g. flies, cockroaches, and rodents) in the domestic environment are altered under higher temperatures and increased humidity. For instance, *Salmonella* in-fections are common in summer and the incidences rise by 5–10% for each 1 °C increase in weekly temperature when the ambient temperature is at least 5 °C (Kovats, Edwards, Hajat, Armstrong, Ebi, et al., 2004). Campylobacter also increases rapidly with rising temperatures and the risk of campylobacteriosis is positively associated with an increase in mean weekly temperatures. **Excessive precipitation** and **flooding** may reduce clean drinking water avail-ability and can overwhelm water-treatment systems. Furthermore, certain food crops and agricultural soil may be contaminated with pathogen-bearing flood waters. A **rise in sea tem-perature** may induce *Vibrio* bacteria production, leading to increased seafood-borne disease risks, such as cholera (National Institute of Environmental Health Sciences, 2010). **Changes in seasonality** such as extended warm weather seasons may enhance food-handling mis-takes. For instance, 32% of food-borne outbreaks in Europe may be linked to 'temperature misuse' (European Centre for Disease Prevention and Control, 2012). Generally, commu-nities have been advised that raw food should not be left out of refrigeration longer than two hours in Europe. However, when the air temperature is over 90 °F (32.2 °C), food safety might be compromised if it was left out of appropriate-temperature storage (e.g. refriger-ation) for only one hour. Unsafe food poses health threats to everyone. However, infants, young children, pregnant women, older people, and those with an underlying illness are particularly susceptible. The risk of food-borne diseases is also greater in developing countries where food supply is insecure, and populations are particularly exposed to more unsafe food without sufficient capacity or public health infrastructures to prevent and treat illness.

Vector-borne diseases

Climate change effects on environmental context and weather patterns may alter the transmission and distribution of vector-borne diseases by influencing the geographic habitable range, population, and seasonality. **Vector-borne diseases (VBDs)** are infectious diseases transmitted by the bite of infected arthropod species, such as mosquitoes, ticks, sandflies, and blackflies. Arthropod species are cold-blooded and sensitive to the local meteorological conditions such as temperature, rainfall, and humidity. Although non-climate factors such as habitat destruction and pesticide spraying also contribute to vector proliferation, climate factors, such as temperature and humidity, play a dominant role in determining: (i) habitat suitability to survive and reproduce; (ii) biting frequency; and (iii) the pathogen's incubation period within the vector organism. For example, vectors require a minimum temperature for activity and breeding. Higher ambient temperatures may increase breeding and a vector's metabolism, causing them to seek for more food (e.g. blood), hence increased biting frequencies. VBDs such as malaria and dengue fever are major causes of illness and death globally (e.g. in tropical and subtropical regions). Climate change may increase health risks from VBDs by altering transmission, the geographical range, and seasonal activity of various vectors.

Population growth, urbanization, change of land use, and environmental context contribute to the alteration of the atmosphere and climate of the Earth, causing general warming, rising sea level, increasing storm intensity, and changing rainfall patterns (IPCC, 2014). These climate-related change phenomena are found to alter existing infectious disease patterns and the re-emergence of some rare vector-borne diseases.

Assessing the future impact of climate change requires a good understanding of countries' capacity to control the disease. The risk for VBDs is much higher in low and lower middle-income countries where people have the least access to effective services for prevention, diagnosis, and treatment. Particularly in poor tropical countries, VBDs place a major public health burden on the poorest and marginalized subgroups. Climate change may exaggerate VBD risks in developed countries by widening the geographic distributions of VBDs such as dengue fever, Lyme disease, and tick-borne encephalitis. For example, disruption of health systems helped the resurgence of malaria in Eastern Europe. Increased international travel and trade has become the means to carry new vector species into new regions; for example, the West Nile virus case in the United States in 1999.

Non-communicable diseases

Non-communicable diseases (NCDs) are diseases that do not transmit from person to person. They tend to progress slowly and their health impact on the individual varies and

may last permanently. With changes in modern lifestyles and nutritional status, the prevalence of NCDs is growing rapidly worldwide. As of 2015, NCDs kill 38 million people
each year (63% of total annual deaths), 28 million of which are in low- to middle-income
countries. Globally, cardiovascular diseases account for 17.5 million deaths, followed by
cancers (8.2 million), respiratory diseases (4 million), and diabetes (1.5 million) per year,
together representing 82% of all NCD deaths. A number of behavioural risk factors, such
as tobacco, alcohol, physical inactivity, and unhealthy diet, are identified to be associated
with the increase in the risk of NCDs. Whilst some risk factors, such as age and sex, are
non-modifiable, most behavioural and environmental factors are modifiable and modification of habits (e.g. smoking) and environment may reduce the risk of developing NCDs.

Although direct scientific linkage remains to be proven, climate change does increase
environmental health risks and exacerbate certain NCD risks. According to the World
Health Organization (WHO, 2014), 24% of the morbidity burden and 23% of all deaths
are caused by environmental factors, such as reduced food production, water scarcity, or
air pollution.

Climate change impacts on non-communicable diseases

Examples of direct and indirect impacts of climate change on four non-communicable
diseases are summarized in the next sections: respiratory and allergic diseases, cardiovascular diseases, cancers, and mental health disorders.

Respiratory and allergic diseases

Major respiratory and allergic diseases include asthma, allergic rhinitis (hay fever), and
chronic obstructive pulmonary disease (COPD). **Asthma** is a chronic inflammation of
the small air passages in the lungs. An estimated 235 million people worldwide currently
suffer, particularly children. The main risk factors for developing asthma are inhaled
substances and particles that trigger allergic reactions (WHO, 2017, August). **Chronic
obstructive pulmonary disease** (COPD) is a lung disease with persistent blockage of
airflow from the lungs. Risk factors for COPD are tobacco, indoor/outdoor air pollution,
occupational dusts, and chemicals (WHO, December 2017). **Allergic rhinitis** (hay fever)
is an inflammation of the nose lining due to inhalation of allergens. Allergic rhinitis can
be triggered by outdoor allergens (e.g. mould or trees, grass, and weed pollens) or indoor
allergens (e.g. animal dander or house dust mites) (WHO, n.d.).

Climate change-related events may increase the risk of mortality and morbidity of
respiratory and allergic diseases. Increasing exposure to risk factors may introduce or
exacerbate pre-existing medical conditions (D'Amato, Cecchi, D'Amato, and Annesi-
Maesano, 2014). The risk of respiratory and allergic diseases is related to reduced outdoor air quality as climate change may: (i) increase concentrations of air pollutants, such
as ozone, particulate matters, and dust; (ii) alter production pattern and allergenicity of
allergens such as pollen and mould spores;(iii) increase the dusts in the air; and (iv) increase the frequencies of wildfires and wildfire smoke consisting of air pollutants (Friel,
Bowen, Campbell-Lendrum, Frumkin, McMichael, et al., 2011).

Increased air pollution

Increased human activities and high-density urban living may lead to more air pollutants (such as ozone, fine particles, and dust) entering the air which may raise the incidence of respiratory illnesses, such as asthma and COPD. The health impact of air pollutants is more apparent with high temperatures. In a multi-city study in Italy, for every 1 °C rise in maximum apparent temperature above the city-specific threshold, the estimated overall change in all-cause mortality was 3.1% in the Mediterranean region and 1.8% in the north-continental region, with a two-to-three times greater effect on respiratory mortality (6.7% and 6.1%, respectively) (Stafoggia, Forastiere, Agostini, Caranci, de'Donato, et al., 2008; Ayres, Forsberg, Annesi-Maesano, Dey, Ebi, et al., 2009; D'Amato, Vitale, De Martino, Giovanni, Maurizia, et al., 2015). Thus, higher incidence of respiratory illness is expected in the future due to the combination of more hot days and higher air pollution. A heatwave in August 2003 in Europe caused approximately 40,000 additional deaths (Ayres et al., 2009; D'Amato et al., 2014). During the heatwave, ground-level ozone concentrations rose above safe air-quality standards (180 μg/m^3) in many monitoring stations in central France and south-western Germany. About one-third of the deaths were attributable to excessive ozone concentrations (Hodzic, Madronich, Bohn, Massie, Menut, et al., 2007).

Changes in allergens

Aeroallergens, such as pollen and moulds, are produced from organisms such as weeds, grasses, trees, and fungus. Mucosal contact with allergens in the eyes, nose, or via inhalation into the lungs may trigger allergic responses, such as allergic rhinitis (hay fever) and asthma. Changes in the numbers of frosty days, temperatures, and carbon dioxide (CO_2) concentration may affect the atmospheric pollen concentration. For example: (i) higher CO_2 level induces more pollen production due to a fertilizing effect on plant growth; (ii) warmer temperatures may affect time and duration of pollen season (e.g. high temperature is associated with an earlier onset of the spring pollen season in the Northern Hemisphere (D'Amato, Cecchi, Bonini, Nunes, Annesi-Maesano, et al., 2007)); and (iii) these changes may introduce pollen allergens in new geographical areas since plants can move into new areas and pollen- and spore-containing dust can be blown to new areas due to changes in atmospheric circulation (Reid and Gamble, 2009). Higher pollen concentrations and longer pollen seasons may also exacerbate allergic rhinitis, particularly in people with existing problems. Furthermore, the prevalence of allergic illness by exposing new populations to new allergens may be increased (IPCC, 2007d). The most susceptible population groups for respiratory and allergic diseases exacerbated by climate change are those suffering from chronic respiratory diseases, people with pre-existing medical conditions such as asthma and cardiovascular problems, and vulnerable population groups such as children and older people (Friel et al., 2011).

Cardiovascular and cerebrovascular diseases

Cardiovascular diseases (CVDs) and cerebrovascular diseases are a group of heart and blood vessel disorders. The WHO (2017, May) reported that CVDs were the leading global cause of death in 2015, leading to 17.7 million deaths (31% of total global mortality). Typical examples include hypertension, coronary disease, heart attack, and stroke. Heart attacks and strokes are acute events resulting from blocked blood supply to the heart or the brain and can lead to death. Over three-quarters of CVD deaths occur in low- to middle-income countries. Climate change may directly or indirectly increase CVD risks through three main pathways: (i) air pollution; (ii) extreme temperatures; and (iii) changes in dietary options (Friel et al., 2011).

Air pollution
Increased exposure to air pollutants may increase CVD-related hospitalization and deaths by triggering heart attacks, strokes, and irregular heart rhythms, particularly in people with pre-existing medical conditions (Gold and Samet, 2013).

Extreme temperatures
Hot and cold weather extremes may increase the risk of CVD-related mortality and morbidity due to the physiological overloading of cardiovascular and respiratory systems. Excessive heat exposure is linked with higher cardiac episodes due to an increase in core body temperature, heart rate, sweating, and dehydration. When extreme heat is combined with high pollution, the CVD risk in susceptible populations may be increased, as the August 2003 heatwave in Europe showed (D'Amato et al., 2014). Seemingly in contradiction to this, global warming may reduce winter CVD mortality, but the net effect of climate change on CVDs is likely to be negative. With more intense and longer duration of heatwaves due to climate change, deaths and hospitalization of CVD patients are expected to increase (De Blois, Kjellstrom, Agewall, Ezekowitz, Armstrong, et al., 2015).

Changes in diet and lifestyles
Changes in diet options and lifestyles as a result of the environmental impact of climate change may increase the risks of CVD indirectly. Some indigenous population may be forced to change traditional lifestyles, hunting, and eating patterns in response to many environmental changes due to climate change (Friel et al., 2011). For example, the Inuit communities in the Arctic region had to change their traditional lifestyle due to the loss of sea ice and permafrost. This adjustment has reduced physical mobility and increased reliance on imported energy-dense processed food, increasing the risk of obesity, diabetes, and CVDs (Dixon, Donati, Pike, and Hattersley, 2009). People with a history of heart attacks, strokes, and with pre-existing cardiac diseases such as angina or irregular heart rhythm, and people who perform heavy physical labour are at higher risk of CVDs (De Blois et al., 2015). Furthermore, age, lifestyle habits, and genetics may also contribute to higher risks, for example smoking, family history of hypertension, or people over 65 years old (Gold and Samet, 2013).

Cancer
Cancer is a group of diseases characterized by the rapid growth of abnormal cells which invade healthy cells in other organs. Cancer is a leading cause of death worldwide, accounting for 8.8 million deaths in 2015 (WHO 2018a). A normal cell becomes a tumour

cell through multistage transformation due to the interaction of various risk factors: *personal* (age, tobacco use, overweight, alcohol use); *chemical* (asbestos, smoking); *biological* (infections from certain viruses); and *environmental* (increased exposure to ultraviolet (UV) radiation). Between 30% and 50% of cancer deaths could be prevented by modifying key risk factors (WHO, 2018a).

Climate change can influence UV radiation level at the Earth's surface and increase skin cancer risk in at least three ways (World Meteorological Organization, n.d.; Arblaster, Gillett, Calvo, Forster, Polvani, et al., 2014): (i) while climate change is not the cause of stratospheric ozone depletion, warming temperature may slow down the recovery of the ozone layer. (ii) Altered precipitation patterns and cloud coverage may change the UV level. UV levels are highest under cloudless skies. Thick clouds may reduce UV level, while thin clouds may augment UV levels because of light-ray scattering. (iii) Warmer climate may change behavioural patterns, for example, increased outdoor activities.

Human behaviour in a warmer climate may be another risk factor for skin cancer. Without appropriate protective measures, this increases UV exposure and skin cancer risks. For example, under high UV levels, in combination with warmer temperature and an increased outdoor lifestyle, the associated skin cancer risk in Australia remains high despite many preventative measures. Around 450,000 Australians suffer from skin cancers each year and UV radiation from sunlight may be responsible for over 95% cases. Hence, many measures to improve sun protection behaviour, such as the use of sunscreen, wearing protective clothing, and avoiding the sun around noon, have been promoted since 1988. These efforts helped reduce sunburn and melanoma incidence among younger people in Victoria (Makin, 2011).

Mental health

The WHO (1946) definition of health includes mental health and emphasizes the importance of positive mental health and well-being (Berry, Bowen, and Kjellstrom, 2010). **Mental health** is defined as 'a state of well-being in which an individual realises his or her own abilities, can cope with the normal stresses of life, can work productively and is able to make a contribution to her or his community' (WHO, 2018b). **Mental well-being** often refers to life satisfaction, a sense of belonging and being supported, and self-esteem. **Mental illness** refers to a diagnosable mental condition that affects an individual's cognitive, emotional, or social abilities. Mental disorders include depression, anxiety, and schizophrenia. Many factors such as socioeconomic, biological, and environmental can be stressors in one's life and affect one's mental health state acutely or chronically. Mental health disorders (WHO, 2018b) are the leading global cause of disability. Mental disorders are risk factors for other diseases such as HIV, cardiovascular disease, and diabetes. The incidence rate of mental disorder doubles after natural disasters.

Climate change-related extreme events may alter social, economic, and environmental determinants of mental health, including destruction of houses or loss of loved ones, increased competition for limited natural resources, and long-term stress on the displaced population. All of these stressors could cause psychological effects, such as anxiety, post-traumatic stress, depression, interpersonal and societal conflict, persistent grief, and child behavioural and developmental problems, and a decline in academic performance.

Vulnerable populations

People with good access to social support tend to have higher mental resilience thus mental health problems can be minimized or avoided. In contrast, for people who have lost or do not have access to resources, social and economic stressors caused by disasters are likely to have cumulative effects on mental well-being. (i) **Individuals who experienced direct impact**: mental disorders tend to increase during and after emergencies (WHO, April 2017; WHO, 2018b). The WHO estimated that between 10% and 15% of the affected population may suffer serious psychological problems after Typhoon Haiyan in the Philippines. People may experience temporary but acute distress in the immediate aftermath of a disaster, which could potentially develop into chronic problems. (ii) **People with compromised access to infrastructure and institutions**: vulnerability is associated with the length of time following a disaster. Two years after Hurricane Katrina, only one-third of childcare centres and schools reopened and a major mental health hospital had not been replaced. These situations may prolong displacement and community fragmentation. (iii) **Individuals with pre-existing physical and mental health disorders**: these are at greater risk of mental illness. Pre-existing physical conditions such as cardiovascular disease could be contributing risk factors for developing serious mental illness. Likewise, pre-existing mental health conditions triple the risk of any-cause mortality during a heatwave (Bouchama, Dehbi, Mohamed, Matthies, Shoukri, et al., 2007). (iv) **Displaced population**: people who are forced to leave their houses and communities tend to lose the sense of connectedness with families, social networks, communities, and cultures (Lundberg, 1998). Population displacement can also increase tensions and conflicts between displaced and host communities, resulting in psychological distress, social isolation, and depression. Moreover, people in refugee camps showed an increased prevalence of domestic violence, suicide, substance abuse, and depression. (v) **Vulnerable population**: Older people, children, and the poor are more vulnerable to poor health outcomes due to limited resources and coping capacities. More than one-third of adult and child disaster victims may suffer from PTSD and from increased risks of substance abuse, anxiety, depression, adjustment disorders, interpersonal problems, suicide, vocational difficulties, long-term physiological changes, and subsequent physical health problems (Norris, Friedman, and Watson, 2002). (vi) **People in regions with ongoing conflict**: due to scarcity of resources, crop failures, economic losses, and population displacement, an increase in violence, conflict, and instability may be triggered which can have serious implications on mental health consequences (Lundberg, 1998). Regions with ongoing unrest, poverty, unequal access to resources, weak institutions, food insecurity, and poor health are at the greatest risk. In Africa, a year-long drought increases the risk of civil war the next year by 50% (Burke, Miguel, Satyanath, Dykema, and Lobell, 2009).

Injuries

About 10% of annual global death (5.8 million people) is attributable to injuries. There are two major categories of injuries, namely **intentional injuries**, which are related to an act of violence- (e.g. suicide, homicide, and war); and **unintentional injuries**, which may be resulted from unintentional events such as traffic accidents. Nearly one-third of the 5.8 million annual deaths from injuries is the result of violence, while almost one-quarter is the result of road traffic crashes. Other main causes of injury-associated deaths are falls, drowning, burns, and poisoning.

Injury is one of the direct non-communicable disease outcomes of the climate change-related events such as flooding and heavy precipitation. Climate change may alter the frequency, timing, intensity, and duration of **extreme weather events**. Droughts, hurricanes, storms, and floods could cost numerous human lives and cause huge economic loss. As an indirect impact of climate change, reports had found association between flooding and increased mental health incidents and suicide rates (Roberts and Hillman, 2005). Each year, approximately half a million of people, including many children, die from drowning. Nearly all these deaths are in low- and middle-income countries, especially in the Western Pacific. It is predicted that climate change will cause further **sea-level rises** of between 18 cm and 59 cm by 2100 (IPCC, 2007d). Populations living proximal to the sea are particularly at risk during storms or cyclones. Meanwhile, increased global temperatures lead to increased evaporation of surface water and many susceptible regions are experiencing more frequent and severe droughts. The lack of access to essential resources like water and food is one of the risk factors in national or regional conflicts.

Responses to climate change

The previous sections are about the challenges brought by climate change. To tackle the impact of climate change, there are two main approaches, namely **adaptation** and **mitigation**.

Adaptation

Adaptation refers to the process of adjustment made according to the actual and expected climate and its effects in order to moderate harm or exploit beneficial opportunities (IPCC, 2012). The adaptive capacity of a country or a region is usually affected by various factors such as economic, social, and human resources. However, an ability to adapt does not mean adaptive measures are accepted and implemented. For example, proactive flood management in Norway was obstructed due to the consideration of interests among different stakeholders (Næss, Bang, Eriksen, and Vevatne, 2005). A partial understanding of the situation or insufficient assessment of the measures needed may lead to poor execution. For example, governments usually meet strong resistance when people have to be relocated because of climate change. Countries or regions may have a high adaptive capacity or can afford to pay for measures to limit the damage of climate change, yet they cannot ensure those measures are effective. For example, although a number of European, North American, and East Asian cities have adopted various adaptation policies to tackle temperature extreme events arising from climate change (Poumadère, Mays, Mer, and Blong, 2005), summer heatwaves still bring severe human health impact. Electricity consumption soars and those who have no shelter can die from the heat.

Adaptation policies

A successful adaptation plan requires cooperation and coordination between health departments and non-health departments. Although measures taken by non-health departments are not directly connected with health, these efforts may reduce the risk of a community's exposure to threat and reduce injuries and health vulnerability by, for instance, setting up an early warning system and building a flood protection dam. Table 3.3 shows some examples of adaptation derived from the Report of the Intergovernmental Panel on Climate Change.

Mitigation

Mitigation refers to basic prevention measures to relieve or stabilize adverse impact of climate change in human living environment. Two main mitigation approaches include: (i) promoting low carbon development to reduce the emission of greenhouse gases from the source by, for example, reducing the demand for activities with high emissions; (ii) strengthening the absorption of greenhouse gases by, for instance, protecting natural carbon sinks (e.g. forests and oceans) or creating new carbon sinks to facilitate the process of carbon dioxide re-absorption (IPCC, 2012).

Mitigation policies

Mitigation measures typically involve multidisciplinary actors and stakeholders to collaborate and reduce greenhouse gases. Table 3.4 illustrates some examples of the mitigation approach.

Limitations of mitigation

The strongest resistance to mitigating climate change always derives from lack of economic means and financial support. Mitigation measures for climate change are usually shelved also because of the lack of immediate results. Both mitigation strategies and measures need long-term planning and a well-trained and skilled workforce to ensure these efforts are launched effectively and continuously. For example, a number of facilitating factors will be required when promoting low-carbon transport. For electric vehicles, supporting charging facilities and repair equipment (e.g. battery exchange) will affect effectiveness of mitigation measures (e.g. measures to reduce carbon dioxide emissions) (IPCC, 2007c).

Table 3.4 Measures and Policies Mitigating the Emission of Greenhouse Gases

Mitigation approaches	Policy options	Mitigation policies
Improving energy utilization efficiency	◆ Enhancing energy supply efficiency ◆ Reducing energy distribution disparities	◆ Setting up performance standards ◆ Voluntary agreements, such as factories agreeing to audit their energy use and improve efficiency voluntarily ◆ Levying tax and fines on carbon emission, e.g. levying carbon and energy tax ◆ Reducing subsidies on fossil fuels ◆ Limiting the emission and consumption levels
	◆ Improving ways of travelling (e.g. increase the use public transport), encouraging walking and cycling ◆ Improving pastoral farming management and paddy planting techniques to reduce the emission of methane	◆ Making the use of ecofuels such as biofuel mandatory ◆ Setting up a carbon dioxide emission standard for transport ◆ Levying tax on buying new vehicles, and introducing registration tax and fuel tax ◆ Establishing financing incentive policies and restrictions for new technology ◆ Improving land use and methods of irrigation
	◆ Using energy-saving electrical appliances and refrigerators ◆ Using building materials that can render the buildings cool in the summer and warm in the winter, so that electrical appliances are used less frequently	◆ Setting up a standard for electrical appliance usage and energy efficiency labelling ◆ Establishing building ordinance and certificate for energy efficiency ◆ Formulating incentives for Energy Service Companies (ESCOs) that design project to reduce costs and save energy
Using substitute energy	◆ Switching from fossil fuels to renewable energy (e.g. hydropower and wind power to generate electricity) ◆ Using clean energy	◆ Lowering the tariffs on renewable energy ◆ Providing financial incentives to encourage new technology ◆ Boosting scientific research
	◆ Using recycled materials and alternative sources	◆ Increasing subsidy and reducing tax on renewable energy
	◆ Incinerating waste to produce renewable energy ◆ Using the organic waste for do composting treatment	◆ Establishing waste and sewage handling financing incentive policies ◆ Establishing renewable energy incentive policies
Afforestation	◆ Improving forest management ◆ Reducing the number of trees that are cut down	◆ Establishing afforestation financing incentive policies ◆ Establishing and carrying out land management regulation

Source: IPCC (2007a).

The interrelationship between adaptation and mitigation of climate change

Adaptation and mitigation approaches should support and complement one another to combat climate change. Not only may these measures reduce the health risks brought about by climate change, but also well-coordinated and planned mitigation and adaptation measures are likely to be more cost-effective. Tables 3.5 and 3.6 show some examples of measures combining adaptation and mitigation.

These examples show integration of adaptation and mitigation measures which can enhance effectiveness, reduce operation complexity, and maximize coordination between environmental and health sectors to protect human well-being.

Health co-benefits of measures responding to climate change

The 'health co-benefits' are measures to tackle climate changes as well as to produce positive health impact. These measures produce both the improvement in the environment and the reduction of health risks. Building green cities that increase the proportion of green space may reduce mortality and the incidence of cardiovascular and respiratory diseases. Green space might also reduce urban heat island (UHI) effect, which occurs when a district becomes significantly hotter than rural areas because of human activity.

Some mitigation measures may not offer direct benefits to human health but, indirectly, they can benefit society, the economy, and the environment. For example, forest protection policies help protect biodiversity, maintain a balance in the ecosystem, and ensure the supply and quality of drinking water. Measures like afforestation can strengthen both nature and human society. Planting mangroves, for instance, protects coastal areas by reducing the erosion caused by floodwater and reduce flood risks and their associated human health impact. Also, eating less red meat reduces an individual's cholesterol and, overall, helps reduce the greenhouse gases produced by farming. Other choices which have indirect benefits include using public rather than private transport which effectively

Table 3.5 Adaptation and Mitigation Approaches

Adaptation measures	Integrated Measures	Mitigation measures:
◆ Enhancement of the hygiene and medical infrastructure	◆ Construction of green roofs and balconies	◆ Utilization of renewable energy
◆ Water quality and water supply monitoring	◆ Conservation of water	◆ Promotion of energy saving vehicles
◆ Provisions of public warning and communication such as haze pollution warning, Air Quality Health Index	◆ Afforestation	◆ Promotion of the use of information technology to reduce unnecessary travels (e.g. air transportation)
◆ Disease vectors control measures	◆ Strengthened efforts of public education	

Source: Center for Clean Air Policy (2015).

Table 3.6 Examples of Integrated Measures Combining Adaptation and Mitigation

Measures	Examples	Effect on mitigation	Effect on adaptation
Green infrastructure	◆ Green roofs ◆ Urban forestry ◆ Permeable pavements	◆ Enhanced natural absorption of carbon dioxide ◆ Water allowed to infiltrate through surfaces and plants given the rooting space to grow	◆ Reduction of the urban heat island effect ◆ Reduction of flooding risks that may be caused by heavy rain
Resilient buildings	◆ Cold-proof and heat-insulated building materials	◆ Reduction of carbon emission caused by energy usage	◆ Maintenance of stability and comfort of indoor temperature to protect well-being
Sustainable transportation planning	◆ Covered pedestrian path and cycling track to enhance use during unfavourable weather context ◆ Low-carbon transportation system	◆ Reduction of carbon emission caused by unnecessary energy usage ◆ Reduction of carbon emission ◆ Reduction of air pollution	◆ Reduction of health risks related to injuries and air pollution

Source: Center for Clean Air Policy (2015).

reduces greenhouse gases and poisonous pollutants, and making more cycling paths to encourage healthy travel (see Table 3.7 and Case Box 3.10).

Global cooperation in climate change and sustainability

Climate change often results in transnational crises (e.g. disasters, migration, and disease transmissions) and requires global cooperation to respond effectively. Formulation and application of global-based approaches are essential to targeting and directing policies, programmes and efforts to reduce adverse impact of climate change. The following are some examples of global policies, programmes, and key stakeholders who are active in the global platform in advocating for and engaging in climate change, environment and health matters.

Policies and programmes

United Nations Framework Convention on Climate Change (UNFCCC)

As an intergovernmental organization having the legal status of global governance, the United Nations had adopted the United Nations Framework Convention on Climate Change (UNFCCC) in 1992. This framework aimed at the 'stabilization of greenhouse gas concentrations in the atmosphere at a level that would prevent dangerous anthropogenic interference with the climate system'. Because of this Convention, the United Nations holds Conferences of the Parties (COPs) every year to assess the progress of relevant policies and to formulate plans to combat the effect of climate change globally in order to reduce the emission of greenhouse gases and establish related policies at a national level.

Table 3.7 Examples of Potential Health Co-benefits and Strategies Responding to Climate Changes

Aspect	Strategies	Potential health co-benefits
Land	Increase in urban green spaces (e.g. parks) ♦ Reducing the building density to relieve the high temperature in urban areas and the potential urban heat island (UHI) effect ♦ Increasing outdoor areas to promote physical activity and social interaction	More exercise encouraged by more green space, which helps reduce cardiovascular disease which can be caused by high temperatures in urban area; Reduction of the risk of such diseases as cardiovascular diseases and cancer caused by a sedentary lifestyle
Energy	Reduction of fossil fuel use ♦ Reducing air pollutants and carbon dioxide emmissions	A reduction in the mortality rate and incidence of cardiovascular and respiratory diseases and associated cancer incidence related to air pollution
Transportation	Using public rather than private transport, or cycle or walk instead ♦ Reducing air pollution in urban area ♦ Increasing one's physical activity level ♦ Improving quality of living in urban context (e.g. reduction of traffic)	Reduction of cardiovascular disease, obesity, diabetes and depression which can be caused by air pollution and a sedentary lifestyle
Pastoral farming	Reduction of the number of ruminants kept for meat, such as cows, and the amount of meat eaten ♦ Reducing the greenhouse gases discharged by ruminants ♦ Cutting the consumption of red meat which usually contains a high level of saturated fat	A reduction in cardiovascular and respiratory diseases related to global warming; a reduction in the risk of colorectal cancer, cardiovascular diseases, and diabetes related to overconsumption of red meat and fat

Source: Remais, Hess, Ebi, Markandya, Balbus, et al. (2014).

Case Box 3.10 Urban Patterns in Health Environmental Co-benefits (HEC) Behaviours: The Case of Hong Kong

A large-scale telephone survey was conducted by Chan, Yue, Lee, and Wang between January and February 2016 (the Hong Kong People's Carbon-reduction Behaviours and Health) in order to understand if and how the local community adopted carbon-reduction behaviour that may reduce carbon emissions and benefit health. A city representational sample from 18 districts of 1,017 Cantonese-speaking local residents of 15 years old or above was selected based on the distribution of the population in terms of age, gender, and district. The results showed that Hong Kong's population exhibited a variation of awareness and practices of environmental behaviours. For example, about 45% of interviewees reduced their electricity consumption and reduced their daily utilization of air-conditioners or heaters as compared with a few years ago. For waste management, approximately 70% of interviewees developed the habit of using less packaging and shopping bags, and 50% followed a home waste separation practice since the government's implementation of plastic bag tax in 2015.

Source: Chan, Yue, Lee, and Wang (2016).

The Kyoto Protocol was adopted in 1997 to limit the emission of greenhouse gases discharged by developed countries. It forms the foundation of a number of global meetings, policies and programmes that were subsequently organized and developed.

Paris agreement

The 2015 United Nations Climate Change Conference (COP21) held in Paris was attended by leaders from 195 countries and representatives from international non-governmental organizations (NGOs) and resulted in the Paris Agreement. This legally binding agreement aims at strengthening the global ability to cope with the threat of climate change through sustainable development. It calls on countries to combat climate change by intensifying the action and investments needed for a low-carbon future, as well as to adapt to the increasing impact of climate change. The main objectives of the Paris Agreement are to limit the global average temperature increase to well below 2 °C above pre-industrial levels and to pursue efforts to limit the temperature increase to 1.5 °C above pre-industrial levels. Recognizing that this effort may significantly reduce the risks and impacts of climate change, the coordinated effort also hopes to increase the ability to adapt to the adverse impacts of climate change and foster climate resilience and low greenhouse gas emissions development in a manner that does not threaten food production. The agreement also facilitates discussion to create financial pathways and availability for low greenhouse gas emissions and climate-resilient development. For example, developed countries should set emission reduction target and developing countries be encouraged to work towards the target gradually. The Paris Agreement has a provision for improving 'transparency of action and support' and developed countries should help developing countries to build in transparency in their efforts to combat climate change (United Nations Framework Convention on Climate Change, 2015). For instance, developed countries are under an obligation to offer financial help to developing countries.

Sustainable development goals

Sustainable Development Goals (SDGs) are a set of global development goals adopted by Member States of the United Nations in 2015 to be achieved by 2030. SDGs include 17 goals and 169 targets that aim at eliminating hunger and poverty, promoting health and education, boosting sustainable development, coping with climate change, and protecting forests and oceans. Specifically, the thirteenth goal advocates taking emergency action to cope with climate change and its impact. Its targets include strengthening the resilience and adaptation ability of countries to tackle climate change and related hazards; integrating climate change measures into national policies, strategies, and planning; strengthening education and raising awareness; increasing the mitigation and adaptation ability of organizations and individuals to cope with climate change; implementing the commitment which developed countries made under the United Nations Framework Convention on Climate Change (UNFCCC). US$100 billion was granted to help developing countries tackle the demand of mitigating climate change and boosting plans and management systems to cope with climate change (United Nations, 2015b).

United Nations International Strategy for Disaster Reduction (UNISDR)— The United Nations Office for Disaster Risk Reduction (UNDRR)

The UNISDR was set up in 1999 'to serve as the focal point in the United Nations system for the coordination of disaster reduction and to ensure synergies among the disaster risk reduction activities of the United Nations system and regional organizations and activities in socio-economic and humanitarian fields'. Since its establishment, the UNDRR (abbreviation changed from UNISDR to UNDRR in 2019) has been working to formulate and update policy frameworks, tools, and global capacity to tackle disasters and alleviate disaster risks.

Sendai framework for disaster risk reduction 2015–30

The Third UN World Conference on Disaster Risk Reduction was held by the United Nations in Sendai, Japan in 2015. The meeting resulted in the Sendai Framework for Disaster Risk Reduction 2015–2030, which identifies a global target for disaster reduction that aims to increase global resistance and resilience. The Sendai Framework focuses on reducing the potential exposure to hazards and the vulnerability of society rather than on management after a disaster. It mainly focuses on disaster risk management; the reduction of risk and loss at various levels including losses in lives, livelihoods, and health; and the economic, physical, social, cultural, and environmental assets of persons, businesses, communities, and countries (United Nations, 2015a).

Key stakeholders

Intergovernmental Panel on Climate Change (IPCC)

The Intergovernmental Panel on Climate Change (IPCC) was established in 1988 by the United Nations Environment Programme (UNEP) and the World Meteorological Organization (WMO) to 'provide the world with a clear scientific view on the current state of knowledge in climate change and its potential environmental and socio-economic impacts'. It is the leading international body for assessing climate change and reviews and assesses the most recent scientific, technical, and socio-economic information produced across the globe that is relevant to understanding climate change. While the IPCC does not conduct any of its own research, as a scientific organization and an intergovernmental international organization, it provides a platform for policy formulation based on scientific findings. It also facilitates policy decision-making by providing access to balanced scientific information for major decision-makers.

World Meteorological Organization (WMO)

The World Meteorological Organization (WMO) was established in 1950 and it is the UN system's authoritative voice on the state and behaviour of the Earth's atmosphere, its interaction with the land and oceans, its weather and climate, and the resulting distribution of water resources. The WMO provides the platform and framework for international cooperation, establishes information networks, facilitates the exchange of data and the formation and the standardization of related data, and assists in technology transfer, training, and research. In the specific case of weather, climate, and water-related disasters, which account for nearly 90% of all natural disasters. The global array of activities and programmes of WMO also provide vital information for advance warnings that save lives and reduce damage to property and the environment. The WMO assesses the climate change phenomenon through meteorological, climatological, hydrological, and geophysical observation and takes a leading role in monitoring and protecting the environment.

World Health Organization (WHO)

The WHO is the directing and co-ordinating authority on international health within the UN system. It provides leadership on matters critical to health; engages in partnership formulation when joint action is needed; formulates research agenda and stimulates the generation, translation, and dissemination of valuable knowledge; sets norms and standards and promotes and monitors their implementation; articulates ethical and evidence-based policy options; provides technical support, catalyses change, and builds sustainable institutional capacity; and monitors the health situation and assesses health trends. The WHO strives to participate in the UN Framework Convention on Climate Change and boost the effective climatic and health policies in order to ensure global health.

National governments and their policies and programmes

To address the climate change phenomenon, national governments formulate and carry out their adaptation and mitigation approaches according to their capacity and the resources available. They leads, coordinates, and encourages various stakeholders to work together to tackle the global climate change problem. National adaptation and mitigation policies are as follows.

Science and technology communities

Scientific research may advance understanding of the potential effects of climate change. It is important to engage in continuous research to fill the knowledge gaps and maximize the technology capacity and application in the construction of a sustainable and liveable country and help cope with the challenges mounted by climate change.

Non-governmental organizations

Non-governmental organizations (NGOs) have significant roles to play in initiating, co-ordinating, and advocating activities and actions that aim to protect the community and the environment. They may provide relevant information, propose initiatives, encourage social and public participation, and contribute to the formulation of new policies and emission-reduction projects. They may also play active roles in advocating protection and adaptation policies for vulnerable groups such as the poor and minorities.

Academia

Academic institutions and research groups produce and identify scientific evidence and policy and programme implications to facilitate national, regional, and global solution identification and decision-making about climate change. They are also involved in education and knowledge transfer to help boost public awareness and the ability to address climate change.

Commercial and private enterprises

Commercial companies and private enterprises play an important role in tackling the effects of climate change. Some of these entities or industries contribute significantly to greenhouse gas emissions and their actions to decrease the level of greenhouse gases in the atmosphere are critical to the effectiveness of climate change actions. Development of new low carbon technology (e.g. electric vehicles) and mitigation measures such as the provision and construction of new infrastructure, and research and development of weather forecasting technology, early warning systems, drought-resistant seeds, and water management infrastructure and technology are some examples of important activities that may enhance human adaptation to climate change.

Individuals and their roles and responsibilities

Individual participation is crucial to reducing the emission of greenhouse gases. People's daily activities produce various greenhouse gases. As a member of the twenty-first century global community, practising health environmental co-benefit (HEC) behaviours may help reduce environmental impact associated with individual behaviours while improving individuals' well-being. Walking (rather than riding cars), using energy-saving light bulbs, adopting water-saving measures, and waste recycling are examples of HEC behaviours (see also Case Box 3.10).

Conclusion

Climate change and its impact on human health and well-being is an important health protection topic for the twenty-first century. As highlighted in this chapter, climate change has affected all aspects of living and human health. With the uncertainties and knowledge gaps, public health policymakers, practitioners, and researchers will need to research and explore approaches to enhance well-being and protect community from potential adverse health impacts brought about by a global changing climate.

References

Arblaster, J. M., Gillett, N. P., Calvo, N., Forster, P. M., Polvani, L. M., et al. (2014). Stratospheric ozone changes and climate. *Scientific Assessment of Ozone Depletion: 2014*. Geneva: World Meteorological Organization. Available at: http://www.wmo.int/pages/prog/arep/gaw/ozone_2014/ozone_asst_report.html.

Associated Press (31 May 2015). Rain brings little relief to southern India as heatwave death toll nears 2,200. Available at: https://www.theguardian.com/weather/2015/may/31/southern-india-heatwave-death-toll-nears-2200-rain-brings-little-relief.

Australian Bureau of Meteorology and Commonwealth Scientific and Industrial Research Organisation (2011). *Climate Change in the Pacific: Scientific Assessment and New Research* (Volume 2: Country reports). Available at: https://www.pacificclimatechangescience.org/publications/reports/report-climate-change-in-the-pacific-scientific-assessment-and-new-research/

Australian Government (August 2012). Tuvalu Annual Program Performance Report 2011. Available at: https://dfat.gov.au/about-us/publications/Documents/tuvalu-appr-2011.pdf.

Ayres, J. G., Forsberg, B., Annesi-Maesano, I, Dey, R, Ebi, K. L., et al. (2009). Climate change and respiratory disease: European Respiratory Society position statement. *Eur Respir J 34*(2) 295–302. doi:10.1183/09031936.00003409.

Baker-Austin, C., Trinanes, J. A, Taylor, N. G, Hartnell, R., Siitonen, A., and **Martinez-Urtaza, J.** (2012). Emerging Vibrio risk at high latitudes in response to ocean warming. *Nat Climate Change 3*(1) 73–7. doi: 10.1038/nclimate1628.

Bedford, R. and Bedford, C. (2010). *Climate Change and Migration. South Pacific Perspectives* (1st edn). Wellington: Institute of Policy Studies, Victoria University of Wellington, New Zealand.

Berry, H. (2009). Pearl in the oyster: Climate change as a mental health opportunity. *Australasian Psychiatry 17*(6) 453–6. doi: 10.1080/10398560903045328.

Berry, H. L., Bowen, K., and **Kjellstrom, T.** (2010). Climate change and mental health: A causal pathways framework. *Int J Public Health 55*(2) 123–32. doi:10.1007/s00038-009-0112-0.

Bouchama, A., Dehbi, M., Mohamed, G., Matthies, F., Shoukri, M., and **Menne, B.** (2007). Prognostic factors in heat wave related deaths: A meta-analysis. *Arch Intern Med 167*(20) 2170–6. doi: 10.1001/archinte.167.20.ira70009.

Burke, M. B., Miguel, E., Satyanath, S., Dykema, J. A., and **Lobell, D. B.** (2009). Warming increases the risk of civil war in Africa. *Proc Natl Acad Sci USA 106*(49) 20670–4. doi:10.1073/pnas.0907998106.

Burton, C. (2015). India's deadly heatwave nears end as monsoon arrives. Available at: https://www.theweathernetwork.com/uk/news/articles/indias-deadly-heatwave-nears-end-as-monsoon-arrives/52420/.

Center for Clean Air Policy (2015). Green Resilience: Climate Adaptation Mitigation Synergies. Available at: http://ccap.org/assets/Green_Resilience_Overview_CCAP-January-2015.pdf.

Centers for Disease Control and Prevention (n.d.). A-Z Index of Water-Related Topics. Available at: https://www.cdc.gov/healthywater/disease/az.html.

Centre for Research on the Epidemiology of Disasters (2015). The Human Cost of Natural Disasters 2015: A Global Perspective. Available at: http://reliefweb.int/sites/reliefweb.int/files/resources/PAND_report.pdf.

Chan, E. Y. Y. (2019a). *Climate Change and Urban Health: The Case of Hong Kong as a Subtropical City*. London: Routledge.

Chan, E. Y. Y. (2019b). *Disaster Public Health and Older People*. London: Routledge.

Chan, E. Y. Y., Goggins, W. B., Kim, J. J., and **Griffiths, S. M.** (2010). A study of intracity variation of temperature-related mortality and socioeconomic status among the Chinese population in Hong Kong. *J Epidemiol Commun Health 66*(4) 322–7. doi:10.1136/jech.2008.085167.

Chan, E. Y. Y., Goggins, W. B., Kim, J. J., Griffiths, S. M., and **Ma, T. K.** (2011). Help-seeking behavior during elevated temperature in Chinese population. *J Urban Health 88*(4) 637–50. doi:10.1007/s11524-011-9599-9.

Chan, E. Y. Y., Goggins, W. B., Yue, S. K., and **Lee, P. Y.** (2013). Hospital admissions as a function of temperature, other weather phenomena and pollution levels in an urban setting in China. *Bull WHO 91*(8) 576–84. doi: 10.2471/BLT.12.113035.

Chan, E. Y. Y., Ho, J.Y., Huang, Z., Liu, S. D., Yeung, M.P. S., and **Wong C.S.** (2016). *Knowledge, Attitude and Practices in Health and Environmental Cobenefits in Hong Kong Population* (CCOUC Working Paper Series). Hong Kong: Collaborating Centre for Oxford and CUHK for Disaster and Medical Humanitarian Response.

Chan, E. Y. Y., Huang, Z., Mark, C. K. M., and **Guo, C.** (2017). Weather information acquisition and health significance during extreme cold weather in a subtropical city: A cross-sectional survey in Hong Kong. *Int J Disastr Risk Sci 8*(2) 134–44. doi:10.1007/s13753-017-0127-8.

Chaves, L. F. and Koenraadt, C. J. (2010). Climate change and highland malaria: Fresh air for a hot debate. *Q Rev Biol 85*(1) 27–55.

Daiss, T. (25 May 2016). Why Vietnam is running dry, worst drought in nearly 100 years. *Forbes.* Available at: https://www.forbes.com/sites/timdaiss/2016/05/25/why-vietnam-is-running-dry-worst-drought-in-nearly-100-years/#4e0a83a974b3.

D'Amato, G., Cecchi, L., Bonini, S., Nunes, C., Annesi-Maesano, I., et al. (2007). Allergenic pollen and pollen allergy in Europe. *Allergy 62*(9) 976–90. doi: 10.1111/j.1398-9995.2007.01393.x.

D'Amato, G., Cecchi, L., D'Amato, M., and Annesi-Maesano, I. (2014). Climate change and respiratory diseases. *Eur Respir Rev 23*(132) 161–9. doi: 10.1183/09059180.00001714.

D'Amato, G., Vitale, C., De Martino, A., Giovanni, V., Maurizia, L., et al. (2015). Effects on asthma and respiratory allergy of climate change and air pollution. *Multidiscip Respir Med 39*(1) 10–39. doi:10.1186/s40248-015-0036-x.

De Blois, J., Kjellstrom, T., Agewall, S., Ezekowitz, J. A., Armstrong, P. W., and Atar, D. (2015). The effects of climate change on cardiac health. *Cardiology 131*(4) 209–17. doi: 10.1159/000398787.

Dixon, J. M., Donati, K. J., Pike, L. L., and Hattersley, L. (2009). Functional foods and urban agriculture: Two responses to climate change-related food insecurity. *NSW Pub Health Bull 20*(2) 14–18. doi:10.1071/nb08044.

European Centre for Disease Prevention and Control (2012). Assessing the potential impacts of climate change on food- and waterborne diseases in Europe (ECDC Technical Report). Stockholm: ECDC. Available at: https://ecdc.europa.eu/sites/portal/files/media/en/publications/Publications/1203-TER-Potential-impacts-climate-change-food-water-borne-diseases.pdf.

Elder, W. (n.d.). Greenhouse effect graphic [online image]. Available at: https:// www.nps.gov/grba/learn/nature/what-is-climatechange.htm.

El-Hinnawi, E. (1985). *Environmental Refugees.* Nairobi: United Nations Environment Programme.

FloodList (22 October 2015). UN report—Floods in Myanmar had devastating impact on agriculture. Available at: http://floodlist.com/asia/un-myanmar-floods-food-security.

Friel, S., Bowen, K., Campbell-Lendrum, D., Frumkin, H., McMichael, A. J., and Rasanathan, K. (2011). Climate change, noncommunicable diseases, and development: The relationships and common policy opportunities. *Ann RevPublic Health 32* 133–47. doi: 10.1146/annurev-publhealth-071910-140612.

Gold, D. R. and Samet, J. M. (2013). Air pollution, climate, and heart disease. *Circulation 128*(21) e411–e414. doi: 10.1161/CIRCULATIONAHA.113.003988.

Hodzic, A., Madronich, S., Bohn, B., Massie, S., Menut, L., and Wiedinmyer, C. (2007). Wildfire particulate matter in Europe during summer 2003: Meso-scale modeling of smoke emissions, transport and radiative effects. *Atmospheric Chem Phys 7*(15) 4043–64.

Hong Kong Observatory (23 March 2015). The weather of March 2014. Available at: http://www.weather.gov.hk/wxinfo/pastwx/mws2014/mws201403.htm.

Intergovernmental Panel on Climate Change (2007a). *Climate change 2007: Mitigation: Contribution of Working Group III to the fourth assessment report of the Intergovernmental Panel on Climate Change.* Cambridge: Cambridge University Press.

Intergovernmental Panel on Climate Change (2007b). *Climate change 2007: Synthesis report. Contribution of Working Groups I, II and III to the fourth assessment Report of the Intergovernmental Panel on Climate Change* [R. K. Pachauri and A. Reisinger (eds)]. Geneva: IPCC.

Intergovernmental Panel on Climate Change (2007c). *Climate change 2007: Impacts, adaptation and vulnerability: Contribution of Working Group II to the fourth assessment report of the Intergovernmental Panel on Climate Change.* (M. L. Parry, O. F. Canziani, J. P. Palutikof, P. J. van der Linden, and C. E. Hanson (eds). Cambridge: Cambridge University Press.

Intergovernmental Panel on Climate Change (2007d). *Climate change 2007: The physical science basis. Contribution of Working Group I to the Fourth Assessment Report of the Intergovernmental Panel on Climate Change* (S. D. Solomon, D. Qin, M. Manning, Z. Chen, M. Marquis, K. B. Averyt, et al. (eds)). Cambridge: Cambridge University Press.

Intergovernmental Panel on Climate Change (2012). *Managing the risks of extreme events and disasters to advance climate change adaptation. A special report of Working Groups I and II of the Intergovernmental Panel on Climate Change* (C. B. Field, V. Barros, T. F. Stocker, D. Qin, D. J. Dokken, et al. (eds)). Cambridge: Cambridge University Press.

Intergovernmental Panel on Climate Change (2013). *Climate change 2013: The physical science basis: Contribution of Working Group I to the fifth assessment Report of the Intergovernmental Panel on Climate Change.* (T. F. Stocker, D. Qin, G.-K. Plattner, M. Tignor, S. K. Allen, et al. (eds)), Cambridge: Cambridge University Press.

Intergovernmental Panel on Climate Change (2014). *Climate change 2014: Impacts, adaptation, and vulnerability: Part A: Global and sectoral aspects: Contribution of Working Group II to the fifth assessment report of the Intergovernmental Panel on Climate Change.* Cambridge: Cambridge University Press.

Jelmayer, R. and Chao, L. (2015). Drought-stricken São Paulo battles dengue fever outbreak. *World Street Journal.* Available at: https://www.wsj.com/articles/drought-stricken-sao-paulo-battles-dengue-fever-outbreak-1425420508.

Kao, E. (31 March 2014). Giant hailstones batter Hong Kong as Observatory warns of heavy rain for days to come. *South China Morning Post.* Available at: https://www.scmp.com/news/hong-kong/article/1461200/giant-hailstones-batter-hong-kong-observatory-hoists-black-rainstorm.

Kovats, R. S., Edwards, S. J., Hajat, S., Armstrong, B. G., Ebi, K. L., and Menne, B. (2004). The effect of temperature on food poisoning: A time-series analysis of salmonellosis in ten European countries. *Epidemiol Infection 132*(03) 443–53.

Lundberg, A. (1998). *The Environment and Mental Health: A Guide for Clinicians.* Mahwah, NJ: Lawrence Erlbaum Associates.

Makin, J. (2011). Implications of climate change for skin cancer prevention in Australia. *Health Promot J Aust 22*(4) 39–41.

National Institute of Environmental Health Sciences (2010). Foodborne diseases and nutrition: Health impacts of climate change. Available at: http://www.niehs.nih.gov/research/programs/geh/climatechange/health_impacts/foodborne_diseases/index.cfm.

Næss, L. O., Bang, G., Eriksen, S., and Vevatne, J. (2005). Institutional adaptation to climate change: Flood responses at the municipal level in Norway. *Global Environ Change 15*(2) 125–38. doi:10.1016/j.gloenvcha.2004.10.003.

Norris, F. H., Friedman, M. J., and Watson, P. J. (2002). 60,000 disaster victims speak: Part II. Summary and implications of the disaster mental health research. *Psychiatry 65*(3) 240–60.

Poumadère, M., Mays, C., Mer, S. L., and Blong, R. (2005). The 2003 heat wave in France: Dangerous climate change here and now. *Risk Analysis 25*(6) 1483–94. doi:10.1111/j.1539-6924.2005.00694.x.

Reid, C. E. and Gamble, J. L. (2009). Aeroallergens, allergic disease, and climate change: Impacts and adaptation. *Ecohealth 6*(3) 458–70.

ReliefWeb (14 April 2016). Viet Nam: Drought and saltwater intrusion (Situation Update No. 2 (as of 14 April 2016)). Available at: https://reliefweb.int/report/viet-nam/viet-nam-drought-and-saltwater-intrusion-situation-update-no-2-14-april-2016.

Remais, J. V., Hess, J. J., Ebi, K. L., Markandya, A., Balbus, J. M. (2014). Estimating the health effects of greenhouse gas mitigation strategies: Addressing parametric, model, and valuation challenges. *Environ Health Perspect 122*(5) 447–55. doi:10.1289/ehp.1306744.

Roberts, I. and Hillman, M. (2005). Climate change: The implications for policy on injury control and health promotion. *Injury Prevent 11* 326–9.

Stafoggia, M., Forastiere, F., Agostini, D., Caranci, N., de'Donato, F., et al. (2008). Factors affecting in-hospital heat-related mortality: A multi-city case-crossover analysis. *J Epidemiol Comm Health 62*(3) 209–15.

Stanke, C., Kerac, M., Prudhomme, C., Medlock, J., and Murray, V. (2013). Health effects of drought: A systematic review of the evidence. *PLopS Currents Disast.* doi:10.1371/currents.dis.7a2cee9e980f91a d7697b570bcc4b004.

Thomson, M. C., Doblas-Reyes, F. J., Mason, S. J., Hagedorn, R., Connor, S. J., et al. (2006). Malaria early warnings based on seasonal climate forecasts from multi-model ensembles. *Nature 439*(7076) 576–9. doi:10.1038/nature04503.

United Nations (1992). United Nations Framework Convention on Climate Change. Available at: unfcc. int/resource/docs/convkp/conveng.pdf.

United Nations (2015a). Sendai Framework for Disaster Risk Reduction 2015–2030. Available at: http:// www.preventionweb.net/files/43291_sendaiframeworkfordrren.pdf.

United Nations (2015b). Sustainable Development Goals. Available at: https://wwww.un.org/ sustainabledevelopment/sustainable-development-goals/.

United Nations Department for Economic and Social Affairs (2009). State of the world's indigenous peoples. Available at: http://www.un.org/esa/socdev/unpfii/documents/SOWIP/en/SOWIP_web. pdf.

United Nations Framework Convention on Climate Change (2015). The Paris Agreement. Available at: https://unfccc.int/sites/default/files/english_paris_agreement.pdf.

United Nations International Strategy for Disaster Reduction (2009). 2009 UNISDR terminology on disaster risk reduction. Available at: http://www.unisdr.org/files/7817_UNISDRTerminologyEnglish. pdf.

United Nations Office for Disaster Risk Reduction (2015). The economic and human impact of disasters in the last 10 years. Available at: http:// www.unisdr.org/files/42862_economichumanimpa ct20052014unisdr.pdf.

Watts, N., Adger, W. N., Agnolucci, P., Blackstock, J., Byass, P., et al. (2015). Health and climate change: Policy responses to protect public health. *Lancet 386*(10006) 1861–914. doi:10.1016/ s0140-6736(15)60854.

World Health Organization (n.d.). Chronic respiratory diseases: Allergic rhinitis and sinusitis. Available at: http://www.who.int/respiratory/other/Rhinitis_sinusitis/en/.

World Health Organization (1946). Preamble to the Constitution of the World Health Organization. Available at: http://www.who.int/governance/eb/who_constitution_en.pdf.

World Health Organization. (2008). *Protecting Hhealth from Cclimate Cchange: World Health Day 2008.* SwitzerlandGeneva: World Health OrganizationWorld Health Organization (2014). Burden of disease from household air pollution for 2012. Available at: http://www.who.int/phe/health_topics/ outdoorair/databases/FINAL_HAP_AAP_BoD_24March2014.pdf?ua=1.

World Health Organization. (2015). *Food safety (Fact sheet No. 399).* Available at: http://www.who.int/ campaigns/world-health-day/2015/fact-sheet.pdf

World Health Organization (2016). Fact sheet: World Malaria Day 2016. Retrieved from http://www. who.int/malaria/media/world-malaria-day-2016/en/.

World Health Organization (April 2017). Mental health in emergencies. Available at: http://www.who. int/news-room/fact-sheets/detail/mental-health-in-emergencies.

World Health Organization (May 2017). Cardiovascular diseases (CVDs). Available at: http://www. who.int/en/news-room/fact-sheets/detail/cardiovascular-diseases-(cvds).

World Health Organization (August 2017). Asthma. Available at: http://www.who.int/en/news-room/fact-sheets/detail/asthma.

World Health Organization (December 2017). Chronic obstructive pulmonary disease (COPD). Available at: http://www.who.int/news-room/fact-sheets/detail/chronic-obstructive-pulmonary-disease-(copd).

World Health Organization (2018a). Cancer. Available at: http://www.who.int/en/news-room/fact-sheets/detail/cancer.

World Health Organization (2018b). Mental health: Strengthening our response. Available at: http://www.who.int/en/news-room/fact-sheets/detail/mental-health-strengthening-our-response.

World Meteorological Organization (n.d.). Global Atmosphere Watch (GAW): UV radiation. Available at: http://www.wmo.int/pages/prog/arep/gaw/UV-radiation.html.

World Meteorological Organization (1992a). *International Meteorological Vocabulary* (2nd edn). Geneva: World Meteorological Organization.

World Meteorological Organization (1992b). Meteoterm. Available at: http://www.wmo.int/pages/prog/lsp/meteoterm_wmo_en.html.

World Meteorological Organization (2012). International glossary of hydrology. Available at: wmo.int/pages/prg/hwrp/publications/international_glossary/385_IGH_2012.pdf.

Chapter 4

Emergency Preparedness and Disaster Response

Emergency preparedness and disaster response to health risks and needs are essential health protection skills and competency to protect community health and well-being in time of crisis. Emergencies and extreme events may disrupt environmental context and destroy essential life- and health-sustaining infrastructures. Crisis often renders a health system ineffective to provide and protect a community from its regular underlying health risks as well as to address the overwhelming health and medical needs associated with the disruption.

In addition, in the twenty-first century, many of the emergencies and disasters transcend national boundaries and require transnational cooperation. Such response requires global involvement to respond effectively and efficiently. Natural disasters that affect multiple nations (e.g. hurricanes/typhoons), global disease outbreaks of old and emerging infectious diseases, and population displacements as results of war, famine, or natural disasters require not just response capacity of a nation; global cooperation and response capacity to ensure well-functioning mechanisms of local, national, and global health risk management and governance can minimise human life loss. This chapter will describe and explain the major principles of disaster preparedness and response in public health.

Definition of disaster

Disaster is an event that may serious disrupt 'the functioning of a community or a society involving widespread human, material, economic or environmental losses and impacts, which exceeds the ability of the affected community or society to cope using its own resources' (United Nations International Strategy for Disaster Reduction [UNISDR], 2009). Disaster may also refer to '[a] situation or [an] event, which overwhelms local capacity, necessitating a request to national or international level for external assistance; An unforeseen and often sudden event that causes great damage, destruction and human suffering' (Centre for Research on the Epidemiology of Disasters [CRED], 2009). Although a disaster with catastrophic consequences may

Essentials for Health Protection. Emily Ying Yang Chan, Oxford University Press (2020).
© Oxford University Press
DOI: 10.1093/oso/9780198835479.001.0001

follow natural hazards, hazard itself might not necessarily result in a disaster event directly.

Classification of disasters and their impact on public health

Disasters and emergencies might originate from natural hazards or human causes. Natural hazards and their associated disasters often have geographic characteristics and predispositions (e.g. being located along tectonic fault lines or volcanic eruption at-risk zones). Human-caused/technological disasters (e.g. nuclear accidents, radioactive contaminations, aircraft accidents) are associated with human activities and use of technology. Another important subgroup of human-caused emergencies that may result in catastrophic consequences is a complex emergency, which often involves violence, conflict, and war.

The medical and public health impacts of disasters can be described in terms of direct health outcomes such as mortality and morbidity, as well as the indirect consequences such as disruption on healthcare services (including the availability of healthcare workers, resources, and technology and the functionality of infrastructure) for immediate disaster response and the increased clinical needs of the affected population (including the injured and the displaced).

Trends and patterns of disasters and health emergencies in the twenty-first century

Asia has always been the region most severely affected by disasters in terms of frequencies and number of people affected globally. In 2014, around 44.4% of natural disasters in the world occurred in Asia and 69.5% of the people affected by natural disasters worldwide resided there (Guha-Sapir, Hoyois, and Below, 2015). Not only are many of these disaster-affected countries of large population, their community members are often with limited disaster risk literacy and measures in disaster preparedness and disaster risk reduction might not be implemented effectively. Moreover, with rise in climate-related disasters, natural disasters will remain a major challenge for health protection in the twenty-first century. In the coming decades, population growth in disaster-prone areas such as coastal cities and urban areas might lead to an increasing number of people at risk and affected by natural disasters.

Causes of the increase in emergencies and disasters in the twenty-first century

A number of reasons have been cited for the increased frequency of disasters in the twenty-first century. **Climate change** poses major challenges to environment and health. Abnormal temperatures and rainfall, sea-level rise, and extreme weather might give rise to health risk and have direct and indirect impacts on the well-being of humans. Global warming accelerates the melting of icebergs, mountain snow and glaciers, exposing some regions to the threat of flooding. Sea-level rise makes the coastal areas susceptible to inland flowing of seawater to flood farmlands. Since seawater is high in salt and other harmful materials that cannot be assimilated by crops, it leads to soil salinization, crop withering and potentially food insecurity crises. Extreme weather like Hurricane Katrina in 2005 and Super Typhoon Haiyan in 2013 causes high casualties and huge economic and property losses. **Urbanization** poses an enormous pressure on society and the environment. High population density requires robust infrastructure and predisposes risk of communicable disease transmission. Although social development brings about the advancement of healthcare technologies, people face new health risks and challenges.

Industrialization and rapid urbanization in developing countries increase the emission of greenhouse gases that accelerate global warming and lead to climate change problems. If disaster response capacity lags behind the pace of urbanization and development and a disaster damages urban infrastructure such as water plants, power plants, communication networks, and the transportation systems essential for food delivery, the health risk of the urban population will be exacerbated. **Globalization** might enable the exchange of technology, information, and resources; yet, it might also enhance the travel opportunities of humans, pathogens, and diseases. Transient movement of people might increase in communicable disease risks. In recent years, pandemic influenza, SARS, Ebola, and Zika virus disease are only some examples of how global population movement may exacerbate risks of disease spreading if responses are not at the global scale. With technology advances and the increasing reliance on lifeline infrastructure (i.e. water, electricity, communication, and transportation infrastructure), there also emerges a new subset of extreme events called *Natech* (natural disaster-triggered technological disaster) that may cause catastrophic human consequences. Natech refers to how natural disasters may exacerbate health risks caused initially by natural disasters but escalated by technology failures (Cruz, Kajitani, and Tatano, 2015) (see Knowledge Box 4.1).

In some regions where socio-economic conditions are poor, the disaster response capacity may be limited due to scant resources. Together with underdeveloped disaster preparedness and relief policies, the casualties in these regions are often heavier than would be the case in richer regions when disasters strike. Moreover, poverty thwarts individuals' chance of receiving education and hinders them from receiving and comprehending health information as well as seeking healthcare services. Weak disaster and health risk literacy in preparedness and awareness among low-income populations make them more vulnerable when facing disasters.

Knowledge Box 4.1 Natech Disasters (Natural Disaster-Triggered Technological Disasters)

Emily Ying Yang Chan and Asta Yi-tao Man

Natural disaster-triggered technological disasters ('Natech' disasters) are technological disasters that are triggered by natural hazard-related disaster events (Girgin, Necci, and Krausmann, 2017). Although Natech incidents do not have to be caused by a major natural hazard event, these often involve cascading events and complex risks that might amplify their adverse impact by two or more types of hazards. Adverse impacts of a natural hazard event might affect lifeline and industrial infrastructure such as water and gas pipelines, chemical installations, and offshore platforms. Much of this infrastructure might involve the processing, storage, or transportation of dangerous substances that can cause fires, explosions, and the release of toxic or radioactive substances, with major health implications for human well-being. Some important incidents in recent years include: the 2002 river flooding in Europe, which caused the release of significant hazardous substances including chlorine; the 2011 Great East Japan earthquake and Tsunami, which caused a nuclear power plant meltdown, raging fires, and explosions at oil refineries; and in 2012, Hurricane Sandy in the United States, which triggered multiple hydrocarbon spills.

Although these Natech accidents have major social, environmental, and economic impacts and features in common with many natural hazards and associated disasters, their impact, preparedness, and risk assessments are often overlooked and not fully understood. In addition, emergency and health responders are often neither equipped nor trained to handle several substance releases at the same time. Because of the inherent multi-hazard nature, Natech risk assessment involves multidisciplinary actors ranging from industry operators and authorities in charge of chemical accident prevention and civil protection, to emergency responders and residents of any potential affected communities. Natech risk assessment and management requires a comprehensive understanding of the interdependencies of human, natural, and technological systems. A Natech accident can result in major unexpected human implications as there may have neither prior risk assessment nor proper preparedness planning for this kind of disaster event and the specific situation.

Myths about disaster

There are many myths associated with disasters and emergencies (Alexander, 2007; Chan, 2017). In particular, as related to human behaviour and post-disaster medical and health response, some of these myths might affect risk perception, disaster preparedness, and response approaches in a country (see Table 4.1).

Table 4.1 Myths and Realities About Disaster

Myth	Reality
Disasters are abnormal events.	Disasters are part of everyday life and often recur with specific characteristics and impact patterns.
Disasters have equal impact on people of different social classes.	Compared to the middle class or the rich, the poor are more vulnerable to disasters.
Earthquakes kill large numbers of people directly.	Most earthquakes do not result in high mortality directly; infrastructure and buildings collapsed in earthquakes do lead to high death toll. Although earthquakes cannot be eliminated, the loss caused by disasters can be alleviated by building seismic-resistant buildings and formulating effective earthquake evacuation plans in advance.
Large numbers of affected people flee from the area struck by disasters.	Usually, there is a 'convergence phenomenon' in a disaster-affected area like a displacement camp or settlement, leading to an overcrowded living environment in the area, which generates other public health problems.
Having experienced a disaster, survivors tend to be dazed and apathetic.	Survivors tend to start reconstruction rapidly. Activism is much more common than fatalism in post-disaster affected communities (formation of a 'therapeutic community'). Only a small portion of the population is affected psychologically.
Looting is common after disasters.	Post-disaster looting is relatively rare and only occurred in specific areas like those facing acute social polarization or other problems.
Epidemics always follow disasters.	Whether there is an epidemic post disaster depends on the actual situations of the disaster-affected area, but the epidemiological surveillance mechanism and healthcare services in the area are usually sufficient to handle any potential epidemics.
Any kind of aid and relief is useful post disaster.	Hasty and ill-considered relief initiatives may create chaos. Types of assistance, goods, and services needed vary with timing and context in the disaster-affected area.
After the occurrence of a disaster not caused by infectious diseases, unburied dead bodies pose a health hazard to other people.	Researches show that, after disasters of non-infectious diseases, unburied dead bodies do not pose a significant health hazard to other people. Proper management of the dead bodies is significant as an act of respect to the deceased, which preserves their dignity.
People should donate used clothes to disaster victims.	Donation items (e.g. clothes) should be based on the 'fit for purpose' principle. Garments may not be suitable for the victims (for reasons like gender, culture, size, etc.) and lack of consideration of their distribution creates pressures on the logistics management in the disaster-affected area (e.g. the accumulation of a huge quantity of garments).
Any kind of medicine is needed in disaster-affected areas.	Medicine should be received with caution. Healthcare needs in the disaster-affected areas should be assessed first and relief medicines be transported to these areas by healthcare organizations. Expired medication and unsolicited drug donations without a specific recipient end should not be encouraged.

Source: Alexander (2007).

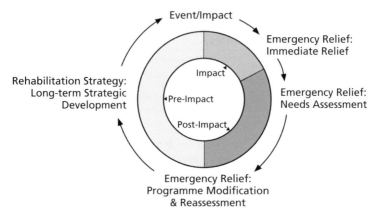

Figure 4.1 Three phases of disaster

Anatomy and structure of disaster

The dynamics and events of a disaster may be understood in three temporal phases: (i) the pre-impact phase; (ii) the impact phase; and (iii) the post-impact phase. The **pre-impact phase** is the period before the occurrence of a disaster. During this phase, there is the greatest potential for preventing the negative health impact of disasters. *Mitigations* are measures taken to reduce the impact and health risk of the population posed by these hazards. Both the natural and built environments can be hazardous if appropriate measures are not taken to protect the population from exposure. *Disaster preparedness* refers to activities taken by professionals to ensure that timely and efficient response systems are in place in times of disaster. It also includes actions taken at the community and individual levels to protect against and minimize physical and emotional damage resulting from disasters. The **impact phase** is the period during and immediately after a disaster, when rapid needs assessment and search and rescue relief work takes place. *Disaster response* is the actions taken to react to an emergency or disaster. These actions include initial assessments as well as search and rescue immediately after the disaster. The **post-impact phase** is the period after the impact of a disaster and relief effort has reached equilibrium, or stabilized. During this phase, efforts typically focus on long-term rehabilitation and recovery. *Disaster recovery* includes the measures taken by national leaders and community stakeholders to help the population return to their 'normal' state before the disaster struck. Both the natural and built environments can be hazardous if appropriate measures are not taken to protect the population from exposure. Post-disaster mitigations measures may be taken to reduce the risk to the health of the population posed by these post-exposure hazards. Figure 4.1 illustrates the interface between the three phases of disasters and disaster response cycle.

Disaster response cycle

An important concept in disaster-related health and medical response is the disaster response cycle (Chan, 2017). Although it is impossible to change the frequency of disasters, it is possible to change the response to a disaster to reduce the human impact. Disaster response should be planned, monitored, and implemented according to the stages of the disaster and a population's associated needs. Figure 4.1 shows the disaster response cycle. The disaster cycle illustrates the five phases at which medical and humanitarian disaster response can take place in a disaster scenario: (i) event or impact; (ii) immediate relief; (iii) needs assessment; (iv) programme modification and reassessment; and (v) long-term strategic development. The disaster cycle will be discussed in more detail in later chapters. Decision-making during the dynamic disaster response cycle should use accepted guiding framework and indicators such as those highlighted in the Sphere guidelines to ensure effectiveness, accountability, and enhancement of response is achieved. A relevant and appropriate disaster response should be planned and organized according to the stage of disasters.

The first phase of the disaster cycle describes the non-disaster or normal state. Development of the country or region often determines the availability of medical services and emergency preparedness for the population. In low-income or developing countries, it is likely that the pre-disaster health services are limited. Even with disaster planning for acute/emergency services, resources may be scarce for non-communicable or chronic diseases during an emergency. At this stage, risk reduction and disaster preparedness programmes are also crucial determining factors that affect future disaster response activities. A key driver of effective emergency preparedness is creating community-based initiatives in all phases of a disaster response including preparedness, protection, and response. Contributing actors including community healthcare workers, trained volunteers, local organizations, and key players from different sectors (e.g. water, shelter, and education) act as the primary human resources for disaster management. In addition, the community is central to post-disaster recovery and a speedy transition back to normality.

Preventive actions are always more effective than restorative ones. Hence, risk reduction is an integral component of the disaster cycle. During times of non-disaster, various actions can help relieve the burden of future disasters.

The second stage of the disaster cycle, immediate relief, is characterized by the event itself and the immediate intervention and relief carried out by local response units. At this stage of the emergency, both government and relief agencies may be strapped for resources due to the immediate surge of emergency cases, mortality cases, and the destruction of health services. Provision of services may be limited to essential life-saving procedures. Except for life-threatening complications of chronic diseases, victims with chronic conditions may be overlooked. A poor baseline health profile of the population and limited available resources could have a detrimental effect on the response capacity. In many developing countries which are facing a double burden of disease (see Chapter 2), the complex health needs of the population are great.

The third stage of the disaster cycle, emergency relief, highlights the importance of obtaining valid information to use for further evidence-based interventions. Initial health-needs assessments should be quickly conducted to aggregate information to assist appropriate and relevant decision-making.

The fourth stage of the disaster cycle, emergency relief, focuses on programme modification based on continuous health-needs monitoring data. Health-needs assessments often use simple measures such as mortality rather than more relevant health determinants that contribute to mortality and morbidity. Such over-simplistic indicators are not sufficient to capture all possible solutions to address real needs. Since ill health can be caused by multiple factors, relief operation recommendations drawn from single sector assessments are inadequate to meet all aspects of underlying health needs. In developing countries, myriad underlying issues may hinder good health and these need to be taken into consideration to set up effective programmes. Due to the target-oriented and short-term nature of most interventions, an exit strategy must be drawn out in the final stage of the disaster cycle, rehabilitation. Community participation and collaboration are essential to the sustainability of post-disaster efforts of a non-acute nature.

Importance of disaster management

Disasters cause extensive losses to human society and the natural environment. Effective disaster management should prepare a community for disasters to minimize losses. Apart from immediate relief, the disaster cycle (see Figure 4.1) describes the several preparedness and response stages pre- and post-disaster, including such measures as situation and needs assessments carried out in a timely fashion after the disaster, relief plan modification, long-term development and disaster preparedness planning, and strengthening disaster education.

Disaster management should aim to control a mortality rate from exceeding the emergency threshold, that is, the rate experienced in normal times. Disaster management is important because people can effectively lessen and reduce the influence and impact of disasters on society through the design and implementation of relevant knowledge, early warnings, emergency responses, and relief programmes.

Public health consequences of disasters

Disasters may result in multiple and long-term problems to a community. In general, there are five major public health consequences after a disaster affects a community. First and foremost, it leads to **morbidity and mortality exceeding the normal rate experienced in non-disaster times**. Disasters cause injures and diseases in vast quantity and variety, compounded by the complex demographic and epidemiological characteristics of the disaster victims, which outs pressure on rescue work. The casualties of disasters often greatly exceed the capacity of the local emergency response system. Second, a disaster may lead to **destruction and disruption of local health systems and normal routine services.** In addition to the direct destruction of the health system by such disasters as earthquakes and typhoons, healthcare needs brought about by disasters also disrupts the local health system. The demand created by the large number of wounded people beyond the capacity of regular healthcare services such as vaccine supply, vaccination services, diagnosis, and maintenance of chronic disease management would need to be addressed. Disaster could

impose grave effects on the environment and residents. Natural disasters like flooding and landslides lead to the destruction and degradation of environment. Disasters may also trigger the emission and release of toxic materials to cause emergent environmental incidents (e.g. the Fukushima nuclear power plant radiation leakage brought about by the April 2011 Japanese earthquake and tsunami). Disasters may also have **profound impacts in psychological and social well-being**. After disasters, survivors may encounter psychological and emotional problems due to their witnessing or experiencing traumatic events and their consequences. **Long-term health problems** associated with extreme events may go beyond the event time period. For people affected by nuclear incidents, they may suffer from increased risks of infertility, cancers, and birth defects in residents affected by nuclear disasters, and famines bring about nutrition and developmental problems.

Health impacts of common emergencies and disasters

Hydrological disasters (floods)

Floods are the most common type of natural disaster. They account for 40% of natural disasters worldwide and are the leading cause of mortality due to natural disasters, with 6.8 million deaths recorded in the twentieth century (Doocy, Dick, Daniels, and Kirsch, 2013). Almost half the flood-related fatalities in the last quarter of the twentieth century occurred in Asia. Generally, floods can be classified into three types: general flood, flash flood, and storm surge/coastal flood (Chan, 2017). **General flood** involves the accumulation of water on the surface due to long-lasting rainfall (waterlogging) and the rise of the groundwater table above the surface. It can be induced by the melting of snow and ice, backwater effects, or special causes such as the outburst of a glacial lake or the breaching of a dam. **Flash flood** is a sudden flooding episode occurs within a short duration. It is typically associated with thunderstorms and can occur in any place. **Storm surge/coastal flood** refers to the rise of the water level of the sea, an estuary, or lake as a result of strong wind driving seawater towards the coast. The areas most threatened by storm surges are coastal lowlands. While not strictly a type of flood, tsunamis are caused by earthquakes or slips on the sea floor generating a series of waves which cause enormous damage to coastal areas. The health impacts of tsunamis are very similar to floods. Different flood types are directly associated with the extent of adverse human impact. For example, flash floods that occur quickly and that leave people with little lead time to respond result in higher mortality rates compared with general floods. In contrast, general floods, despite the slower onset, affect larger populations and a wider area. Floods with higher water depth and greater flow velocity result in greater damage.

Although rainfall is one of the main determinants of flooding event, **human factors** (e.g. lack of structural flood control measures such as embankments, obstruction of river water flow due to debris and wastes, and **lack of drainage basins in urban areas**), **meteorological factors** (e.g. solidified ground surface after a drought reducing the ability of soil to absorb excessive rainwater quickly, and excessive precipitation over a prolonged period oversaturating the soil and increasing overland run-off) and **topographical**

factors (e.g. a lack of vegetation or woodland of trees and plants to intercept precipitation when a river bank bursts, leading to the water overflowing onto the **floodplain**) (Associated Programme on Flood Management [APFM], 2013) may all affect the outcomes of a flooding event.

The health impact of floods is complex and is difficult to generalize across contexts. Drowning and traumatic injuries are common causes of death during floods as fast-flowing flood water carries vehicles, trees, or building materials that cause orthopaedic injuries, trauma, and lacerations. In addition to drowning, victims are prone to **hypothermia**, especially in cold weather, injuries, and animal bites while being under floodwater from rivers and other water bodies that may host snakes or other dangerous animals. Floods may comprise fresh or salt water. Each type has particular health implications. For instance, freshwater floods leave mud and soil when the waters recede and they contaminate drinking water sources. Saltwater can affect the salinity of groundwater, make it undrinkable, and harm aquatic animals (Smith, 2009). Floodwater also destroys power lines, submerges electrical equipment, causes **electrical shocks**, and increases fire risks. Floods cause **water contamination** by bacteria and viruses. Floods in Mozambique in 2000 caused a rising number of diarrhoea cases, those in Mauritius in 1980 triggered an outbreak of typhoid fever, and those in West Bengal in 1998 created a cholera epidemic (Gayer and Connolly, 2005). Cholera is an infectious diarrheal disease, caused by *Vibrio cholerae*. It is estimated that there are 3–5 million cases of cholera annually, and 100,000–200,000 deaths due to cholera per year (De Cock, Simone, Davison, and Slutsker, 2013). Studies show that *V. cholerae* is native to coastal ecosystems, particularly in the tropics and subtropics (Colwell, Kaper, and Joseph, 1977; Lipp, Huq, and Colwell, 2002). Coastal flooding increases the risk of cholera infections. Furthermore, stagnant water, remaining for days or weeks after the initial flood, increases the risk of vector-borne illnesses by providing new breeding sites for vectors.

In general, the key health risks associated with flooding events include injury (drowning) and trauma, increased communicable disease risks (due to water source contamination), and suboptimal water quality, sanitation, and waste management (Ahern, Kovats, Wilkinson, Few, and Matthies, 2005; Chan, 2017). The psychological impact of floods is also well-documented and the potential large scale of internally displaced people might lead to multiple psychosocial issues that affect well-being in the recovery period and beyond.

Geophysical disasters (earthquakes, tsunamis, and volcanic eruptions)

When compared to flooding, geophysical events are more likely to involve massive death than injury. Depending on seismic factors (magnitude and intensity), demographic characteristics (e.g. extremes of age), disaster preparedness, living environment (e.g. building constructions and codes), and community resilience (emergency response system in place), the risk of mortality and morbidity varies with time and location (Ramirez and Peek-Asa, 2005; Chan, 2017).

The majority of the health impacts of an earthquake stem from the collapse of buildings and infrastructure (Chan, 2017). Search and rescue are fundamental to the immediate earthquake response. Falling debris and entrapment may directly cause trauma, crush injuries, and fractures in victims. Cuts and bruises can be expected in most of the patients presented during the first week. Other associated health risks of entrapment include hypoxia (lack of oxygen), hypothermia (especially during winter), and electrocution. The fall of debris may also cause dust inhalation, which in turn may trigger acute respiratory distress and cardiovascular complications. A high volume of injuries and fractures are expected in the first weeks after an earthquake, therefore orthopaedic surgeons and anaesthesiologists are vital. Nephrologists or physicians specializing in renal care are also needed at the initial phase of disaster relief as patients with crush injuries may develop acute kidney failure. In Haiti, after the earthquake in January 2010, kidney failure became one of the most urgent public health concerns (Portilla, Shaffer, Okusa, Mehrotra, Molitoris, et al., 2010). Surged health needs and re-organization of injury medical services are also needed to manage. Since earthquakes bring huge destruction and damage to buildings, management of displaced and homeless populations is also crucial. Physical disability and psychosocial support for earthquake survivors often require long-term management.

Biological disasters

Common emergencies associated with biological agents include disease outbreaks and food poisoning incidents. Depending on the availability of service and treatment to manage the disease impact, these events might potentially lead to high case-fatality rate and high demand of health service needs. An **outbreak of infectious disease** can be defined as an increase in the number of cases of a disease beyond what is normally expected in a specific population and area within a short period of time. An **epidemic** occurs when an outbreak spreads through a larger geographical area with a higher proportion of infected people. Epidemics are classified under the biological category of natural hazards (International Federation of Red Cross and Red Crescent Societies [IFRC], n.d.). They are considered as disasters as they affect large quantities of people and result in public health emergencies.

An epidemic may occur due to a recent increase in amount or virulence, or an enhanced mode of transmission of the pathogens. While different diseases have specific characteristics and risks to become epidemic, in general, epidemic risk increases when the interaction of host, disease agent, and environment becomes abnormal. Poverty is a potential determinant for epidemic and may be associated with malnutrition and low vaccination uptake. Moreover, it may hamper access to healthcare facilities and services and result in lack of resources for disease control. The risk of an epidemic may also increase after the occurrence of other types of disaster. Altered environments might favour the proliferation of pathogens and/or decreases the immunity of the host population. Particularly in those disasters with large-scale population displacement, the consequent of overcrowding in temporary settlements and disruption of water supplies and sanitation render people vulnerable to water-borne and other infectious diseases (Watson, Gayer, and Connolly, 2006; Spiegel, Le, Ververs, and Salama, 2007). Climate change alters the environment of disease transmission vectors thus becoming another risk factor. Epidemics may happen due to the introduction of new pathogens in a setting that previously did not have the disease. People in the region might not have previous immunity, which favours the proliferation of disease transmission. Diseases with high epidemic potential include pandemic influenza, cholera, dengue fever, malaria, measles, etc.

The immediate health impact of epidemics include diseases and death. The consequences of infections range from respiratory illness to diarrhoea and severe dehydration, depending on the type of disease. Severe cases may be fatal. Major epidemics and disease outbreaks cause social and political disruptions and economic losses, as well as affect human health both physically and psychologically. Notably, animal epidemics should not be ignored, especially when 61% of human infectious pathogens are zoonotic (Taylor, Latham, and Mark, 2001). Some animal epidemics may be transmitted across animal species to human populations. For example, swine influenza, which normally circulates among swine species, caused a human pandemic in 2009.

Specific control measures depend on the route of transmission of disease agent and setting. The World Health Organization (WHO) and other public health agencies have developed guidelines for handling different types of epidemics (WHO, 2014, 2017). Principles for epidemic response include enhancing disease surveillance, controlling or eliminating agents at the source of transmission, improving environmental conditions, and increasing the host's defence mechanisms. Common responses include safe water supply in order to prevent water-borne disease spread, practising rigorous hygiene to protect humans from contaminated sources, vaccination campaigns to boost immunity, and isolation and quarantine to prevent further contact with infected people.

In summary, infectious diseases outbreaks are characterized by an unexpected, sudden, severe disease occurrence in a geographical location. They occur when the interaction of host, disease agent, and environment become unbalanced. Health impacts vary among different epidemic agents, but often the consequence is severe and fatal. Continual surveillance and appropriate infection control measures targeting specific epidemic agents and settings help reduce the further spread of disease and alleviate the health impact.

Human-caused disasters: technological disasters and complex emergencies

Human-caused disaster is defined as 'an event which, either intentionally or by accident cause severe threats to public health and well-being. Because their occurrence is unpredictable, man-made disasters pose an especially challenging threat that must be dealt with through vigilance, proper preparedness and response' (CrisisTimes, 2015). Human-caused disaster is a broad category that is characterized by the presence of human factors as a cause of the event. Some common human-caused disasters include technological disasters, bioterrorism, famine, complex emergencies, and others. **Technological**

disasters include disasters that result as a consequence of human error or breakdown of technological systems, which can be further categorized into: (i) industrial accidents; (ii) transport accidents; and (iii) miscellaneous accidents. Industrial and technological disasters might be caused by a range of factors and causes. They can be related to non-intentional technological and mechanism failure, human error, and a failure in safety regulations. Some of these incidents might have long-term health and environmental consequences and last for more than one generation and extend beyond a single country (e.g. nuclear accidents and chemical spills).

Natural and human factors may affect the severity and outcome of the human impact of technological disasters. Natural factors include context, location, extreme events, and technological failure, and human factors include human error, system failures, and policy. The severity and outcome of human-caused disasters vary with these factors. The natural factors are predominantly uncontrollable and/or unpredictable by humans. Some of these factors include location, the trigger (e.g. forest fire triggered by extreme temperature and low humidity), and the type/nature of the technological failure itself. The severity and extent of the outcome is affected by human-related factors. These include factors associated with humans at the individual level, such as lack of skill and training in machine operations, fatigue, performance instability, occupational hazards, and also systems and policies at the societal level.

For chemical incidents or radiation emergencies, specific guidelines and training should be implemented in industries, such as scenario analyses and impact assessment, planning for training and practising the response, and training and equipping responders to deal with loss of containment and its community impact (WHO, United Kingdom Health Protection Agency [HPA], and partners, 2011a).

War and conflicts are complex emergencies that disrupt the social fabric, generate massive violence, and lead to large-scale emigration. Not only do these events accumulate large number of casualties, the consequences may also have far-reaching impacts on the affected community. Complex emergencies are 'humanitarian crises in a country, region or society where there is total or considerable breakdown of authority resulting from internal or external conflict and which requires an international response that goes beyond the mandate or capacity of any single agency and/or the on-going United Nations country program' (Inter-Agency Standing Committee [IASC], 1994). Many people leave their homes to seek safety and shelter to escape from complex emergencies, destruction of homes, hunger, disease, and persecution. These people become **refugees** or Internally Displaced Persons (IDPs). Complex emergencies often occur in settings where there have been protracted community disputes and disruptions to livelihoods (threats to life produced by warfare, civil disturbance, and large-scale movements of people). In these settings, the fragile or failing economic, political, and social institutions may fuel violation of **human rights**. Complex emergencies may emerge and continue over a period of time, sometimes exacerbated by natural disasters (WHO, n.d.-a). However, countries at war or experiencing chronic conflict may or may not be reported as complex emergencies.

What is risk?

The potential occurrence and impact of hazard events or disaster outcomes might be conceptualized through the concept of 'risk' and its mathematical description in the risk formula, which shows the relationship between four components, **risk**, **hazard**, **exposure**, and **vulnerability**.

Risk = hazard × exposure × vulnerability

Risk is the potential for damage, loss, injury, death, or other negative consequences as a result of events such as war, natural or human-made disasters, and the like. **Hazard** is a dangerous physical phenomenon, substance, or human activity/condition that may cause loss of life, injury, or other health impacts, property damage, loss of livelihoods and services, social and economic disruption, or environmental damage. **Exposure** describes people, property, systems, or other elements present in hazard zones, which are thereby subject to potential losses. **Vulnerability** describes the characteristics and circumstances of a community, system, or asset that make it susceptible to the damaging effects of a hazard. Some policymakers argue that there is another important dimension, **manageability**, for conceptualizing risk, at least in relevant discussions in public health (Chan, 2017). Manageability describes how well and effective an organization or response consortium may respond to the hazard. Notably, manageability can be subsumed within the concept of 'vulnerability' since a better managed and supported population subgroup or community has less vulnerability.

Risk is thus the product of three factors: hazard, exposure, and vulnerability. Risk exists only if there is the presence of a hazard. Vulnerability and exposure affect how a community might be affected by the hazard. Thus, the same triggering event that resulted in a disaster in one community may not become a disaster in another if vulnerability and exposure are managed differently. The risk may vary with community-specific characteristics and resilience. Risk might be quantified as the degree of loss (from 0% to 100%) resulting from a potentially damaging phenomenon. This mathematical description might also be helpful to quantify and justify the needs for disaster preparedness programmes and education.

The concept of 'emergency thresholds'

Emergency threshold is an indicator to signify if a region or an area is in an emergency situation. Typically, it is judged by the mortality rate of a population in a specific period of time. **Mortality rate** is a measure of the frequency in death occurrences among a defined population during a specified time interval and might be used as a potential monitoring indicator for emergency thresholds (Chan, 2017). Different organizations may set the emergency threshold according to their operational and policy standards. According to the definition of the Office of the United Nations High Commissioner for Refugees, the crude mortality rate (CMR) of a country in non-disaster condition is set at 0.5 death per

10,000 people per day, whereas the under 5 mortality rate (U5MR) is set at 1 death per 10,000 people per day. When either of these two figures doubles, the emergency threshold is considered to be exceeded and implementation of emergency response actions is required. When the mortality rate hikes and exceeds the threshold, the emergency response measures will be activated; when the mortality rate falls back below the threshold, the emergency response will be called off. Two of the common mortality rates used to set the emergency threshold include the **CMR**, describing the death rate of the entire population, regardless of age, gender and cause, and the **U5MR**, describing the death rate among children below five years in the population.

General public health response in disasters

The public health impact of disasters includes direct impact (such as mortality and morbidity) as well as indirect impact (such as the effect on healthcare services, including the availability of healthcare workers, the functionality of infrastructure, the availability of resources and technology for immediate disaster response, etc.). In addition, as basic lifeline services might be affected, indirect needs for maintaining health and well-being might also arise as a consequence of disasters (such as loss of access to water, sanitation, and relevant information, and physical displacement). In principle, the public health response to any disaster or crisis has three basic objectives: (i) securing the basic resources that human beings require to maintain health; (ii) determining the current and likely health threats to the affected community, given the local environment and community's resources and knowledge, and enabling health-maintaining behaviours; and (iii) finding and providing the resources required to address the first two principles (Chan, 2017).

Securing basic requirements for health

To secure health and well-being of a population affected by a disaster or emergency, five basic requirements for health maintenance must be supported (Sphere, 2011; Bolton and Burkle, 2013; Chan, 2017). Related relief programmes may consider the provision of (i) clean water and sanitation; (ii) food and nutrition; (iii) shelter and clothing; (iv) health services; and (v) information. Health risks and adverse health outcomes may be prevented or minimized if relevant responses are mounted for at risk populations. Rapid needs assessment in these areas can help responders understand what is required and so plan appropriate and immediate assistance accordingly.

Water Supply, Sanitation, and Hygiene Promotion (WASH)

'WASH' stands for water, sanitation, and hygiene. WASH is a core component affecting health outcomes. WASH programmes are not only important during emergency situations but also in the normal routine of everyday life. Water supply facilities are usually damaged seriously during disasters such as earthquakes, or contaminated in human-caused disasters such as chemical spills. In these, the public water system can no longer support the distribution of water to the affected population nor supply a sufficient amount of water to perform daily activities. Water is essential for human life, and without an adequate quantity, or acceptable quality, it can pose health threats to humans. In disasters, people are often challenged by substandard sanitation, inadequate water supplies, and poor hygiene that make affected people more vulnerable to **water and sanitation-related illnesses**, such as diarrhoeal diseases, measles, cholera, and malaria. In refugee camp situations in particular, more than 40% of deaths are due to diarrhoeal diseases, with more than 80% of these deaths occurring in children under two years old (Connolly, Gayer, Ryan, Salama, Spiegel, et al., 2004). Factors related to the spread of these preventable infectious diseases are contaminated water, lack of water, unwashed hands, and flies. **Vector-related diseases** such as malaria, dengue fever, filariasis, and skin irritation can also occur in emergency settlements (WHO, HPA, and partners, 2011c). Mosquitoes, flies, fleas, or lice are the most common vectors identified in overcrowded situations with poor hygiene. **Acute respiratory infections** such as pneumonia and bronchitis are also the major cause of death in disasters. Poor shelters, and overcrowding of the population in situations with indoor air pollution may contribute to the development of these illnesses.

Food and nutrition

Food and nutrition are the cornerstones of survival. Food shortages are associated with some emergencies and food security is crucial to ensure well-being of a disaster-affected population. During the emergency phase of a disaster, rapid nutritional needs assessments are needed at different levels (individual, family, vulnerable groups, and the general population levels) (WHO, HPA, and partners, 2011b). As nutritional needs are different for particular groups such as older people and pregnant women (who may need various micronutrients for the healthy growth of the foetus), analysis of food and nutritional needs should be undertaken by sex and age so as to examine the needs of vulnerable groups appropriately. Nutritional interventions might be organized and targeted at high risk subgroups (WHO, HPA, and partners, 2011d). Optimizing infant and child feeding, improving food security, and ensuring the access to healthcare are all ways to reduce the risks of malnutrition. With appropriate infant and child feeding, including promotion of breastfeeding, mortality can be reduced (WHO, HPA, and partners, 2011e). In general, programmes targeting food and nutrition can be classified into two types: **general feeding programmes** and **selective feeding programmes**. In an emergency setting where a large number of people have been affected, ensuring basic food and nutrition is of utmost importance for survival. The general feeding programme aims to provide the affected population with minimum energy, protein, fats, and micronutrient requirements for light physical activity.

Shelter and non-food-related health-maintaining supplies

Disasters may bring massive destruction and causes loss of shelter and personal assets. Shelter and clothing provide physical protection and offer living **comfort** (e.g. thermal comfort) to a person. Non-food-related health-maintaining supply may **protect** people from weather changes and offer **personal safety**, **privacy**, and **dignity**. Inadequate shelter and clothing, especially in extreme weather, can increase the risk of getting sick. Suboptimal shelter results in inadequate protection (e.g. temperature) and health risks (**vector-borne diseases**). Non-food supplies help protect dignity and facilitate psycho-social well-being of a community.

Health services

Both natural and human-caused disasters create problems for health services. **Damage to health infrastructure** disrupts the existing health services while the **mass influx of injured victims** and a **shortage of health workers** and facilities may cause chaos in health service provision. At the early stage of disasters, the access to and provision of life-saving healthcare services is a critical determinant for survival. With limited resources during and after disasters, how medical and health services should be organized becomes a subject of important research and effort. In the emergency situation, with the limited time, services, and human resources, it is not possible to do everything for everybody and the aim therefore is to achieve the best possible results for the greatest number of people. **Triage** may help sort and prioritize victims for medical attention based on the severity of injury/illness and expectations for survival. There may also be specific health needs of population subgroups (e.g. older people) that need to be supported (Chan, 2019).

Information

Access to information is one of the human basic needs. However, the need for information is often neglected and underestimated. In a disaster, people require information about the current and predicted situation. For instance, if there is a tsunami following an earthquake and there is no announcement made to the affected population, they may miss the opportunity to take appropriate action to avoid the risks. In addition, by knowing what is happening and who is providing assistance, disaster victims can look for help to fulfil their basic needs. Well-established communication network and promotion of evidence-based message may help discredit myths and rumours that can cause insecurity and mistrust among the affected population (Bolton and Burkle, 2013; Chan, 2017).

Determining the current and potential health threats

Understanding the current and potential health threats to the affected community strengthens disaster management and minimizes negative health impacts (Chan, 2017). Overall, direct health impacts from disasters include deaths, injuries, and other negative physical and psychological short- and long-term effects. Indirect impacts may arise from the effects on systems, such as disruption to livelihoods and communities, loss of services, social and economic disruption, and environmental degradation (Watts, Adger, Agnolucci, Blackstock, Byass, et al., 2015). For example, disasters can disrupt existing health systems and provision of services by damaging healthcare infrastructure and delivery systems. Some disasters may have long-term consequences such as instance, famine's effect on child development or nuclear accidents on the affected populations. According to Bolton and Burkle (2013), each incident has different consequences depending on demography, size, and general condition of the affected population, environmental condition, security issues, size of the vulnerable population, coping capacity, impact severity of a disaster. Table 4.2 provides an overview of the public health consequences of various disasters.

Table 4.2 Overview of Public Health Consequences of Various Disasters

Impact	Earthquake	High wind	Flood	Flash flood/ Tsunami	Complex emergency
Deaths	Many	Few	Few	Many	Many
Severe injuries	Many	Moderate	Few	Few	Varying
Increased risk of communicable diseases	Small	Small	Varying	Small	High (in IDPs and refugees)
Food scarcity	Rare	Varying (depending on landuse and season)	Varying	Common	Common
Water security	Possible	Rare	Possible (contamination)	Possible (contamination)	Common
Population displacement	Common	Rare	Rare (only in badly flooded areas)	Rare (only in badly flooded areas)	High

Source: Adapted from Chan (2017); Sphere (2011).

Finding and providing the resources required to address the needs and protect from threats

A rapid assessment based on these two principles will identify the resources the affected population needs most. Common stakeholders who can provide required resources and emergency responses include donors, governments, communities (via fundraising), and non-governmental organizations (local, national, and international). As there are many stakeholders, it is important to determine and understand each organization's capacities and objectives. In order to gain their cooperation and avoid duplication of effort, a cluster approach is often used to coordinate humanitarian actors by sector. The cluster approach aims to improve the effectiveness, predictability, and accountability of humanitarian responses (Fredriksen, 2012). Basic needs include the five essential domains illustrated in Figure 4.2.

Humanitarian principles

When responders provide humanitarian aid, the main objective is to ensure the affected population can live with dignity and suffering might be alleviated. Humanitarian actions and responders should adhere to four key humanitarian principles when implementing their projects and programmes.

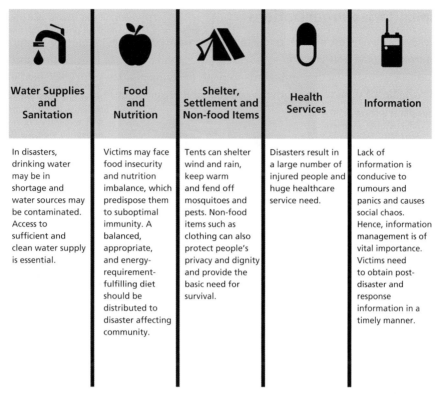

 Water Supplies and Sanitation	 Food and Nutrition	 Shelter, Settlement and Non-food Items	 Health Services	 Information
In disasters, drinking water may be in shortage and water sources may be contaminated. Access to sufficient and clean water supply is essential.	Victims may face food insecurity and nutrition imbalance, which predispose them to suboptimal immunity. A balanced, appropriate, and energy-requirement-fulfilling diet should be distributed to disaster affecting community.	Tents can shelter wind and rain, keep warm and fend off mosquitoes and pests. Non-food items such as clothing can also protect people's privacy and dignity and provide the basic need for survival.	Disasters result in a large number of injured people and huge healthcare service need.	Lack of information is conducive to rumours and panics and causes social chaos. Hence, information management is of vital importance. Victims need to obtain post-disaster and response information in a timely manner.

Figure 4.2 Five Basics Required for Health
Sources: Bolton and Burkle (2013); Sphere (2011).

Humanity

Human suffering should be addressed to protect the life, health, and dignity of human beings.

Impartiality

Humanitarian action should be taken based on need alone, giving priority to the most needy regardless of nationality, race, gender, religion, belief, class, or political stance.

Neutrality

Humanitarian organizations and their work must not favour any group of a political, racial, religious, or other ideological nature.

Independence

The policies and actions formulated and implemented by humanitarian organizations must be autonomous from political, economic, military, or other objectives.

Humanitarian organizations

Whenever a disaster occurs, actors and responders from governments, inter-governmental organizations, and non-governmental organizations should aim to provide the most appropriate care to the victims in accordance with the humanitarian principles mentioned earlier. Table 4.3 shows some of the institutions and organizations that promote humanitarian principles.

Disaster risk reduction and preparedness

A disaster event may result after the occurrence of a natural hazard. Disasters caused by hazards, regardless of whether they are human-induced or nature-induced, are increasing in frequency, magnitude, and cost. The severity of human and environmental impact of a disaster, however, depends on how the specific hazard may affect a society and its living environment. Thus, the potential impact intensity of the hazard may differ because of the decisions and choices a society make regarding land use, food production, governance,

Table 4.3 Selected Organizations Promoting the Humanitarian Principles

Inter-governmental organizations
Formed by various nations, they can coordinate all countries in the world to respond to disasters and their derived threats via a transnational platform.

United Nations (UN)	World Health Organization (WHO) (https://www.who.int)	World Bank Group (https://www.worldbank.org)
The United Nations takes action on the series of issues confronted by human beings in the twenty-first century, specifically peace and security, climate change, sustainable development, human rights, disarmament, terrorism, humanitarianism and health emergency, gender equality, governance, food production, and the like. Examples of UN funded, agencies and programmes include: ♦ United Nations Children's Fund (UNICEF) (https://www.unicef.org) ♦ Office of the United Nations High Commissioner for Refugees (UNHCR) (https://www.unhcr.org) ♦ World Food Programme (WFP) (https://www.wfp.org) ♦ United Nations Development Programme (UNDP) (https://www.undp.org)	The World Health Organization is the specialized agency in the United Nations system directing and coordinating international health issues. Its duties include providing leadership on matters critical to health and engaging in partnerships where joint action is needed; shaping the research agenda; and stimulating the generation, translation, and dissemination of valuable knowledge; setting norms and standards and promoting and monitoring their implementation; articulating ethical and evidence-based policy options; providing technical support, catalysing change, and building sustainable institutional capacity; and monitoring the health situation and assessing health trends.	♦ The World Bank Group has set two broad goals that the world needs to achieve by 2030: Ending extreme poverty and reducing the proportion of people living on less than US$1.90 a day to no more than 3% ♦ Promoting shared prosperity and fostering the income growth of the poorest 40% of people in each country

Table 4.3 Continued

Non-governmental organizations (selected examples) Directly involved in disaster response and launching targeted response programmes in various regions.		
International Federation of Red Cross and Red Crescent Societies (IFRC) (https://www.ifrc.org)	**Médecins Sans Frontières (MSF) (https://www.msf.org)**	**Oxfam (http://www.oxfam.org)**
Providing assistance to victims of natural disasters and healthcare crises based on humanitarian principles.	Providing emergency healthcare relief to distressed people without discrimination as to race, religion, gender, and political affiliation, based on the principles of neutrality and impartiality.	Alleviating poverty and redressing injustice that causes poverty by such means as assisting victims to resume their livelihood and global policy initiatives in poverty reduction. Engaging in food, water, sanitation, and hygiene management in disasters.

preparedness, and responses. **Disaster risk reduction** (DRR) is the concept and practice of reducing disaster risks through systematic efforts to analyse and reduce the causal factors of disasters (UNISDR, n.d.). DRR-related activities aim to reduce the damage caused by natural hazards like earthquakes, floods, droughts, and cyclones based on an ethos of prevention. Examples of disaster risk reduction activities are hazard exposure reduction, human and physical structure (e.g. housing) vulnerability reduction, hazard risk awareness raising in land and environment management, disaster preparedness, and early warning systems establishment.

Resilience is the power or ability to recover readily from an adverse event and situation. Human health as defined by the WHO (1946; see Chapter 2) incorporates physical, behavioural, social, and environmental health and well-being. The foundation of disaster resilience building is to address the interest in preserving human health and welfare. **Community resilience** expands the traditional preparedness approach by encouraging actions that build preparedness while also promoting strong community systems and addressing the many factors that contribute to health. Key preparedness activities—such as continuity of operation plans for organizations, reunification plans for families, compiling disaster kits and resources, building social connectedness, and improving everyday health, wellness, and community systems—may enhance community resilience.

Community health resilience (CHR) is the ability of a community to use its assets to strengthen public health and healthcare systems and to improve the community's physical, behavioural, and social health to withstand, adapt to, and recover from adversity (United States Department of Health and Human Services, 2015). A resilient community are likely to be socially connected and have an accessible and robust health system to withstand disaster and foster community recovery. Developing community resilience offers benefits to disaster planners and community members alike. Resilient communities promote individual and community physical, behavioural, and social health to strengthen their communities for daily, as well as more extreme, challenges.

Bottom-up resilience: individual, household, and community disaster resilience

Bottom-up resilience is the concept suggesting that resilience actions and activities might be undertaken by individuals, households, and the community. Instead of the traditional approach of relying on top-down resilience decision-making process (such as the national agenda, policies, and institutional programmes), bottom-up resilience emphasizes actions taken by those directly involved or affected individuals or stakeholders (Chan 2013, 2017, 2018) (see Case Box 4.1).

Case Box 4.1 A Rethink of the Bottom-up Resilience with the Use of Technology

During the 2008 China Wenchuan earthquake, 13 million volunteers were reported to have taken part in the relief efforts and 3 million of those were working on the frontline in Sichuan Province. As of 2011, an estimated community volunteer population of over 60 million were reported in China while only about 20 million were registered under various government-led community volunteer systems. As one of the most disaster-prone and populous countries in the world, China has ample opportunities to engage this volunteer community. However, volunteer engagement and roles have not been explicitly targeted in the current disaster response policies. A surge of uncoordinated, untrained volunteers with no clearly defined role and no protection or accountability for their actions could hamper the overall response effectiveness and efficiency.

Finding ways to identify and mobilize unregistered volunteers in a useful way remains a significant challenge. The Internet and social media can facilitate civil society participation in disaster response. There are over half a billion Internet users in China and the Internet could provide an effective platform for early warning and a powerful mechanism to recruit and mobilize volunteers and resources. The Internet also serves as an education tool to disseminate information about disasters and associated health risks. Furthermore, it provides a medium for tracking issues that could be easily overlooked in the myriad of top-down approaches. The fate of thousands of children in the Wenchuan earthquake, as well as that of many older and injured people, seems to be unrecorded and forgotten. The Internet could be a tool to track populations of affected people and empower local communities, households, and individuals in large-scale relief operations. It should serve as an essential component of disaster resilience and response.

Effective disaster rescue and response also require contributions from the local community and the volunteer sector. Disaster health risk literacy cultivation, emergency health and medical preparedness training, and managing effective information technology and communication platforms in facilitating bottom-up resilience strategies are important evidence gaps in current literature.

Source: Chan (2013).

Individual level

Disaster preparedness at the individual level mainly focuses on raising awareness, increasing knowledge, and promoting behaviour adaptation. Promotion and education efforts may help raise individuals' disaster health risk literacy, that is, the capability to acquire, process, and make use of disaster-related information, including understanding disaster prevention and preparedness measures that can reduce the impact of disasters. Guidelines for disaster response, basic first aid knowledge, and activities such as drills and exercises are other key activities in disaster resilience building to strengthen individuals' capacity to help themselves after a disaster (Chan, Huang, Mark, and Guo, 2017).

Household level

Disaster preparedness at the household level mainly focuses on the fundamental social unit and the ability of community to be self-sufficient temporarily after a disaster strikes. Household-level disaster preparedness is particularly crucial for families in remote areas where access to external relief is more challenging and faces more difficulties (Chan, Guo, Lee, Liu, and Mark, 2017). Relevant provisions for household disaster preparedness include basic first aid supplies and medication, a fire extinguisher, emergency food and drinking water, a light blanket for keeping warm, a torch for illumination and seeking help, a whistle, a portable radio for receiving disaster information, a functional communication device like a mobile phone for keeping contact with the outside world, and spare batteries (Chan, 2017, 2018; Pickering, O'Sullivan, Morris, Mark, McQuirk, et al., 2018).

Community level

Disaster preparedness at the community level typically involves the organization of education and training programmes related to disaster risk reduction efforts (e.g. establishing disaster early warning systems) (Chan and Shi, 2017). Education and training programmes may shift their focus from post-disaster emergency response to disaster risk reduction and disaster impact mitigation via strengthening of pre-disaster preparedness like contingency exercises and drills. The operation of an early warning system involves the collection of long-term disaster data and continuous disaster risk assessment, the surveillance and forecast of disaster threats, the provision of information related to long-term disaster risk, and disaster threat surveillance inthe public and the emergency departments. The establishment of a systematic community disaster preparedness education programme that includes various stakeholders (e.g. older people) may help develop the national and local disaster response capabilities (Chan, 2019).

Global level

Global disaster preparedness includes planning, supporting, and implementing the macro international-based policy and schemes that can be applied in the global level to reduce disaster risk, such as the two international disaster risk reduction policy documents endorsed by the United Nations World Conference on Disaster Risk Reduction: the Hyogo

Framework for Action 2005–2015 and the Sendai Framework for Disaster Risk Reduction 2015–2030. The Hyogo Framework for Action is the first international document that explains and describes what measures organizations in various sectors are required to adopt in order to reduce disaster losses. It is a common disaster risk reduction coordination system developed after negotiation with all disaster risk reduction partners, including governments, international agencies, disaster experts, and many others. Its goal is to substantially reduce disaster loss of life and social, economic, and environmental assets by strengthening the resilience of nations and communities to disasters. The current Sendai Framework for Disaster Risk Reduction further suggests four priorities for action, which are: understanding disaster risk; strengthening disaster risk governance to manage disaster risk; investing in disaster risk reduction for resilience; and enhancing disaster preparedness for effective response and to 'Build Back Better' in recovery, rehabilitation, and reconstruction.

Challenges for emergency and disaster health responses in the twenty-first century

There are a number of challenges for public health disaster response in the coming decades (Chan, 2017). Populations who are of 'extremes of age' (e.g. infant/children and older people) are often more vulnerable during emergencies and disasters. In addition to demographic health needs, a number of other important issues may also pose new challenges for emergency preparedness and response. New treatments (e.g. drug and intervention) developed to respond to newly emerging/re-emerging diseases in emergency (e.g. Ebola outbreaks) are urgently required. With technological advancement, effectiveness evaluation is needed to understand the appropriate application of fit-for-purpose technology in disaster response and health risk communication. Global burden of non-communicable diseases will require the further development of guidelines and protocols for chronic disease management in the emergency context. With global population ageing and the multiple morbidity associated with the elderly, how older people's health needs might be addressed effectively will be an important disaster response need for the twenty-first century. Not only are new approaches needed to address medical and physical health responses but other major areas in disaster management also require response development. The management of mental and social health needs of various stakeholders (patients, families, medical/relief workers, volunteers, and bystanders), how rehabilitation service may be organized in suboptimal health systems, health protection and security issues for internally displaced populations, assessments of health impacts and health risk reduction of secondary and Natech disasters are examples of key issues to be examined.

Health Emergency and Disaster Risk Management (Health-EDRM)

Disaster prevention refers to 'the outright avoidance of adverse impacts of hazards and related disasters through actions taken in advance.' (United Nations International Strategy for Disaster Reduction [UNISDR], 2009). The notion suggests that it is always possible to minimize the adverse impact of disasters. Even with limited resources and capacity in post-disaster settings, there are always ways to support populations with chronic conditions following disasters.

'Health' is recognized as an outcome in the four landmark UN agreements adopted in 2015–16. These global agreements include: the Sendai Framework for Disaster Risk Reduction 2015–30; the 2030 Sustainable Development Goals (SDGs); the Paris climate agreement; and the New Urban Agenda (Habitat III). As a key goal of disaster risk reduction, the broad intersection of health and disaster risk reduction is captured in the concept of Health Emergency and Disaster Risk Management (Health-EDRM) which encompasses various fields (Chan and Murray, 2017; Lo, Chan, Chan, Murray, Abrahams, et al., 2017). The focuses of Health-EDRM research include an all-hazards approach that incorporates the full spectrum of hazards; a holistic all-needs approach, including physical, mental, and psychosocial health and well-being; research and interventions facilitated during all phases of a disaster; disaster risk identification for populations with specific health needs such as children, people with disabilities, and older people; and research on and the building of health resilience in all communities. Some health services, such as health advice, incur almost no operation costs but have potential long-term implications for disease prevention. For instance, not only can smoking cessation advice prevent potential adverse clinical outcomes such as heart diseases, stroke, and cancer but health advice may also reduce spending on cigarette consumption. In order to implement chronic disease preventative-based relief programmes, it is pertinent to emphasize the need to collect relevant demographic profiles, health information, knowledge, attitudes, and behaviour information during needs assessment so as to design and implement relevant programmes according to the project needs.

Knowledge Box 4.2 discusses a review of evidence related to Health-EDRM interventions in rural communities in Asia. Figure 4.3 shows how the prevention of a potential cholera outbreak in a displaced population might be conceptualized in Health-EDRM.

Conclusion

Hazard risks, extreme events, emergency incidents, disasters, and crises may all present significant threats to health and well-being at local, national, and global levels. With the increasing complexity and new risks associated with modern living, strengthening

Knowledge Box 4.2 Adequate Evidence of Health-EDRM Activities in Disaster- and Hazard-Prone Rural Communities?

Chan, Man, and Lam (2019) conducted a literature review of published English language reports and papers retrieved from PubMed, Google Scholar, Embase, Medline, and PsycINFO on rural disaster and emergency responses, and relief, health impact, and disease patterns in the 10 most disaster-prone countries in Asia from January 2000 to January 2018. Of the few disaster risk reduction and health emergency and disaster risk management (EDRM) prevention interventions documented, there is a general absence of consistency (e.g. intervention durations, outcome measures, and disasters or hazard categories) and of evaluations of interventions under different disaster/hazard categories. Interventions that target households, such as oral rehydration solution (ORS), are more widely implemented and used as secondary disaster risk reduction interventions in floods, cyclones, and earthquakes. However, as only cross-sectional studies and immediate pre/post education survey-based studies have been published on those topics for rural areas, and even with the plethora of recommendations that are offered in these surveys (e.g. preparation of homemade ORS and household-based disaster preparedness kits, warning and evacuation drills, psychological first-aid training, and improvement in disaster health literacy through health education), there remain major gaps and inconsistencies in results of the efficacy of these interventions. As climate change-related disasters increase in frequency and severity, evidence is needed for disaster risk reduction interventions to address the health risks specific to rural populations.

capacities in preparedness and response for these emergency events could help minimize suffering and protect health and well-beings of humans. Developing relevant preparedness and responses for many of these events might require specific technical knowledge and considerations, as described in other chapters in this book such as those on infectious diseases and environmental health. Nevertheless, the common public health and disaster response principles discussed in this chapter may be useful and applicable universally when examining emergency health needs and facilitating response planning to protect and reduce potential adverse impacts of these events to human health, lifeline infrastructure, and related health systems in an affected community.

Health-Emergency and Disaster Risk Management

Defined as: the systematic analysis and management of *health risks* surrounding emergencies and disasters by *reducing the hazards* and **vulnerability** along with extending preparedness, response, and recovery measures.

Guilding Principles from the Sendai Framwork (UNISDR) on DRR that may be applied to Health-EDRM
1. Shared responsibility between central governments and relevant national authorities, sectors, and stakeholders.
2. All-of-society engagement and partnership
3. Cross-sector stakeholder coordination mechanisms with evidence-based approach
4. Multi-hazard approach with easily accessible and science-based risk information
5. Effective and strengthened global partnership and international coorperation

Case: Potential cholera outbreak after mass population displacement

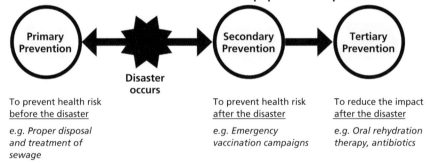

Primary Prevention	Disaster occurs	Secondary Prevention	Tertiary Prevention
To prevent health risk <u>before the disaster</u>		To prevent health risk <u>after the disaster</u>	To reduce the impact <u>after the disaster</u>
e.g. Proper disposal and treatment of sewage		*e.g. Emergency vaccination campaigns*	*e.g. Oral rehydration therapy, antibiotics*

Figure 4.3 Prevention of potential cholera outbreak in population displacement conceptualized in health emergency and disaster risk management
Sources: Chan and Murray (2017); Lo et al. (2017).

References

Ahern, M., Kovats, R. S., Wilkinson, P., Few, R., and Matthies, F. (2005). Global health impacts of floods: epidemiologic evidence. *Epidemiol Rev 27*(1) 36–46.

Alexander, D. E. (2007). Misconception as a barrier to teaching about disasters. *Prehosp Disast Med 22*(2) 95–103.

Associated Programme on Flood Management (2013). What human factors contribute to flooding ? Available at: http://www.floodmanagement.info/what-human-factors-contribute-to-flooding/.

Bolton, P. and Burkle, F. M. (2013). Emergency response. In C. Guest, W. Ricciardi, I. Kawachi, and I. Lang (eds), *Oxford Handbook of Public Health Practice* (3rd edn). Oxford: Oxford University Press.

Centre for Research on the Epidemiology of Disasters (2009). EM-DAT glossary. Available at: https://www.emdat.be/Glossary.

Chan, E. Y. Y. (2013). Bottom-up disaster resilience. *Nat Geosci* 6(5) 327–8. doi:10.1038/ngeo1815.

Chan, E. Y. Y. (2017). *Public Health Humanitarian Responses to Natural Disasters*. London: Routledge.

Chan, E. Y. Y. (2018). *Building Bottom-Up Health and Disaster Risk Reduction Programmes*. London: Oxford University Press.

Chan, E. Y. Y. (2019). *Disaster Public Health and Older People*. London: Routledge.

Chan, E. Y. Y., Guo, C., Lee, P., Liu, S., and **Mark, C. K. M.** (2017). Health Emergency and Disaster Risk Management (Health-EDRM) in remote ethnic minority areas of rural China: The case of a flood-prone village in Sichuan. *Int J Disast Risk Sc* 8(2) 156–63.

Chan, E. Y. Y., Huang, Z., Mark, C. K. M., and **Guo, C.** (2017). Weather information acquisition and health significance during extreme cold weather in a subtropical city: A cross-sectional survey in Hong Kong. *Int J Disast Risk Sc* 8(2) 134–44.

Chan, E. Y. Y., Man, A. Y. T., and **Lam, H. C. Y.** (2019). Scientific evidence on natural disasters and health emergency and disaster risk management in Asian rural-based area. *Br Med Bull* 129(1) 91–105. doi:10.1093/bmb/ldz002.

Chan, E. Y. Y. and **Murray, V.** (2017). What are the health research needs for the Sendai Framework? *Lancet* 390(10106) e35–e36. doi: 10.1016/S0140-6736(17)31670-7.

Chan, E. Y. Y. and **Shi, P.** (2017). Health and risks: Integrating health into disaster risk reduction, risk communication, and building resilient communities. *Int J Disast Risk Sc* 8(2) 107–8.

Colwell, R. R., Kaper, J., and **Joseph, S. W.** (1977). *Vibrio cholerae, Vibrio parahaemolyticus*, and other vibrios: Occurrence and distribution in Chesapeake Bay. *Science* 198(4315) 394–6.

Connolly, M. A., Gayer, M., Ryan, M. J., Salama, P., Spiegel, P., et al. (2004). Communicable diseases in complex emergencies: Impact and challenges. *Lancet* 364 1974–83.

CrisisTimes (2015). Surviving disasters. Available at: http://crisistimes.com/urban_disasters.php.

Cruz, A. M., Kajitani, Y., and Tatano, H. (2015). Natech disaster risk reduction: Can integrated risk governance help? In U. Fra-Paleo (ed.), *Risk Governance*. Dordrecht: Springer, pp. 441–62.

De Cock, K. M., Simone, P. M., Davison, V., and **Slutsker, L.** (2013). The new global health. *Emerg Infect Dis* 19(8) 1192.

Doocy, S., Dick, A., Daniels, A., and **Kirsch, T. D.** (2013). The human impact of tropical cyclones: A historical review of events 1980–2009 and systematic literature review. *PLoS Currents Disasters*.

Fredriksen, A. (2012). *Making humanitarian spaces global: Coordinating crisis response through the cluster approach* (Doctoral dissertation). Available at: Columbia University Academic Commons: http://hdl.handle.net/10022/AC:P:14511.

Gayer, M. and Connolly, M. A. (2005). Communicable disease control after disasters. In E. K. Noji (ed.), *Public Health Consequences of Disasters* (2nd edn). Oxford: Oxford University Press.

Girgin, S., Necci, A., and Krausmann, E. (2017). Natech hazard and risk assessment. In S. Safaie (ed.), *Words Into Action Guidelines: National Disaster Risk Assessment: Governance System, Methodologies, and Use of Results*. Geneva: UNISDR, pp. 90–8. Available at: https://www.unisdr.org/files/52828_nationaldisasterriskassessmentwiagu.pdf.

Guha-Sapir, D., Hoyois, P., and **Below, R.** (2015). *Annual Disaster Statistical Review 2015: The Numbers and Trends*. Brussels: CRED.

Inter-Agency Standing Committee (IASC) (9 December 1994). *Working paper on the definition of complex emergencies*. New York, NY.

International Federation of Red Cross and Red Crescent Societies (n.d.). Biological hazards: Epidemics. Available at: http://www.ifrc.org/en/what-we-do/disaster-management/about-disasters/definition-of-hazard/biological-hazards-epidemics/.

Lipp, E. K., Huq, A., and Colwell, R. R. (2002). Effects of global climate on infectious disease: The cholera model. *Clin Microbiol Rev 15*(4) 757–70. doi:10.1128/CMR.15.4.757.

Lo, S. T. T., Chan, E. Y. Y., Chan, G. K. W., Murray, V., Abrahams, J., et al. (2017). Health Emergency and Disaster Risk Management (Health-EDRM): Developing the research field within the Sendai Framework paradigm. *Int J Disast Risk Sc 8*(2) 145–9.

Pickering CJ, O'Sullivan TL, Morris A, Mark C, McQuirk D, et al. (2018). The promotion of 'grab bags' as a disaster risk reduction strategy. *PLoS Currents Disasters* Jul 6(1). doi:10.1371/currents.dis.223ac 4322834aa0bb0d6824ee424e7f8.

Portilla, D., Shaffer, R. N., Okusa, M. D., Mehrotra, R., Molitoris, B. A., et al. (2010). Lessons from Haiti on disaster relief. *Clin J Am Soc Nephrol 5*(11) 2122–9. doi: 10.2215/CJN.03960510.

Ramirez, M. and Peek-Asa, C. (2005). Epidemiology of traumatic injuries from earthquakes. *Epidemiol Rev 27*(1) 47–55.

Schull, M. J. and Shanks, L. (2001). Complex emergencies: Expected and unexpected consequences. *Prehosp Disaster Med 16*(4) 192–6.

Smith, M. (2009). Lessons learned in WASH response during urban flood emergencies (The Global WASH Learning Project). New York, NY: Global WASH Cluster. Available at: http://www.bvsde. paho.org/texcom/desastres/washurbfl.pdf.

Sphere (2011). Humanitarian charter and minimum standards in disaster response. Available at: http:// www.ifrc.org/PageFiles/95530/The-Sphere-Project-Handbook-20111.pdf.

Spiegel, P. B., Le, P., Ververs, M.-T., and Salama, P. (2007). Occurrence and overlap of natural disasters, complex emergencies and epidemics during the past decade (1995–2004). *Confl Health 1*(2). doi:10.1186/1752-1505-1-2.

Taylor, L. H., Latham, S. M., and Mark, E. J. (2001). Risk factors for human disease emergence. *Philos Trans R Soc London B 356*(1411) 983–9.

United Nations International Strategy for Disaster Reduction (2009). *Terminology on Disaster Risk Reduction*. Geneva.

United Nations Office for Disaster Risk Reduction (n.d.). What is Disaster Risk Reduction?. Available at: https://www.unisdr.org/who-we-are/what-is-drr

United States Department of Health and Human Services (2015). Community resilience. Available at: https://www.phe.gov/Preparedness/planning/abc/Pages/community-resilience.aspx.

Watson, J., Gayer, M., and Connolly, M. A. (2006). Epidemic risk after disasters. *Emerg Infect Dis 12*(9) 1468–9.

Watts, N., Adger, W. N., Agnolucci, P., Blackstock, J., Byass, P., et al. (2015). Health and climate change: Policy responses to protect public health. *Lancet 386*(10006) 1861–914.

World Health Organization (n.d.-a). Complex emergencies. Available at: https://www.who.int/ environmental_health_emergencies/complex_emergencies/en/.

World Health Organization (1946). Constitution of the World Health Organization: Principles. Available at: https://www.who.int/about/mission/en/.

World Health Organization, United Kingdom Health Protection Agency, and partners (2011a). Disaster risk management for health: Chemical safety (Disaster Risk Management for Health Fact Sheets). Available at: http://www.who.int/hac/events/drm_fact_sheet_chemical_safety.pdf.

World Health Organization, United Kingdom Health Protection Agency, and partners (2011b). Disaster risk management for health: Child health (Disaster Risk Management for Health Fact Sheets). Available at: http://www.who.int/hac/events/drm_fact_sheet_child_health.pdf?ua=1.

World Health Organization, United Kingdom Health Protection Agency, and partners (2011c). Disaster risk management for health: Communicable diseases (Disaster Risk Management for Health Fact Sheets). Available at: http://www.who.int/hac/events/drm_fact_sheet_communicable_ diseases.pdf?ua=1.

World Health Organization, United Kingdom Health Protection Agency, and partners (2011d). Disaster risk management for health: People with disabilities and older people (Disaster Risk Management for Health Fact Sheets). Available at: http://www.who.int/entity/hac/events/drm_fact_sheet_disabilities.pdf?ua=1.

World Health Organization, United Kingdom Health Protection Agency, and partners (2011e). Disaster risk management for health: Sexual and reproductive health (Disaster Risk Management for Health Fact Sheets). Available at: http://www.who.int/hac/events/drm_fact_sheet_sexual_and_reproductive_health.pdf?ua=1.

Chapter 5

Communicable Disease and Control

According to World Health Organization (2015b), the number of deaths due to communicable diseases reduced from 12.1 million in 2000 to 9.5 million in 2012, a partial success of the Millennium Development Goals (MDGs). However, malaria, tuberculosis, HIV/AIDS, and the neglected tropical diseases remain challenges for the global community and the targets of Sustainable Development Goals (SDGs). For the coming decades, with the impact of globalisation, changing of behavioural patterns, lifestyle, urbanisation, and technological outcomes will pose major challenge to communicable disease control. Socioeconomic, environmental, and ecological determinants, as well as risks of antimicrobial resistance will affect effectiveness of control and management.

Overview of infectious diseases

Globally, infectious diseases contribute to 11 million deaths in low-and middle-income country annually (WHO, 2010) and are the causes of major mortality in childhood and adolescent. Also known as communicable diseases, infectious diseases are illnesses caused by different pathogens that infect people through various modes of transmission. After invading the human body, the pathogens can replicate or release toxins, and can spread to other people, causing outbreaks and even mass casualties. Currently, humans have achieved a certain level of progress in the prevention and management of infectious diseases. In high-income countries and areas, infectious diseases are no longer the main cause of death. Unfortunately, the main burden of infectious disease threats remains significant in low-income countries. Infectious diseases continue to create serious disease burdens for these societies, especially when various forms of emerging and re-emerging infectious diseases appear.

Categorization of infectious diseases

Infectious diseases may be classified in various ways. In clinical medicine, infectious disease might be named after anatomical sites (e.g. upper respiratory infections and gastrointestinal infections). In public health, infectious disease may be categorized according to the public health approach which might support disease prevention, control, and management such as by route of transmission (e.g. water-borne diseases, sexually transmitted diseases, nosocomial (see Knowledge Box 5.1), and vector-borne), or whether the disease might be **vaccine preventable**. **Emerging infectious disease** refers to diseases that have never been reported nor found in humans, or that have only occurred in remote areas with sporadic cases. **Re-emerging infectious disease** refers to infectious diseases that

Essentials for Health Protection. Emily Ying Yang Chan, Oxford University Press (2020).
© Oxford University Press
DOI: 10.1093/oso/9780198835479.001.0001

Knowledge Box 5.1 Nosocomial Infection

Nosocomial infection refers to healthcare-acquired infections (HCAIs). Patients are infected as a result of healthcare services/interventions and typical examples of such pathogens include *Clostridium difficile*, Methicillin-resistant *Staphylococcus Aureus* (MRSA), Glycopeptide-resistant enterococci (GRE). Studies indicated 30% of the general population in the United Kingdom (Henderson, 2016), 56.8% of general population in Asia (Stefani, Chung, Lindsay, Friedrich, Keams, et al., 2012) and 30.1% of older people living in residential care homes in Hong Kong (Chen, Au, Hsu, Lai, Myint, et al., 2018) were colonized by MRSA. Risks factors associated with HCAIs include susceptibility of patients (e.g. people who are sub-immune, with non-communicable disease, of extremes of age, in immunosuppressive therapy, etc.); medical procedure involved (e.g. invasive, or with long-term use), environmental context (e.g. poor infection control in hospital); and community behavioural practices (antibiotic utilization and practice pattern). Infection control measures such as universal precaution, hand washing, guidelines in antibiotics prescription, surveillance, treatment, and isolation have been advocated for HCAIs.

have a history of transmission throughout a country or even globally, and that were once under control but are reappearing in human community (NIH, 2012).

Communicable disease transmission

Human health outcome of infectious disease varies with the interaction and disease control in the affected community. In principle, three factors affect communicable disease transmission. These are the host, pathogen, and the environment or vector that are interacting with and affecting each other (Mausner and Kramer, 1985).

Host

The host is a person or animal that provides an organic environment for pathogens to survive and thrive. If the host has a strong immune system, the pathogen is less likely to infect the host and this host may even be able to get rid of or destroy the pathogen quickly. However, for the hosts with weaker immune systems such as those at the extremes of age (i.e. children and older people) and people with chronic diseases, they are more susceptible to succumbing to infection and therefore develop diseases.

Pathogen

Pathogens are microorganisms and agents that might cause disease in a human host. Typical pathogens include bacteria, viruses, parasites, fungi, and prions. **Bacteria** are microscopic unicellular organisms with a high replication rate and often cluster together in colonies. Examples of diseases caused by bacteria include pneumonia, tuberculosis, and salmonellosis. **Viruses** consist of genetic materials wrapped within an outer coating of protein. Viruses cannot exist independently and require a host's cellular machineries in order to replicate. Examples of diseases caused by viruses include influenza, hepatitis, and SARS (severe acute respiratory syndrome). **Prions** are a type of specialized infectious protein. Although a prion might be conceptualised as a slow virus, it is also called an unconventional virus because it does not completely fit the definition for a virus. These protein substances cause central nervous system illnesses in humans and livestock. Examples of diseases caused by prions include mad cow disease (bovine spongiform encephalopathy) and Creutzfeldt–Jakob disease (CJD). **Parasites** live inside or on the surface of hosts, while consuming nutrients and harming the host. Examples of diseases caused by parasites include malaria and intestinal worms. **Fungi** are eukaryotes that survive through parasitic or saprophytic behaviour. Examples of diseases caused by fungi include tinea manus and tinea pedis. In the human physiological environment, a special subgroup of infection is called **opportunistic infection**. These infection episodes refer to how non-pathogenic microorganisms might become a major health and life threat when the host immune system is compromised. Affected individuals may become seriously ill due to pathogens that might otherwise be harmless to a healthy individual. Potentially, such infections might even be fatal for immunocompromised individuals. For instance, many infections found in HIV-infected patients with a compromised immune system are common pathogens among healthy people.

Environment or vector

The environment is the physical context where the hosts and pathogens may interact and change the dynamics of the transmission rate of pathogens. An environment can be categorized into three subsets, namely physical, social, and biological. A **physical** environment may affect human and their risks of infection. Some examples include temperature, humidity, water, and air. A **social** environment that renders a person vulnerable to disease transmission includes population density, living and working environments, etc. A **biological** environment describes the physiological medium (e.g. a living organism that is infected by a pathogen) or reservoir serving as a vehicle for the pathogen to infect another host. A **reservoir** refers to any medium where pathogens can live and reproduce. Notably, if a living organism (e.g. a mosquito) has been infected by a pathogen, the organism might serve as a vehicle for the pathogen to infect another host. After a pathogen infects a host, it can reproduce within the host and can even make the host into a reservoir to continue transmitting infections.

Determinants of human infectious diseases

Pathogens by themselves cannot cause an infection of disease. The clinical manifestation of infectious diseases in the human body depends on the interaction among host, pathogen, its specific mode of transmission, and environment. **Exposure** refers to the contact between pathogens and a host through a specific mode of transmission. **Infection** refers to the occurrence of pathogens replicating or growing inside a host. **Disease** refers to a host's symptomatic reaction(s) caused by the pathogens inside their body.

Different pathogens invade a host through their specific **modes of transmission**. Whether or not a person gets sick depends on the person's immune response's capacity to eliminate the pathogen or the pathogen's ability to cause a disease. Sometimes, the body's immune system and the pathogen's ability to cause a disease is in equilibrium, which means that the infected host shows no clinical symptoms of an illness, yet the pathogen is still growing and replicating. In this case, the host will be an asymptomatic carrier, where the pathogen can spread within a crowd but may not cause any illness. However, when the immune response of the host diminishes, the immune system and the pathogen's infectiousness will no longer be in balance and the host may eventually succumb to illness. Thus, pathogen transmission may not lead to an infection, and the host infection may not necessarily lead to an illness.

The level of population immunity and the transmission dynamics may be associated with population structure, microorganism pathogenicity, and the environmental contexts (e.g. an urban highly densely populated context that relies on lifeline infrastructure is more vulnerable). A population's immunity to a communicable disease is the summation of immunity of all individuals in the society (Lee, 2012). As pathogenicity of microorganisms is a function of virulence, dose, host immunity, and infection control, intervention may change the course of the interaction between hosts, pathogen, and population.

Disease transmission

Infectious disease might be classified according to the timing, anatomical site of infection, route of transmission, or context of acquisition. **Acute infectious disease** refers to infectious diseases which have a short incubation period, or those with a rapid onset of clinical symptoms. Examples include influenza, cholera, and typhoid. **Chronic infectious disease** refers to infectious diseases with a relatively long incubation period, insidious onset and non-specific symptoms. Disease treatment, if available, tends to require longer period than an acute one and some of this disease can only be managed with suboptimal symptomatic control. Examples include hepatitis B, hepatitis C, AIDS (acquired immune deficiency syndrome), and tuberculosis.

The specific means for pathogens to infect the hosts are called the **transmission routes**. An infectious disease may have multiple transmission routes. An example is influenza, which can be transmitted through contact with excreta as well as through droplets. The transmission routes of infectious diseases are categorized as **direct** and **indirect**. Direct transmission refers to the pathogens that travel directly from one host to another host without any intermediary factors. Often, this transmission process is short and occurs over a close distance. Direct transmission routes include contact, droplets, and mother-to-child transfers. Indirect transmission refers to the transmission of pathogens from one host to another host involving an intermediary factor such as the air, a vector, or inanimate objects. Air, vector, as well as food and water transfers are types of indirect transmission route. Some pathogens might have more than one route of disease transmission. For instance, the transmissions of blood or bodily fluids can be both direct and indirect. Sexually transmitted infections are examples of direct transmissions, while needle sharing during intravenous drug use is an example of indirect transmissions. Knowledge Box 5.2 describes characteristics of some main routes of transmission.

Some human disease infections might have multiple routes of transmission. Zika infection is an example of communicable disease that might have multiple routes of

Knowledge Box 5.2 Transmission Route for Common Human Pathogens

Direct transmission

Contact

Transmission of infectious disease is through direct physical contact with an infected organism or an inanimate object that contains infectious agents. Examples of such infection include tinea pedis and Ebola virus disease.

Droplets

Transmission is through contact with droplets from coughs, sneezes, spitting, or any other droplets sprayed from an infected individual. The pathogen-containing droplets can infect the host directly or indirectly through touching the mucous membranes of the mouth, nose, and eyes with hands that are contaminated with the infective agents. Influenza is an example.

Mother-to-child

A pregnant woman who is infected with the pathogens may transmit them to her foetus, thus causing an infection. Congenital rubella syndrome that affects foetal development is an example.

Blood or bodily fluid

Infected people can transmit the pathogen to another host through the blood or other bodily fluids, thus causing an infection. Examples include hepatitis B and HIV/AIDS.

Indirect transmission

Air-borne

Infection occurs through breathing in the pathogens that can survive in the air. Examples include measles and TB.

Vector-borne

Transmission occurs through a bite or prick from a vector that is already infected with the pathogen. Such vector may be a mammal, a bird, or an insect. Examples include dengue fever and Japanese encephalitis spread by mosquitoes.

Food-borne or water-borne

Infection occurs through consuming contaminated food, substances, or beverages that contain the pathogens. Examples include cholera and hepatitis A.

Case Box 5.1 Zika Virus: A New Global Threat

Zika virus infection is a vector-borne disease spread by the mosquitoes *Aedes aegypti* and *Aedes albopictus*. While Zika virus infection to human received global attention in 2015, periodic outbreaks of Zika virus infection in monkey and human populations have been reported in literature since 1947 (WHO, 20 July 2018). Although human infection was mostly reported with mild and transient symptoms, if infection occurs during pregnancy, the foetus may suffer from complications that affect foetal brain development and result in microcephaly and other congenital malformations, known as congenital Zika syndrome. Infection with Zika virus is also associated with other pregnancy complications including pre-term birth and miscarriage. An increased risk of neurologic complications, including Guillain–Barré syndrome, neuropathy, and myelitis, is also associated with Zika virus infection in adults and children.

Notably, Zika virus disease, as a vector-borne disease, shares the same vector with yellow fever, dengue fever, and chikungunya. It might also be transmitted sexually and from mother to child. Until 2015, infected humans experienced mild and transient symptoms, but no other major clinical symptoms were reported. In 2015, a number of babies were found to be born with microcephaly, other neurologic complications, and brain damage in Brazil. In 2016, the WHO reported 46 countries, including most countries in South America, reported their first cases of Zika virus transmission, with implication of clinical complications and foetal brain malformation in about 12 countries.

Currently, there is no vaccination and a lack of effective treatment for Zika virus infection. Prevention remains the best option for Zika virus control. In addition to potential avoidance of travel to high risk locations among at-risk populations such as pregnant women, control strategies for other vector-borne diseases such as vector control (e.g. elimination) and mosquito bed net distribution (for avoiding exposure to mosquito bites) are key strategies. Due to the possibility of sexual transmission, safe sex practices and use of condom are also advocated.

transmission, which requires a complex array of control measures for the protection of susceptible population (see Case Box 5.1).

Host immunity

Immunity refers to the ability of organisms to defend themselves from the invasion of external factors. At the personal level, immunity refers to a human's ability to maintain health through the immune system. In general, intact immunity will protect the host from infection but a defective or an overwhelmed immunity system in the host will result in extensive dissemination of disease in the body.

Innate versus acquired immunity

Depending on whether or not the immunity is present at birth, it can be classified as innate immunity or acquired immunity. The **innate immune system** is the immune system of the individual since birth. This is the natural defence system that prevents pathogens from invading and breeding by destroying them. As the first line of defence, it is non-specific and broad in nature. Innate immune systems include the skin, mucus, phagocytes, neutrophils, and lysozymes, etc. Physical barriers (e.g. skin, mucous members in the respiratory tract, gut, and reproductive tract) are the first line of defence in the human body for the potential invasion of infectious diseases invaders. For example, injury and trauma may destroy the physical barriers (skin), and external agents and the physiological state may trigger a range of physiological defences that aim to prevent infective agents from settling and growing in the human body. As **innate immunity** is pathogen-non-specific, it includes the production of cells (such as macrophages and phagocyte) and enzyme agents (such as lysozyme for bacteria and interferons for virus) that attempt to eliminate and stop microorganisms from direct contact with the sterile body environment and cause medical problems.

When people are infected by pathogens, apart from creating antibodies to fight them, the **acquired immune system** is being formed. This system enables the future recognition of pathogens. If a specific pathogen infects a person again, the acquired immune system can quickly and more efficiently fight back against the pathogen. However, during the initial contact with a new pathogen, the human immune system is often unprepared and can only wait for help while being attacked. **Vaccination** is an example of proactive early intervention that gives the body the ability to eliminate pathogens or lower their virulence, before making contact with an intruder (see also the section Vaccination and Immunization p105). With prior knowledge about the intruder, the human body should be able to identify the pathogen, and the immune system may be able to respond quickly and prevent adverse health outcomes from ever occurring. Most acquired immunity will develop gradually over time, and it has the ability to recognize specific pathogens and to trigger a tailored response. The release of antibodies (also known as immunoglobulins/Ig) is the acquired immune system's main weapon of choice. **Adaptive immunity** is the target-specific immune response in the host body and consists of the production of proteins and cells to fight against pathogens, including antibodies (also known as immunoglobulin which is part of humoral immunity) and the T and B lymphocytes (as specific types of white blood cell, and related to the cellular pathway that responds to infection). Specifically, vaccination strategies are often associated with the boosting of immunogenicity that are associated with antigens, which are molecules recognized by an antibody. Moreover, adaptive immunity might acquire naturally or artificially.

Natural and artificial immunity

Acquired immunity can be further divided into natural and artificial immunity. **Natural immunity** is immunity acquired passively through previous exposure, such as through maternal transfer (i.e. passing from mother to her foetus). **Artificial immunity** may be developed through patient treatment (e.g. infusion of gammaglobulins, antibodies which typically act in an electrophoresis process) (see Knowledge Box 5.3).

> ### Knowledge Box 5.3 Potential Sources of Antibody in Human Body
>
> Human antibody may be developed through four main mechanisms, namely:
> 1. Natural active immunity: Antibodies created by the host after an infection.
> 2. Natural passive immunity: Antibodies obtained from mother-to-child transfer during pregnancy or breastfeeding.
> 3. Artificial active immunity: Antibodies created by the host after a vaccination.
> 4. Artificial passive immunity: Antibodies obtained from receipt of an injection that has immunoglobulins.

Active versus passive immunity

Furthermore, how the antibodies are acquired can be categorized into active and passive processes. Active immunity may be acquired when human body is exposed to the pathogen or via artificial process such as immunization which stimulates the body to build its defence towards the pathogens. **Natural active immunity** describes antibodies created by the host after an infection while **natural passive immunity** is acquired from another individual. An example of passive immunity would be mother-to-child transfer of antibodies during pregnancy or breastfeeding. **Artificial active immunity** delineates antibodies that are created by the host after vaccination while **artificial passive immunity** refers to the receipt of an injection that contains immunoglobulins (Centers for Disease Control and Prevention [CDC], 2017) (see also Knowledge Box 5.3).

Pathogen transmissibility and pathogenicity

Transmissibility refers to the pathogen's ability to infect and reproduce within the host. The ability for pathogens to be transmitted varies in time, environment, and population. Notably, population structure might affect the effectiveness of control interventions. Within a population or community, each individual might have a different immunity level and individuals at higher risk of infections are typically of a weaker immune system, such as older people, children, and people with chronic diseases. If the number of these high-risk individuals is high within a population, the chance of a large-scale outbreak will also increase. An example of a disease prevention intervention would be to encourage an at-risk population to receive vaccinations to lower the proportion of the vulnerable population, which also increases herd immunity. The basic reproduction number (R_o) is a key indicator for a pathogen's transmissibility. For example, within a population where no-one has immunity, the R_o number indicates, on average, the number of individuals that a single infected person will infect. $R_o > 1$ indicates that the pathogen has the ability to infect more people continuously. During the 2003 SARS outbreak, the R_o number was 2.7 (excluding the extreme incidents at the hospital and the community housing where concentrated outbreaks occurred).

Pathogenicity refers to a pathogen's ability to cause disease. Disease development in a host after being infected by the pathogen depends not only on the host's immunity but also on the pathogen's pathogenicity. Pathogenicity mainly depends on the virulence and amount of the pathogens. Virulence refers to the degree to which the pathogens can cause and develop a disease. The higher the virulence, the easier it is for the disease to develop. Pathogens with a low virulence can often lead to diseases with minor symptoms. Inside the host, pathogens rarely survive as individual organisms. Instead, they live in clusters: the larger the cluster, the higher the pathogenicity and the more effective the pathogen transmissions.

Treatment of communicable diseases

Treatment of communicable diseases mainly includes three components: (i) specific treatment for a targeted microorganism aiming to inhibit the growth of the pathogens or eliminate them; (ii) treatment for clinical symptom management aiming to relieve the patient's discomfort; and (iii) treatment of related medical complications aiming to address the symptom's complications rather than addressing the microorganisms that have initially caused the symptoms.

For treatment targeting specific microorganisms, pharmacological agents might seek to suppress or eliminate the disease-causing infection. Chemotherapeutic agents might include **non-therapeutic agents** such as antiseptics (substances which, applied on the surface of living tissue, reduce infection opportunity) and disinfectant (substances applied on the surface of non-living tissue) as well as **therapeutic agents** such as antimicrobials (chemical substances which act against microbes), antibacterial agents and antibiotics (antibacterial substances that are produced by the microorganism of concern), and antivirals. The treatment regimen might be based on single or multiple agents that target a specific or various stages of the life cycle of the infection agent. It might be a single dose, lasting for days/months (e.g. DOTS treatment for TB/MDR-TB) or require life-long regular consumption (highly active antiretroviral therapy (HAART) for HIV patients).

Antibiotics, one of the most important medical discoveries of the twentieth century, are the main type of medication used to treat bacterial infections. They have saved countless lives but, due to their significant efficacy, many people are misled by the ability of antibiotics and believe they can cure any disease. Antibiotics have been readily prescribed for symptoms such as swollen throats, coughs, and runny noses even when the disease was caused by non-bacterial pathogens. The misuse of this drug not only fails to relieve the symptoms but also leads to bacteria adapting and ultimately developing resistance to the antibiotics. In recent years, with the continued and inappropriate use of antibiotics, some of the traditional antibiotic treatments are no longer as effective due to drug resistance such as antimicrobial resistance (AMR). Examples of antibiotic-resistant species include methicillin-resistant *Staphylococcus aureus* (MRSA) and drug-resistant tuberculosis (DR-TB) (see Knowledge Box 5.4).

In addition to relieving physiological discomfort and exertion, **symptomatic treatment** helps support the patient from further exacerbating their conditions. Particularly

Knowledge Box 5.4 Antimicrobial Drug-Resistant Infections

In the modern world, common use of medications and antibiotics for treatments (for both humans and animals), suboptimal treatment management (e.g. inappropriate prescriptions and incomplete drug regimen adherence), and non-medical use for growth promotion or enhancement (in food production) have led to major changes of the physiological process in responding to treatment and medication. Drugs that have been useful in treating certain conditions may no longer be as effective as cells have become less responsive, which leads to the emergence of antibiotic-resistant bacteria strains such as multidrug-resistant *Mycobacterium tuberculosis* (leading to multidrug-resistant tuberculosis, MDR-TB), *Clostridium difficile* (C. diff), and methicillin-resistant *Staphylococcus aureus* (MRSA). These antimicrobial drug-resistant bacteria cause serious concerns because infections with these microorganisms can be lethal. Antibiotic resistance has also threatened the effectiveness of prophylactic treatment for important global health-affecting infections like malaria. *Plasmodium falciparum*, the most lethal species of Plasmodium that causes malaria, has developed resistance to most antimalarial treatments in recent decades. Such a resistant pattern hampers health protection effort and control for vulnerable populations who tend to be at the extreme ends of the age spectrum, live in less developed countries, and often in poverty.

Sources: WHO, 2011; WorldWide Antimalarial Resistance Network (n.d.).

if specific treatment is not available, supportive treatment will be as important to control symptoms. Some common symptomatic medications are antipyretics (reducing fever/temperature), anti-cough, anti-diarrhoeal, painkillers, and products to combat dehydration. Although these drugs are often available over-the-counter, as these pharmaceutical agents will supress symptoms, they make diagnosis and monitoring of treatment challenging.

Treatment of complications might be associated with superimposed conditions (e.g. opportunistic infection for HIV/AIDS patients) and infection that might potentially predispose the patient to malignancies (e.g. chronic hepatitis B infection to liver cancer).

Currently, some infectious diseases do not have a treatment; thus, preventive measures are especially important. Preventive measures for infectious diseases can be implemented both before and after exposure to the disease. Using rabies as an example, the vaccine for rabies can be used both before and after exposure to a suspected canine. Even though Hong Kong is a rabies-free city, there are post-exposure measures implemented when an animal suspected of having rabies bites or scratches a person. Rabies vaccinations for pre-exposure prevention are also given to people at high risk of getting an infection such as veterinarians, rabies researchers, and animal caretakers.

Moreover, as discussed earlier, when a person is infected with an organism, he/she is not necessarily in a state of ill health. Although clinical diseases should always be treated and symptoms should be relieved when possible, some treatments might affect normal flora in the human physiological environment and thus lead to drug-related -complication (e.g. antibiotic-associated diarrhoea).

Prevention and control of infectious diseases

The world has become increasingly interconnected through increasing international trade and the exponential growth in global travel. However, such phenomena have also increased the risk of disease outbreaks: a shorter time frame is required for pathogens to travel from one end of the world to another which, as a result, speeds up the speed of transmission. Preventing and controlling a major outbreak is still very challenging. Mega cities often attract migrant populations for the jobs, education, and service access they offer. High-density living is the ideal environment for pathogens to spread. In addition, if an outbreak does occur in this context, the pathogen can spread rapidly, and containing and controlling the outbreak will prove difficult.

Communicable disease prevention and control require a coordinated effort throughout the entire pathway of care and approaches to disease prevention (see Knowledge Box 5.5 and Chapter 2). Specifically, if the hierarchy of prevention is applied to infection control, primary, secondary, and tertiary prevention might be applied to address the three major phases of infection control, namely exposure, infection, and disease (Lee, 2012).

Knowledge Box 5.5 Common Terminology in Communicable Disease Control

Emerging infectious diseases refers to diseases that have never been found in humans or have only occurred in remote areas with sporadic cases.

Re-emerging infectious diseases refers to infectious diseases that in the past were commonly found throughout a country or even globally, were then under control, but are currently reappearing.

Endemic describes an area that routinely experiences cases of a specific infectious disease.

Epidemic describes an area where the number of infected people with a specific infectious disease suddenly increases past the expected rate.

Pandemic refers to a scenario where an epidemic is spreading and affecting people in multiple countries or across several continents

At the *primary prevention level*, exposure avoidance might be achieved through simple but effective approaches such as promotion and practice of personal and environmental hygiene as well as the avoidance of risky behavioural that might enhance pathogen transmission. Lack of hand and food hygiene is the most common form of health risk that can be reduced through personal awareness, knowledge, and behavioural adaptation. **Personal hygiene measures** such as **handwashing** (i.e. proper way to wash with soap and clean water before and after meals and toilet use, when visiting clinics and public facilities, and handling livestock), **respiratory etiquette** (e.g. covering mouth and nose when coughing and sneezing, refraining from spitting, and wearing facemask when experiencing respiratory symptoms), and **food hygiene and safety** (consuming only clean water and food, hygienic food handling, proper storage, using separate utensils for raw and cooked food, and using proper utensils in meal-sharing practices) are common effective approaches (Lee, 2012; WHO, 2014).

Treatment of disease is also an important step in the control of infection. Apart from relieving the symptoms of the disease, it can also prevent the spread of the pathogens in some cases. However, treatment alone is not sufficient to stop the spread of disease as many pathogens do not necessarily reproduce inside human bodies (e.g. plasmodium). Furthermore, the medication used for treatment is usually only useful for humans and may not be effective to protect against vectors and thus, the source or vector of infection is not addressed or controlled. In addition, some infectious diseases may not have effective treatment options (e.g. hepatitis B and hepatitis C); therefore, prevention is the main method to stop the spread of these diseases. Hence, the fight against infectious disease requires both treatment and prevention measures.

Methods of communicable disease control

In principle, there are seven methods for communicable disease control in a community. These include universal precautions, immunization, source removal, isolation, decontamination, quarantine, and chemoprophylaxis. Table 5.1 highlights the key methods of communicable disease control according to the hierarchy of prevention (see Chapter 2). Depending on the context, situation, and the system, the approaches that are described in Table 5.1 may be implemented alone or together.

Host protection

Host protection involves actions and interventions that aim to increase the immunity of potentially affected populations. Because contact with pathogens does not necessary lead to infection, raising the host's immunity and awareness of disease risks are crucial to avoiding future infections. Maintaining a balanced diet and taking sufficient exercise and rest are helpful in raising a person's immunity and improving the overall functioning of the immune system. Meanwhile, strengthening the acquired immune system involves acquiring a defence mechanism for specific pathogens. One of the most effective methods is to provide prophylaxis or prevention through interventions such as vaccines, drugs, and physical protection.

Table 5.1 Application Hierarchy of Prevention in Communicable Disease Control

Level of prevention	Approach	Examples of activities
Primary prevention	Health management	Health promotion (i.e. promoting health protection practices): healthy habits, food safety, waste management, healthy diet, etc.
	Universal precaution	Avoiding contact of bodily fluids (use of protective gears such as PPE, gloves, goggles, and facemask, needle injury prevention, and handwashing)
	Vaccination	Vaccine prophylaxis immunizing people with high risk of exposure
Secondary prevention	Source removal	Closing down of restaurants (e.g. during food-related outbreaks); product recall
	Isolation	Avoiding spread from infected individuals (e.g. negative pressure room for source isolation, and positive pressure room for protection and isolation of immunocompromised patients)
	Decontamination	Disinfection of equipment, environment, contacts, and families
	Quarantine	Isolation of people or animals who might have been in contact with the infected sources
	Chemoprophylaxis	Medications/antibiotics prescribed to people who have been exposed to sources of infection (e.g. individuals or materials infected by meningococcal meningitis)

Vaccination and immunization

Vaccines are one of the most important inventions used to prevent infections. When people are infected by pathogens, apart from creating antibodies to fight them, the acquired immune system is able to recognize and remember the pathogens. This means if a specific pathogen infects a person again, the acquired immune system can quickly and more efficiently fight back against the pathogen. However, during the initial contact with a new pathogen, the immune system is often unprepared and can only wait for help while being attacked. Being vaccinated is an early intervention method that gives the body the ability to eliminate pathogens or to lower their virulence before the pathogen is encountered. With prior knowledge about the intruder before the contact is made, the whole body is alert and able to spot the pathogen. If the pathogen does appear again, the immune system will then be quick to respond and to prevent harm from occurring.

Although vaccination and immunization are terms usually used interchangeably, they describe two related, but different health protection concepts. **Vaccination** refers to the administration of a **vaccine** which is a biological preparation designed for inducing immunity against specific diseases. Medically, vaccines are being developed as strategies for health protection towards infection, allergy, and cancer (Lee, 2012). Most vaccine for communicable disease control is infection target-specific and its effectiveness might depend on a number of factors. **Immunization**, also known as **immunoprophylaxis**, is the achievement of immunity artificially through or after the vaccination process. It is an acquired immunity rather than genuine immunity acquired through natural infection. **Inoculation** is the process of injecting external agents into the body to allow the agent to grow and induce an immune response in the host body. **Passive immunization** describes the immunity induction by administrating a pre-formed antibody. Notably, people who receive a vaccine might not necessary develop the relevant or enough immune response to prevent disease manifestation.

Vaccinations are not only a personal form of health precaution but also a public health protective approach at the population level. Overall benefit of a vaccination campaign may yield greater benefit for the community than the individuals who have received the vaccination. Using the highly contagious disease of measles as an example, the vaccination coverage within a population has to reach 95% or greater to achieve herd immunity to protect an at-risk community (World Health Organization Regional Office for South-East Asia, 2013). Therefore, vaccine accessibility and accurate information dissemination to ensure a high vaccination coverage, as well as population acceptability, are important to ensure herd immunity can be achieved. The World Health Organization (WHO) has recommended the immunization schedule as summarized in Table 5.2 (WHO, 2018).

Even though vaccines are an effective means of infection control, many infectious diseases currently have no available vaccine. One of the main reasons for this is a lack of profitability. Nowadays, most vaccine developments are dependent on private pharmaceutical companies in developed countries, yet the main incidence of infectious disease happens within poverty-struck countries like Sudan, Democratic Republic of the Congo, and Uganda. These low-income countries have a very low purchasing power, which means that in a profit-driven market, the pharmaceutical companies are often not motivated to pursue technology that has a high risk or a low rate of return. The incentive of pharmaceutical companies that operate purely using a business model may not align with the global effort to prevent the transmission of infectious disease. This phenomenon is not confined only to vaccine development but is also seen in the research for treatment drugs and other similar disease prophylactics. To develop a vaccine programme that protects against health risks associated with communicable diseases, relevant scientific evidence, programme strategy, administration structure and finances, vaccine management (purchase, storage, and distribution), community organization, communication, education, and informatics all facilitate monitoring and follow-up. With competing priorities and resource limitation, prioritization of prevention and treatment modalities must be given to local epidemiology, risks, efficacy of the vaccine (according to the target age group and underlying health risks), funding, and implementation system availability.

Typically, a vaccine is developed with the idea of presenting as an antigen to the individual in order to stimulate an immunological response. Using live attenuated, inactivated, component, and recombinant vaccines are four main approaches of vaccines in

Table 5.2 World Health Organization's Recommendations for Routine Immunization

Antigen	Children	Adolescents	Adults
Bacille Calmette–Guérin (BCG)	1 dose		
Hepatitis B	3–4 doses	3 doses (for high-risk groups if not previously immunized)	
Diphtheria, tetanus, and pertussis containing vaccine (DTPCV)	3 doses + 2 boosters: 12–23 months (DTPCV) 4–7 years (Td/DT containing vaccine)	1 booster 9–15 years (Td)	
Polio	3–4 doses with DTPCV		
Haemophilus influenza type b	Option 1: 3 doses, with DTPCV		
	Option 2: 2 or 3 doses, with booster at least 6 months after last dose		
Pneumococcal (conjugate)	Option 1: 3 doses, with DTPCV		
	Option 2: 2 doses before 6 months of age, plus booster dose at 9–15 months old		
Rotavirus	2–3 doses depending on product with DTPCV		
Measles	2 doses		
Rubella	1 dose	1 dose (adolescent girls and women of child-bearing age if not previously vaccinated)	
Human papillomavirus (HPV)		2 doses (females)	

Source: WHO (2018).

modern vaccination development (refer to Table 5.3). A vaccine can be monovalent, actively targeting a single or single strain of microorganisms (e.g. hepatitis B), or poly-valent/multivalent, addressing more than one pathogens (e.g. mumps–measles–rubella (MMR) and seasonal influenza). To improve response, an adjuvant, a substance such as aluminium or compounds that support immunomodulatory actors, may be adminis-trated in conjunction with the vaccine antigen component.

When vaccines target individual patients, they protect from an infection and safeguard against ill health. When they are used systematically and at the societal level, they can control disease transmission and promote public health and well-being. Although most

Table 5.3 Four Main Types of Vaccines in Modern World

	Type	Description	Examples
1	Live attenuated	Attenuation of live microorganism	BCG, mumps, measles, rubella, polio, yellow fever
2	Inactivated	Killed microorganism	Pertussis, typhoid, influenza
3	Component	Fraction of microorganism/its product (e.g. toxoid)	Pneumococcus, meningococcus, haemophilus influenzae, tetanus (toxoid)
4	Recombinant	Involving a carrier organism (vector) in combination of a component (e.g. peptide synthesis by gene)	Hepatitis B

vaccines may aim at offering life-long protection or immunity, in reality, with the changes of pathogen presentation, transmission dynamics, and emerging and re-emerging of existing disease, to ensure effectiveness and protection, a majority of them are constantly under regular redevelopment and the population might require re-immunization to sustain the intended protection.

Despite its potential effectiveness, vaccination is constantly subject to debate and controversy. Community acceptance of vaccination often depends on many factors. Public perception of how good a specific vaccine is depends on **effectiveness** (degree of protection against microorganism), **safety** (potential adverse reaction which majority of people might experience after receiving the vaccination), and **stability** (the potential usefulness and application in various context). At the public health level, **cost** (resources required to implement the vaccine at a societal level to ensure effectiveness), **coverage**, and **herd immunity** are also determinants to ensure population protection. In addition to a country's general strategies in immunization, to address the health risks of specific subgroups, target vaccination programme may be implemented. Target-specific vaccination programmes might be required and implemented for travellers (e.g. hepatitis A and yellow fever), occupational subgroups (hepatitis B), people affected by outbreak incidents (e.g. meningitis C), and global strategies of disease management (e.g. eradication of smallpox and elimination of polio).

Immunization approaches in public health protection

Herd immunity

Vaccines are one of the most important inventions used to prevent infections. When the number of vaccinated people within a population reaches a certain threshold, it will strengthen the herd immunity, which means that unvaccinated individuals will also be less susceptible to infections (John and Samuel, 2000). Thus, vaccinations are not only a personal form of health precaution but can be protective at population level. This means the overall benefit is greater than the sum of each individual vaccination. As mentioned earlier, when the vaccination coverage against measles within a population has to reach 95% or above to achieve herd immunity (Lee, 2012). Therefore, whenever possible, health departments around the world should provide free vaccinations and disseminate accurate information to the local residents to ensure a high vaccination coverage, as well as to rid the population of any concerns and dispel misinformation about the vaccine.

Gap in vaccination strategies

Even though vaccines are an effective means of infection control, many infectious diseases lack the relevant vaccine for protection. As mentioned earlier, drug companies are reluctant to pour significant funds into developing new treatments where their rate of return is uncertain or low. Unfortunately, this affects low-income countries disproportionately.

Prophylaxis treatment

There are two main type of prophylaxis, pre-exposure and post-exposure, to prevent infection associated with exposure. Pre-exposure prophylaxis is the use of therapeutic agents before exposure. A typical example would be to provide antibiotic prophylaxis to some high-risk patients (immunocompromised individuals) before surgical procedure to avoid potential infection due to suboptimal immunity. Post-exposure prophylaxis (PEP) is the use of therapeutic agents after exposure to a pathogen. This might be used before infection is confirmed and in healthcare settings to prevent infection after medical incidents (such as needle-stick injury).

A range of vaccines are available and each of these approaches have its own characteristics and impact. These include live attenuated, inactivated (i.e. killed), conjugate, polysaccharide subunit, and toxoid vaccines. The **live attenuated** vaccine contains live microorganisms whose virulent components have been disabled. Examples of such vaccine include BCG, MMR, yellow fever, polio (Sabin), rotavirus, and influenza (see Knowledge Box 5.6). An **inactivated vaccine** contains microorganisms that have been killed. Examples include hepatitis A, influenza, inactivated polio (Salk), cholera, rabies, and plagues. A **conjugate vaccine** is created by covalently attaching a poor antigen to a strong antigen, thereby eliciting a stronger immunological response in the host body. The advantages of the conjugate vaccines are their ability to elicit immunological memory and to reduce asymptomatic carriage of the bacteria, resulting in marked herd immunity (WHO, 2013). Examples include meningitis C, Haemophilus influenzae type b (Hib), meningococcal vaccine, and pneumococcal vaccine. For the **polysaccharide vaccine**, only the sugar part of the bacteria, the capsule, is included as the antigen to stimulate the immune response. Pneumovax 23 (PPV-23) and typhoid vaccines are common examples. The **subunit vaccine** contains only a fragment of the microorganism and examples include hepatitis B, human papilloma virus (HPV), and acellular pertussis. A **toxoid vaccine** contains inactivated toxic compounds and examples include tetanus and diphtheria.

In addition to the choices of vaccine, programmes and policies for immunization strategies need to consider the potential side-effects of the vaccines, age of the recipients, immunization schedule (dose interval and need for booster doses), implementation and

Knowledge Box 5.6 Vaccine Development for Seasonal Influenza and Avian Influenza

Seasonal influenza (flu) is by no means the same as the common cold. It is caused by influenza viruses that cause acute respiratory illnesses (WHO, 30 March 2018). The influenza virus has a very high pathogenicity and can easily mutate, and the illness has comparatively severe symptoms. According to the target of the infection, influenza can be divided into human, avian, and swine strains, to name a few. The strains that are prevalent in animals tend not to be easily transmitted to humans. However, if there is a large-scale outbreak in animals, like the H5N1 avian flu, the risk of humans being infected will no doubt increase.

The influenza virus is constantly mutating. If the genetic composition of the virus changes dramatically, it can greatly increase the chance of a new virus being transmitted from one person to another. Such scenarios may lead to a global pandemic (CDC, 2016) (see also Knowledge Box 5.5). Two international conferences are held each year where the top influenza experts meet and discuss which strains of the influenza virus may be prevalent in the northern and southern hemispheres, as well as deliberate on which strains should be included in the seasonal influenza vaccine (CDC, 2016; CHP, 14 June 2018). The conference for the northern hemisphere usually convenes in February and the conference for the southern hemisphere is held in September. The suggested mixtures of influenza strains for the vaccine also differ between the hemispheres.

Although the seasonal influenza vaccine is a safe and reliable means of protection against seasonal influenza, it is not an absolute guarantee and it cannot prevent avian influenza. Meanwhile, even though a vaccine exists for poultry to prevent avian influenza, a vaccine against avian influenza for humans has yet to be developed (see also Case Box 5.2). Several groups of people are at a higher risk of being infected with seasonal influenza, and thus need to be vaccinated against the virus. These include pregnant women, older people, long-term residents of institutions for the disabled, people with chronic illnesses, children aged 6 months to 11 years, poultry workers, pig farmers, and people who work in the pig slaughtering industry (CHP, 10 September 2018). Other occupations that require the influenza vaccination include healthcare workers. In this way, the chance of spreading influenza to high-risk patients in hospitals is lowered.

surveillance system support and monitoring, and potential related outbreak responses (e.g. the need to stockpile additional vaccines).

Health and risks literacy education

Prevention of communicable diseases also involves education and health risk awareness raising in the general and at-risk community. To be effective, these attempts might have to be target- and location-specific. For example, for sexually transmitted infections, health and sex education, counselling, availability of condoms, early detection, access to effective treatment, contact and treatment tracing, and opportunistic screening are important aspects of communicable disease control measures.

Managing the source of infection

Infectious disease reporting system, early detection, isolation, and clinical management of a disease are important measures to protect public safety. During a disease outbreak, the early screening and investigation of suspected cases should be performed, suspected cases be put under close observation, and suitable treatment be concurrently offered for the affected people. When indicated, isolation or even the quarantine of specific susceptible populations may be required.

Domestic pets, livestock, or wild animals are common animal reservoirs harbouring pathogens that might have serious consequences for human health. Pet and farm owners must ensure that their pets and livestock are vaccinated against diseases and manage their living context systematically. Vaccines for rabies (among dogs) and influenza (among chickens) are important methods to prevent disease outbreaks in animals and protect human owners.

Mosquitoes, rats, and ticks are other vectors that may cause major health hazards and epidemics. Public environmental measures such as vector control and elimination efforts are essential to protecting public health. For example, *Aedes aegypti* and *Aedes albopictus* are vector mosquito species that might transmit dengue fever. With global warming, urban environments become more suitable for mosquito breeding and risk of dengue fever transmission increases. It is estimated that by 2085, there will be 5.2 billion people globally at risk of becoming infected with dengue fever (Hales, Wet, Maindonald, and Woodward, 2002). Currently, as there is no known drug for effective treatment of dengue, vector control and prevention of mosquito bites are the most important methods of disease control. Preventive vector control measures against dengue fever include the routine disposal of waste, regular house cleaning, the removal of stagnant water, and dredging ditches to reduce the breeding grounds for mosquitoes. Other human health protection measures also include using mosquito nets, coils, and repellents to prevent bites (see also Case Box 3.6 on malaria).

Interrupting transmission routes

Overall, one of the most cost-effective ways of interrupting the disease transmission routes involves cultivating good personal hygiene and food safety practices. Maintaining personal hygiene practices include the use of liquid soap or alcohol hand-rub for handwashing, especially before handling or eating food, after going to the toilet, after coughing or sneezing, after touching public items, and after touching animals or birds; proper waster management; and good food safety practices such as separating raw and cooked food, managing food storage, and observing food expiration dates and colling requirements.

For human-infected communicable diseases, if human is the only infection route for the outbreak and epidemic (see Knowledge Box 5.5), effective treatment of infected individuals might disrupt further transmission. However, many communicable diseases involve complex interaction between human, vectors, and the environment. Although treatment of patients might restore the well-being of the individual and save him/her

Case Box 5.2 Public Health Approach to Address the Transmission of Avian Influenza: 'Central Slaughtering'

Hong Kong SAR, China experienced confirmed cases of people being infected by H7N9 on separate occasions in 2013, 2014, 2016, and 2017. Although H7N9 avian strain of influenza is only transmitted among birds, direct contact with infected birds (dead or alive) or their faeces, or indirect contact with a contaminated environment (such as a wet market or live poultry market) may lead to human infection (CHP, 3 April 2018). One of the most important measures to reduce the risk of the transmission of avian influenza to humans is lowering the chances of direct human contact with live and slaughtered poultry. As retail poultry butchering is a common practice in marketplace in Hong Kong, central slaughtering system was suggested as a way to reduce the direct contact between humans and live poultry. When there is an outbreak of avian influenza, it is a common infection control measure to enforce central mass slaughter of chickens to avoid further transmission. Nevertheless, livelihood of poultry farmers and wholesale retailers are seriously affected if people prefer consuming frozen chicken to fresh chicken. In addition, some of the opponents of a central slaughtering site argue that avian influenza outbreaks would still occur even after its implementation. Thus, the views on central slaughtering are still controversial and subject to heated public debates whenever such measures are called for.

from adverse health outcomes, it might not be effective to stop the pathogen from moving from person to person (see Case Box 5.3).

Surveillance of infectious diseases

Disease surveillance and reporting are crucial prevention and intervention measures. They involve the ongoing systematic collection, analysis, interpretation, and dissemination of information generated for disease prevention. Because medical conditions and standards for diseases vary from place to place, the same type of disease may have different diagnostic criteria. Case definition is usually based on clinical or microbiological criteria. The sources of case detection may come from primary, secondary, and tertiary care. In addition to a reporting system of notifiable diseases, reports from laboratory, clinic statistics, and various standardized reporting systems (e.g. vaccination coverage systems) are often used. Data collection tools and systems must be standardized, ideally to include the time, place, person, and diagnostic criteria so that decision-makers can assess the situation and grasp the specifics of the outbreak. Analysis of data and summary statistics should be developed for monitoring and as feedback to data providers. The outcome of the surveillance aims to detect trends, evaluate prevention and control measures, and alert appropriate stakeholders for potential outbreak threats.

Surveillance refers to the examination of a population subset (e.g. a particular at-risk groups or a subgroup of a geographic location of interest). There are several types of surveillance. **Passive** surveillance involves data from routine sources (laboratory reports). It

Case Box 5.3 Surveillance and Monitoring of Antimicrobial Use and Resistance

Kin-on Kwok

Antimicrobial use is an effective approach to treat a broad range of life-threatening infections. However, the inadvertent use of antimicrobials among the human population, coupled with few new antibiotics in research and development, has escalated the widespread resistance to these treatments (Fair and Tor, 2014) which jeopardized their clinical efficacy and increased treatment costs. Antimicrobial resistance (AMR) is currently a top global public health concern (Ciorba, Odone, Veronesi, Pasquarella, and Signorelli, 2015). To echo the World Health Organization's efforts to foster AMR knowledge through surveillance and monitoring (WHO, 2015a), global communities should mobilize through international collaboration to develop a nationwide surveillance system to mitigate the AMR risk and protect the health of global citizens. In addition to the human population, AMR is also attributable to animals and the environment. One health surveillance approach is to integrate data from different domains and analyse it in an optimal cross-disciplinary AMR framework (McEwen and Collignon, 2018). This integrated system would provide policy-makers with insights in: (i) identifying both human and animal population at risk; and (ii) understanding how and why antimicrobials are used and their consumption patterns. This information helps formulate the infection control policies for high-risk subgroups, inform better antimicrobial therapy decision, assess the impact of possible resistance containment interventions, and facilitate the commitment amongst different stakeholders to implement successful campaigns to contain resistance in the future.

is the simplest automatic collection of data for trend patterns but might be incomplete in terms of assessing a specific situation. **Active** surveillance targets diseases for reporting. As it is an active effort (e.g. follow-ups to ensure completion and accuracy), frequently, negative reporting including 'no case' may be involved. A subtype of active surveillance is called '**enhanced** surveillance' which involves additional data about cases. This may be used when research studies or specific tasks (e.g. when establishing or evaluation of guideline) might be conducted. **Syndromic** surveillance, which is commonly used in emergencies or during the investigation of an outbreak, is the surveillance of clinical symptoms rather than confirmed cases. Case Box 5.3 discusses the global monitoring of antimicrobial use and resistance, which illustrates how various global platforms might support health protection against infectious diseases and other health risks in the twenty-first century.

Communicable disease outbreak and control

Disease outbreak investigations can be divided into four stages: the description of outbreak, determination of the cause, implementation of control measures, and the communication of the risks (Lee, 2012; WHO, 2014). An **outbreak** is defined as an event where the number of disease incident (or case) within a defined area and time period suddenly increases. The number of infected cases alone may not determine whether an event is an outbreak. The decision is made through an analysis of whether the number of infected cases is higher than the norm or typical pattern. Based on the transmission pattern, there are multiple ways of describing an outbreak including common-source, propagated, mixed, and others (CDC, 2012). **Common-source** transmission refers to a disease outbreak in a group of infected people who have all had contact with the same transmission source. Examples include food poisoning incidents like consumption of contaminated food that results in an outbreak of salmonellosis and the sharing of water sources that leads to cholera outbreak. **Propagated** transmission refers to an outbreak that originates from a single host but subsequently transmits to another or multiple hosts in a chain reaction manner. Notable examples include HIV transmission through needle sharing and infections that occur due to pathogen-infected droplets entering the body. **Mixed** transmission pattern refers to infections by pathogens through the same transmission source and spread among various hosts. An example is dysentery. **Others** refer to pathogenic infections that have different sources of transmission and do not spread directly from person to person.

Three main objectives of an outbreak control are: (i) to minimize the number of primary cases (illness) and secondary cases with appropriate action of prevention; (ii) identification of potential hazards and eliminate or minimize the risks which these hazards might pose to the affected community; and (iii) implement prevention measures for future incidents. Knowledge Box 5.7 describes the key elements in outbreak control. An example of the development of the infectious disease outbreaks reporting system in Guangdong–Hong Kong–Macao Greater Bay Area in China after the 2013 SARS outbreak is described in Case Box 5.4.

Case Box 5.4 Infectious Disease Outbreaks Reporting System for Guangdong–Hong Kong–Macao Greater Bay Area

During the 2003 SARS outbreak in Mainland China and Hong Kong, the Hong Kong and Guangdong health authorities established a series of notification mechanisms for sharing disease surveillance information on cases of human infection and disease. Later on, this reporting system also evolved and included Macau and was subsequently known as the Guangdong–Hong Kong–Macau infection disease notification mechanism. After years of hard work, these three places have provided the essential platform and standards for controlling major infectious diseases such as avian influenza, hand, foot and mouth disease, MERS, and dengue fever. This three-way partnership has also created opportunities for information sharing, research collaborations, and exchange programmes between the infectious disease experts.

Apart from a monthly exchange of statutory reports on infectious diseases, the Guangdong–Hong Kong–Macau partnership also reports to each other the outcomes during emergencies or when needed.

Knowledge Box 5.7 Approaches in Communicable Disease Outbreak Control

To investigate and control of disease outbreak, the following subsections describe the principles and efforts. Notably, with the exception of epidemiological sequences of case management that should be done in a serial manner, most of these tasks are done concurrently to address the public health protection objectives.

Convening an Outbreak Control Group

Although disease control relies on clinical and public health expertise, successful outbreak control requires multidisciplinary actors and collaboration. A coordinating group should be convened to examine diseases that occur in large numbers of cases and may pose immediate health hazards and have serious implications for the local population.

Determination of the Cause and Epidemiological Sequence/ Approach

In outbreaks, case definition and mechanisms for case confirmation need to be established to monitor background disease progress. The team needs to investigate and determine the cause of a disease. Epidemiological characteristics of cases (time, place, persons, clinical characteristics, and laboratory confirmation) need to be described. Epidemic curves is an example of skill tools which helphypothesis generation of disease transmission pattern with all the known and available information. Hypothesis will be further tested by analytic studies and via statistical analysis. Correlations such as contact with the reservoir and the presence of symptoms will be identified to establish an association between certain factors and the disease.

Implementation of Control Measures

Controlling the epidemic and reducing the number of incident cases is the priority in any disease outbreak investigation. Important goals for any outbreak control measures include the control of disease spread, protection of at-risk population, coordinating and communicating with public and stakeholders, and proposing measure to prevent future outbreaks.

Risk Communication

Effective risk communication includes regular and timely public reports of the ongoing situation, the transparency of already-known information, accuracy, and presenting the next steps in the response procedures. Choice of media of communication to the specific target audiences is also an important consideration.

Case Box 5.5 Control of SARS Outbreak in Hong Kong

During the 2003 Hong Kong SARS outbreak, the two main disease control actions were undertaken. Multiple quarantine measures included facility quarantine (e.g. hotel), building isolation (where the confirmed cases of SARS patients reside), and relocation (the remaining residents being relocated to a temporary quarantine camp). For the incident, residents were quarantined for ten days and were assessed daily by clinicians.

Another important outbreak control measure was advocating the use of facemasks, which may prevent droplets and bodily fluids from the mouth and nose from spreading into the environment. In general, the 2003 SARS outbreak has led to major changes in public health awareness and practices for local citizens.

Global partnerships for the prevention and control of infectious disease

Under the influence of globalization, the active cross-border exchanges and people movement have greatly increased the chances of infectious disease transmission across states and countries. As an example, the 2003 SARS epidemic was first officially reported in March 2003, yet within a month it had affected areas including the United States and Canada in North America; England, Ireland, France, Germany, Switzerland, Spain, and Italy in Europe; and Thailand, Viet Nam, Singapore, China, Taiwan, and Hong Kong in Asia (WHO, 2003a, 2003c). By the time when the outbreak halted after four months, it had spread to nearly 30 countries with over 8,000 cases recorded (WHO, 2003b). This is an example showing how infectious disease transmission is borderless and the prevention and control have to be a global effort (see Case Box 5.5). Knowledge Box 5.8 introduces the International Health Regulations.

While surveillance systems established by national authorities work within single countries, international surveillance systems serve as early warning systems for potential global epidemics and may facilitate and coordinate public health interventions and responses.

Port health

Population movement and global trade increases the risks of the global transmission of infectious diseases. Port and border health management is crucial to protect modern communities from communicable disease risks as a result population movement and global trade. Management of travellers' health, control of outbreaks related to food- and water-borne diseases in travelling vessels, pest control, and health risk communication are all important health protection measures at borders and ports. Even before the Industrial Revolution, **quarantine** and **trade embargoes** have been key interventions that have helped control communicable disease transmission beyond national boundaries.

Knowledge Box 5.8 International Health Regulations

The cholera epidemics of the 1830s in Europe were catalysts for intensive infectious disease diplomacy and multilateral cooperation in public health. This led to the first International Sanitary Conference in Paris in 1851. After the WHO constitution had entered into force in 1948, WHO Member States adopted the International Sanitary Regulations in 1951 which were subsequently renamed as the International Health Regulations in 1969. The 1969 regulations were subject to further minor modifications in the next few decades. By 2000, the resurgence of some well-known epidemic diseases, such as cholera and plague, and the emergence of new infectious diseases, such as Ebola haemorrhagic fever and SARS, resulted in a major updated to its current format. The International Health Regulations (2005) (IHR (2005)) are established as international legal instrument that facilitates countries to work together to protect lives and livelihoods caused by the international spread of diseases and other health risks. The agreement binds 194 countries to work together and contribute to global disease surveillance and commitment of control in emergency.

According to the IHR (2005), a public health emergency of international concern refers to an extraordinary public health event that is determined, under specific procedures: (i) to constitute a public health risk to other states through the international spread of disease; and (ii) potentially to require a coordinated international response.

Overall, IHR aims to prevent, protect against, control, and respond to the international spread of diseases while avoiding unnecessary interference with international traffic and trade. It supports the international community prevent and respond to acute public health risks that might cross national boundaries. The agreement requires countries to report specific disease outbreaks and public health events to the WHO. Building on the unique experience in global disease surveillance, alert, and response, the IHR (2005) define the rights and obligations of countries to report public health events and establish a number of procedures that the WHO must follow in its work to uphold global public health security.

Source: WHO (2016a).

In 2007, the WHO ratified the International Health Regulations (2005) (WHO, 2007b) and this international legal document was agreed by 194 Member States in an attempt to prevent the spread of infectious disease outbreaks within a country and across international borders (WHO, 2007a). According to the International Health Regulations (2005), Member States bear responsibility to alert the WHO of any public health incidents that may pose an international threat within 24 hours of their discovery.

The WHO will be responsible for collecting reports from various places and confirming the received intelligence before distributing the information globally. Member States should adopt an open and transparent attitude to the situation and report outbreaks that are confirmed. Apart from having a well-coordinated global alert mechanism, the international community's ability to prevent diseases also relies on the capacity of individual Member States to protect and prevent outbreaks on their own. Each Member State is responsible for evaluating and strengthening its own surveillance and response systems in case an outbreak occurs. These systems should include the accurate monitoring of the situation to allow for timely decision-making, outbreak controls, and disease containment. If the systems of the Member States do not meet the standards of the 2005 International Health Regulations, they may request the support of the WHO. To prevent outbreaks from spreading across or within state borders, proper surveillance mechanisms should be established at the entry points such as international airports, ports, and ground crossings. At the entry and exit points of each of these countries, the member states have to establish medical and surveillance facilities that will ensure measures such as the diagnosis, quarantine, and transportation of suspected patients to a medical facility for treatment.

Global Outbreak Alert and Response Network (GOARN)

The Global Outbreak Alert and Response Network (GOARN) is a technical and operational resources network that gathers over 200 global, regional, and country-level organizations. It includes networks of public health experts, infection control, and biomedical scholars, laboratory scientists, the United Nations, and various international non-governmental organizations (INGOs) (WHO, n.d.-c). It aims to improve efficiency in global health responses and the WHO uses resources identified in this network to coordinate response to global disease outbreaks. Case Box 5.6 describes the challenges and gaps identified for Ebola management.

Case Box 5.6 The Failures during the Ebola Outbreak and the WHO Reform

In 2014, three countries in West Africa (Guinea, Liberia, and Sierra Leone) experienced an unprecedented outbreak that crossed the borders of many countries; it was the Ebola virus disease. This Ebola outbreak involved over 28,000 cases and caused the deaths of 11,300 people (WHO 10 June 2016). The first Ebola patient was confirmed in March 2014 in Guinea and within two months, the outbreak had already spread to the neighbouring countries of Liberia and Sierra Leone. However, it was only in August of that year that the WHO announced the outbreak to be a Public Health Emergency of International Concern (PHEIC). By then, there were over 3,000 cases and 1,500 deaths attributed to the disease (WHO 29 August 2014). During this time, the WHO was over-reliant on the capacity of local governments and NGOs to handle the epidemic. Taking Médecins Sans Frontières (MSF) as an example, healthcare workers were tasked with managing one-third of all the cases in the three West African countries mentioned (MSF, 2016), far beyond the capacity and the level of responsibility they could handle.

Case Box 5.6 The Failures during the Ebola Outbreak and the WHO Reform *(continued)*

The 2014 Ebola outbreak also exposed the shortcomings of the WHO's ability in responding to epidemics and managing emergencies. Inadequate resources, inability to provide ground-level assistance, slow deployments during crises, a lack of independence, overly political responses, and a poor working relationship with other organizations, are some key issues identified (WHO, 2016b).

The inadequacies led to the following internal reforms and restructuring within the WHO (WHO, August 2015).

1. Unified WHO Programme for Outbreaks and Emergencies

To ensure the employment of a transparent and rapid reporting system during emergencies, the WHO established an integrated surveillance, data, and information management system. The WHO also established pre-negotiated agreements with UN agencies, funds and programmes, and other partners to ensure the rapid mobilization of resources.

2. Global Health Emergency Workforce

To improve response capacity among local and international stakeholders, the WHO has established a global health emergency workforce that may respond to international emergencies. The workforce comprises national and international emergency responders and various UN agencies. This set-up can strengthen the capability of the supporting member states, especially those who have higher risks of emergencies, as well as assist their national alert and response systems to achieve a rapid response during a disease outbreak.

3. Accelerated Research and Development

The WHO agreed that vaccine development for Ebola was a priority and partnership among the WHO, the Norwegian Institute of Public Health, Médecins Sans Frontières, and the Guinean authorities was formed. The preliminary clinical trials conducted with participants from Guinea showed promising results when using the rVSV-EBOV vaccine. Apart from the vaccine development, the WHO also supported advancements for the rapid diagnostic testing of suspected Ebola cases, as well as assessment tools for the clinical trials involving samples of the convalescent plasma from recovered Ebola patients. Furthermore, guidelines are being developed for surveillance and testing policies in all the Member States.

4. WHO Contingency Fund

To ensure there are enough financial resources to respond to a large-scale outbreak and other emergencies, the WHO established a WHO Contingency Fund for Emergencies. The aim is to have US$100 million USD that is fully funded by voluntary contributions.

Infectious disease and development: Sustainable Development Goals

In 2015, global community adopted a new set of goals called the Sustainable Development Goals (SDGs), with targets to be met by 2030 to replace the previous Millennium Development Goals (MDGs, 2000-2015). The 8 broad goals of MDG were expanded to the 17 goals to create a sustainable global living context and protect health and well-being of citizens around the world comprehensively. Health is at the centre of the Sustainable Development Goals (WHO, n.d.-a). Specifically, the third SDG goal is to 'ensure healthy lives and promote well-being for all at all ages'. Examples of communicable disease control-related targets include 'end[ing] the epidemics of AIDS, tuberculosis, malaria and neglected tropical diseases and combat[ing] hepatitis, water-borne diseases and other communicable diseases [by 2030]' (United Nations, n.d.).

As highlighted in the SDGs, AIDS (acquired immune deficiency syndrome), the disease caused by HIV (the human immunodeficiency virus), is transmitted through the exchange of bodily fluids. In 2017, there were more than 35 million people living with HIV globally, and 940,000 deaths were attributed to HIV-related complications. The region most affected by HIV/AIDS was Africa (WHO, 19 July 2018). Tuberculosis (TB) is caused by the mycobacterium tuberculosis bacteria and is an airborne disease transmitted between humans. In 2017, there were 10 million people falling ill with TB, and over 95% of TB cases and deaths occurred in developing countries (WHO, 18 September 2018). Malaria is a vector-born disease caused by plasmodium and transmitted by mosquitoes. In 2016, there were an estimated 216 million cases of malaria in 91 countries (up by 5 million over the previous year), of which African countries were disproportionally burdened with issues relating to the disease, with 90% of cases and 91% of deaths (WHO, 11 June 2018). Neglected tropical diseases (NTDs) refer to an assortment of diseases that are endemic to tropical and sub-tropical regions (e.g. dengue, rabies, and trachoma). Over 1 billion people worldwide are affected by these diseases, which also cause over US$1 billion of annual economic losses in developing countries (WHO, n.d.-b).

Conclusion

Control of communicable diseases is one of the main areas in the health protection practice. As highlighted previously, new emergent and re-emerging diseases constantly present new health risks to population. The increasingly urbanized lifestyle and high-density-based living will also render most city-based communities vulnerable to communicable disease risks and challenges in disease control. This chapter has described some key concepts and principles related to communicable diseases and their management. Effectiveness of future communicable disease control relies on global coordination and cooperation. With globalization, re-emergences of infectious diseases, new infections, resistance developed for therapeutic agents, chronic burden (HIV/AIDS), and causation of certain cancers, communicable infectious diseases will continue to be a topic of major public health importance in the years to come.

References

Centers for Disease Control and Prevention (2012). Lesson 1: Introduction to epidemiology. Available at: https://www.cdc.gov/ophss/csels/dsepd/ss1978/lesson1/section11.html.

Centers for Disease Control and Prevention (2016). Selecting viruses for the seasonal influenza vaccine. Available at: https://www.cdc.gov/flu/about/season/vaccine-selection.htm.

Centers for Disease Control and Prevention (2017). Immunity types. Available at: https://www.cdc.gov/vaccines/vac-gen/immunity-types.htm.

Chen, H., Au, K. M., Hsu, K. E., Lai, C. K. C., Myint, J., et al. (2018). Multidrug-resistant organism carriage among residents from residential care homes for the elderly in Hong Kong: A prevalence survey with stratified cluster sampling. *Hong Kong Medical Journal 24*(4) 350–60. doi: 10.12809/hkmj176949.

Ciorba, V., Odone, A., Veronesi, L., Pasquarella, C., and Signorelli, C. (2015). Antibiotic resistance as a major public health concern: Epidemiology and economic impact. *Annali di Igiene: Medicina Preventiva e di Comunità 27*(3) 562–79.

Department of Health of the Government of the Hong Kong Special Administrative Region, Centre for Health Protection (3 April 2018). Avian influenza. Available at https://www.chp.gov.hk/en/healthtopics/content/24/13.html.

Department of Health of the Government of the Hong Kong Special Administrative Region, Centre for Health Protection (14 June 2018. Seasonal influenza. Available at: https://www.chp.gov.hk/en/healthtopics/content/24/29.html.

Department of Health of the Government of the Hong Kong Special Administrative Region, Centre for Health Protection (10 September 2018). Frequently asked questions on seasonal influenza vaccine 2018/19. Available at: https://www.chp.gov.hk/en/features/100764.html.

Fair, R. J. and Tor, Y. (2014). Antibiotics and bacterial resistance in the 21st century. *Perspect Med Chem* 6(6) 25–64.

Hales, S., Wet, N. D., Maindonald, J., and Woodward, A. (2002). Potential effect of population and climate changes on global distribution of dengue fever: An empirical model. *Lancet 360*(9336) 830–4.

Henderson, R. (2016). Methicillin-resistant *Staphylococcus aureus*. Available at: https://patient.info/doctor/methicillin-resistant-staphylococcus-aureus-mrsa.

John, T. J. and Samuel R. (2000). Herd immunity and herd effect: New insights and definitions. *Eur J Epidemiol 16*(7) 601–6.

Lee, S. S. (2012). *Public Health in Infectious Disease*. Hong Kong: Stanley Ho Centre for Emerging Infectious Diseases, The Chinese University of Hong Kong.

Mausner, J. S. and Kramer, S. (1985). *Epidemiology: An Introductory Text*. Philadelphia, PA: WB Saunders Company.

McEwen, S. A. and Collignon, P. J. (2018). Antimicrobial resistance: A One Health perspective. *Microbiology Spectrum 6*(2). doi: 10.1128/microbiolspec.ARBA-0009-2017.

Médecins Sans Frontières (2016). Ebola: 2014–2015 facts & figures. Available at: http://www.msf.org/sites/msf.org/files/ebola_accountability_report_low_res.pdf.

National Institutes of Health (2012). Emerging and re-emerging infectious diseases. Available at: https://science.education.nih.gov/supplements/nih_diseases.pdf.

Stefani, S., Chung, D. R., Lindsay, J. A., Friedrich, A. W., Keams, A. M., et al. (2012). Methicillin-resistant *Staphylococcus aureus* (MRSA): Global epidemiology and harmonisation of typing methods. *Int J Antimicrob Ag 39*(4) 273–82. doi: 10.1016/j.ijantimicag.2011.09.030.

United Nations (n.d.). Goal 3: Ensure healthy lives and promote well-being for all at all ages. Available at: http://www.un.org/sustainabledevelopment/health/.

World Health Organization (n.d.-a). Health in the SDG era [infographic]. Available at: http://www.who.int/topics/sustainable-development-goals/test/sdg-banner.jpg?ua=1.

World Health Organization (n.d.-b). Neglected tropical diseases. Available at : http://www.who.int/neglected_diseases/diseases/en/#.

World Health Organization (n.d.-c). Partners: Global Outbreak Alert and Response Network (GOARN). Available at: http://www.who.int/csr/disease/ebola/partners/en/.

World Health Organization (2003a). Emergencies preparedness, response: Cumulative number of reported cases (SARS). Available at: http://www.who.int/csr/sarscountry/2003_03_24/en/.

World Health Organization (2003b). Emergencies preparedness, response: Summary table of SARS cases by country. Available at: http://www.who.int/csr/sars/country/2003_08_15/en/.

World Health Organization (2003c). Emergencies preparedness, response: Update 95-SARS: chronology of a serial killer. Available at: http://www.who.int/csr/don/2003_07_04/en/.

World Health Organization (2007a). International Health Regulations 2005: Area of work for implementation. Available at: http://apps.who.int/iris/bitstream/10665/69770/1/WHO_CDS_EPR_IHR_2007.1_eng.pdf?ua=1.

World Health Organization (2007b). Notification and other reporting requirements under the IHR (2005): IHR brief no.2. Available at: http://www.who.int/ihr/publications/ihr_brief_no_2_en.pdf.

World Health Organization (2010). Global status report on noncommunicable diseases 2010. Available at: http://www.who.int/nmh/publications/ncd_report_full_en.pdf.

World Health Organization (2011). Global plan for artemisinin resistant containment (GPARC). Available at: https://apps.who.int/iris/bitstream/handle/10665/44482/9789241500838_eng.pdf;jsessionid=ACB921EE921A8FD628EE67EF4A4E94EC?sequence=1.

World Health Organization (2013). Vaccine safety basics: More about conjugate vaccine [e-learning course]. Available at: http://vaccine-safety-training.org/about-conjugate-vaccines.html.

World Health Organization (2014). Infection prevention and control of epidemic- and pandemic-prone acute respiratory infections in health care: WHO guidelines. Available at: http://apps.who.int/iris/bitstream/handle/10665/112656/9789241507134_eng.pdf?sequence=1.

World Health Organization (29 August 2014). WHO: Ebola response roadmap situation report 1. Available at: http://apps.who.int/iris/bitstream/handle/10665/131974/roadmapsitrep1_eng.pdf?sequence=1.

World Health Organization (2015a). Global action plan on antimicrobial resistance. Available at: http://www.wpro.who.int/entity/drug_resistance/resources/global_action_plan_eng.pdf.

World Health Organization (2015b). Health in 2015: From MDGs to SDGs. Available at: http://apps.who.int/iris/bitstream/handle/10665/200009/9789241565110_eng.pdf;jsessionid=DB5C96205449EDB8309FDB0CA9114154?sequence=1.

World Health Organization (August 2015). WHO Secretariat response to the report of the Ebola Interim Assessment Panel. Available at: http://www.who.int/csr/resources/publications/ebola/who-response-to-ebola-report.pdf?ua=1.

World Health Organization (2016a). International Health Regulations (2005) (3rd edn). Available at: http://apps.who.int/iris/bitstream/10665/246107/1/9789241580496-eng.pdf?ua=1.

World Health Organization (2016b). Second report of the advisory group on reform of WHO's work in outbreaks and emergencies. Available at: http://www.who.int/about/who_reform/emergency-capacities/advisory-group/second-report.pdf?ua=1.

World Health Organization (10 June 2016). Situation report: Ebola virus disease. Available at: http://apps.who.int/iris/bitstream/10665/208883/1/ebolasitrep_10Jun2016_eng.pdf?ua=1.

World Health Organization (2018). Table 1: Summary of WHO positions papers – Recommendations for routine immunization. Available at: https://www.who.int/immunization/policy/Immunization_routine_table1.pdf?ua=1.

World Health Organization (30 March 2018). Influenza (seasonal): Ask the expert: Influenza Q & A. Available at: http://www.who.int/en/news-room/fact-sheets/detail/influenza-(seasonal).

World Health Organization (11 June 2018). Malaria. Available at: http://www.who.int/en/news-room/fact-sheets/detail/malaria.

World Health Organization (19 July 2018). HIV/AIDS. Available at: http://www.who.int/en/news-room/fact-sheets/detail/hiv-aids.

World Health Organization (20 July 2018). Zika virus. Available at: https://www.who.int/news-room/fact-sheets/detail/zika-virus.

World Health Organization (18 September 2018). Tuberculosis. Available at: http://www.who.int/en/news-room/fact-sheets/detail/tuberculosis.

World Health Organization Regional Office for South-East Asia (2013). Measles elimination by 2020. Available at: http://www.searo.who.int/mediacentre/releases/2013/pr1565/en/.

WorldWide Antimalarial Resistance Network (WWARN) (n.d.). Available at: https://www.wwarn.org.

Chapter 6

Environmental Health

Human health is closely linked to natural environments and behavioural and policy context. Environmental health is the branch of public health that focuses on the interrelationships between people and their environment, promotes human health and well-being, and fosters healthy and safe communities. Environmental threats to health require rapid and urgent action to protect the environment for both present and future generations. This chapter describes key concepts in environmental health.

Environment and health

Many aspects of human health are affected by the environment, with approximately 23% of global deaths are related to modifiable environmental factors (Prüss-Üstün, Wolf, Corvalán, Bos, and Neira, 2016). Ambient and indoor air quality and water, sanitation, and hygiene are all important issues. Environmental factors cause common diseases such as cardiovascular diseases, diarrhoeal diseases, and lower respiratory infections. Environmental risks can play different roles in the occurrence, development, treatment, and rehabilitation of many diseases. The interaction between humans and the environment is an important part of public health and medical research (Moeller, 2005). Changing environmental factors and contexts may reduce disease risks.

According to the World Health Organization (WHO): environmental health

> addresses all the physical, chemical, and biological factors external to a person, and all the related factors impacting behaviours. It encompasses the assessment and control of those environmental factors that can potentially affect health. It is targeted towards preventing disease and creating health-supportive environments. This definition excludes behaviour not related to environment, as well as behaviour related to the social and cultural environment, as well as genetics. (WHO, n.d.-a)

Environmental stewardship refers to protection of the environment. This is to prevent environmental degradation and its resulting impacts on health.

Environment and its influence on human health and well-being are associated with human activities (Martens and McMichael, 2009). Diseases and health are products of a combination of environmental factors, many of which are influenced by individual behaviours and lifestyles. **Environmental health** is a branch of public health that focuses on how environmental factors may be associated with human health and what can be done to prevent or minimize the negative impacts.

Essentials for Health Protection. Emily Ying Yang Chan, Oxford University Press (2020).
© Oxford University Press
DOI: 10.1093/oso/9780198835479.001.0001

Exposure, hazard, and risk

Exposure, hazard, and risk are important concepts for understanding the dynamics of environmental health (see Chapters 2–5 for other related concepts). **Exposure** is any direct contact between an individual and a substance, whether by contacting, touching, inhaling, or swallowing the substance from a source. While *exposure* happens outside the physical body (or at the interface between the environment containing the hazard substance and the human body), *dose* refers to the amount of hazardous substance absorbed into or inside the body. As it is difficult to measure the dose, the magnitude, frequency, and duration of exposure are often used as proxiese and these two terms are often used interchangeably. A **hazard** is a source of danger and a **risk** is the quantitative probability that a health effect will occur after an individual has been exposed to a specified amount of a hazard. *Acute toxicity* is the adverse effects (including death) observed within a short time of exposure to a hazardous substance while *chronic toxicity* is the adverse effects observed following repeated exposure to a substance. People are constantly exposed to a range of environmental health hazards, such as flu viruses, ultraviolet rays from the sun, and various chemicals. Once the hazard enters the human body (e.g. through ingestion, dermal absorption, and inhalation), the individual will experience the potential impact of such hazard (University of Washington, 2005). When the dose of that hazard exceeds the limit that the human body can manage or eliminate, it becomes 'toxic' and may cause harm to the human body.

Relationship between human health and environment

The relationship between human health and the environment is complex and subject to multiple modifications. Although exposure to environmental hazards can be the direct cause of adverse health effects, frequently, exposure to environmental health risks may involve various simultaneous chains of events and thus human health and disease outcomes vary with hazard exposure.

Causal chain

The primary concern in environmental health is to identify the relationships between environment (as a source of exposure to hazards or access to resources) and human health. These relationships comprise causes and effects and typically involve multiple linkages and associations. They are best represented, therefore, in the form of a causal chain or web (also known as the 'full impact chain'), which shows the links between sources and impacts, via a series of steps. The concept of causal chain is fundamental to integrated environmental health impact assessment (IEHIA), and one of its defining principles (Integrated Environmental Health Impact Assessment System, n.d.-a). There are multiple ways to conceptualize or depict causal relationships. A simple causal chain for pollution-based hazards may be represented in the following way:

> Sources → releases → environmental concentrations → human exposure and intake → health effects → physiological impacts

Framework for linkages in health, environment, and development

Population growth, economic development, and technological advancement are all **driving forces** for the development of human society, but these driving forces may exert a huge **pressure** on the environment. High density living, uncontrolled emission, and excessive industrial development are examples of forces that change the **state** of the environment, which will result in problems such as air, soil, and water pollution, thereby posing serious environmental hazards. If humans are **exposed** to these environmental hazards, they are at risk of developing single or multiple adverse health implications. The extent of these effects will be associated with the toxicity of the hazard and the dose to which individuals are exposed. Understanding the links between development, the environment, and human health thus help assess risks and establish and implement appropriate measures or **actions** to prevent and control the adverse health effects of environmental hazards (von Schirnding, 2002).

Conceptual frameworks have been developed with the aim to summarize the relationships between environment and health. They help identify and select appropriate environmental health indicators for monitoring, build research studies, and guide policy planning. The WHO developed the DPSEEA (driving forces, pressures, state, exposures, health effects, and actions) framework for environmental health indicator identification. It hypothesizes that health impact as originating from driving forces (D) (e.g. population growth, economic development, and technology advancement), which exert pressures (P) on the environment in the forms of production, consumption, waste generation, etc., and their releases into the environment. These external factors lead to changes in the state (S) of the environment, (e.g. in the forms of environmental pollution and increased risks of natural hazards). Exposure (E) occurs when humans come into contact with these hazards, resulting in potential health effect (E). Actions (A) like policies, implementations, awareness raising, and treatment targeting at different points in the casual chain are taken to mitigate adverse health effects. Although later-stage interventions that reduce exposures or mitigate the health impacts may appear to be more effective and sometimes cheaper because they can target more directly at specific population groups and health outcomes, preventive measures often have the major overall advantages as they prevent and mitigate problems at source and may often offer other environmental and social benefits if implemented effectively (see Figure 6.1).

At-risk community

Economically underdeveloped areas are exposed to a greater burden of disease than the developed world. Major environmental hazards in under-developed areas affect health and well-being. Poor quality in air and water, suboptimal food safety and sanitation standard are typical causes for diseases that affect extremes of age (Smith, Corvalan, and Kjellstorm, 1999) (see also Figure 6.2). Globally, children under the age of five are most affected by environmental hazards (WHO, n.d.-b).

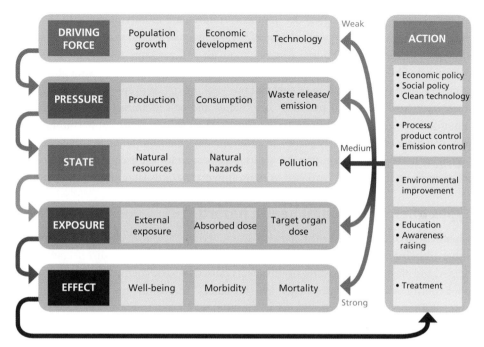

Figure 6.1 The DPSEEA Framework

Source: Adapted from Integrated Environmental Health Impact Assessment System (n.d.-b), Open Access.

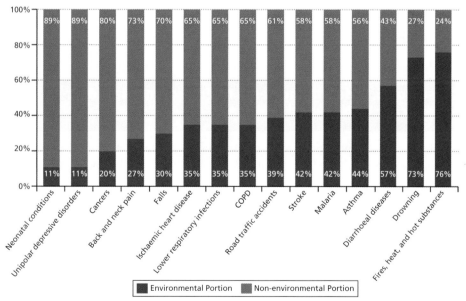

Figure 6.2 Diseases with the strongest environmental contributions globally in 2012

Reproduced with permission from Prüss-Üstün, A., et al. (2016). Preventing disease through healthy environments: A global assessment of the burden of disease from environmental risks. Copyright © 2016 WHO. Available at: <https://apps.who.int/iris/bitstream/handle/10665/204585/9789241565196_eng.pdf?sequence=1>

Due to stages of physiological development, children are more vulnerable to environmental health hazards than adults (Bearer, 1995) and are at greater risk when exposed to environmental hazards. Children respirate more air and consume more water and food per pound of body weight than adults. They are more likely to engage in suboptimal hygiene practices (e.g. defecating openly and not washing hands properly), play around in unsanitary conditions, and put their dirty hands and/or contaminated objects in their mouths. Their immature immune systems may not be able to get rid of harmful organisms that enter or invade their bodies. In addition, many environmental health conditions take years to develop and children have a longer life span for these conditions to develop when compared with adults exposed to environmental hazards later in life (CDC, 2017c).

Types of environmental health hazard

Chemical environmental health hazards are caused by hazardous chemicals that can be either entirely natural (such as lead and mercury) or synthetic (such as disinfectants, pesticides, and plastics). The adverse health effects caused by toxic chemicals often arise from poor control or improper use of chemical substances. Therefore, improving the management and monitoring of toxic chemical utilization is the key to prevent and control the health risks of chemical environmental health hazards (see Case Box 6.1).

Biological environmental health hazards generally refer to microorganisms, such as bacteria, viruses, and parasites, that may cause harm to human health (Schweihofer and Wells, 2013). When humans are exposed, these disease-causing microorganisms infect humans via various modes of transmission. For example, areas with intense biological environmental health hazards (e.g. vectors) are often at high risk of infectious diseases (see Case Box 6.2).

Case Box 6.1 Health Incidents of Environmental Toxic Chemicals: USA (1940s) and Japan

A photochemical smog appeared in Los Angeles, the United States in the summer of 1943. The culprit was the large volume of vehicle exhaust gas. When chemical compounds in the exhaust gas reacted under the influence of sunlight, a toxic, coloured haze was formed. Many Los Angeles residents were reported to suffer from clinical symptoms such as red eyes and headache.

In the 1950s and 1960s, mines in Toyama Prefecture, Japan, discharged wastewater during mining. As a result, heavy metal cadmium in the wastewater was accumulated in rivers. Local population in the prefecture suffered from cadmium poisoning due to long-term drinking of contaminated river water and consumption of cadmium-containing food. In addition to poisoning, some reported skeletal deformity and susceptibility to premature fractures and permanent physical handicaps (Nishijo, Nakagawa, Suwazono, Nogawa, and Kido, 2017).

Case Box 6.2 Dengue Fever

The breeding speed and activity of mosquitoes increase in specific temperature range and humanity. The gradually warming climate widens the geographic distribution of areas that are suitable for mosquito growth and expands the prevalence of diseases such as dengue fever, Japanese encephalitis, Zika virus infection, and other mosquito-borne diseases. In areas with both high densities of vector (i.e. mosquito) and human populations, a small number of people infected may be enough to transmit major vector-borne diseases (e.g. dengue fever) among the human population (see also Figure 6.3).

Physical environmental health hazards refer to physical elements, phenomena, or processes in the environment that may cause damage to human health, including damage caused by physical factors such as noise, radiation, fire, electricity, and machinery (see Case Box 6.3).

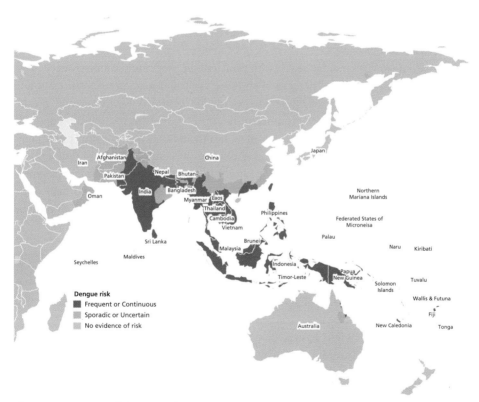

Figure 6.3 Dengue risk in Asia and Oceania

Adapted with permission from Centers for Disease Control and Prevention. (2017b). CDC Yellow Book 2018: Health information for international travel. New York, NY: Oxford University Press. Copyright © 2018 OUP.

Case Box 6.3 Tianjin Industrial Accident in 2015

Multiple warehouses exploded simultaneously on 12 August 2015 in Tianjin, a major port city in North China near Beijing. The incident caused 158 deaths and 698 hospital admissions, injured hundreds more, and devastated large areas (Chan, Wang, Mark, and Liu, 2015; Mcgarry, Balsari, Muqueeth, and Leaning, 2017). The fires caused by the explosions were finally put out after 72 hours. Since the warehouse contained hazardous and flammable chemicals, long-term environmental hazards in the air, soil, and water may affect the health of nearby residents for years to come.

Social environmental health hazards are potential health risks caused by social factors such as living context (e.g. suboptimal infrastructure support), socioeconomic status (e.g. poverty and low education level), and behavioural habits (e.g. smoking and alcohol addiction). In general, people living in poorer and less developed areas are more likely to be exposed to social environmental hazards in the living and working environment than their counterparts who live in wealthy developed areas (Kjellén, 2001). Associations and hypotheses have been developed to explain how social determinants may influence environmental hazards and context that may be linked to poor human health outcomes (see Knowledge Box 6.1).

Safeguarding environmental health with policies and programmes may reduce chemical and other environmental hazards in air, water, soil, and food, protect residents, and provide communities with healthier environments (National Environmental Health Association, 2016). Tracking environmental hazard exposures in communities and potential links with disease outcomes can protect health and well-being of susceptible communities. In a healthy community, homes should be safe, affordable, and healthy places for families to gather. Workplaces, schools, and childcare centres should be free of exposures that negatively affect the health of workers or children. Nutritious, affordable food should be safe for all community members. Access to safe and affordable multimodal

---

Knowledge Box 6.1 Socio-Economic Status and Health

The link between socio-economic status and unhealthy behaviours (such as smoking, alcoholism, and lack of exercise) has been extensively studied in the fields of sociology and public health (Pample, Krueger, and Denney, 2010). Research study results have shown that poor and uneducated people are more likely to fall ill than wealthy and highly educated people. Lack of financial sources to ensure safe access to essential materials for well-being (e.g. water, air, and food), the unavailability of health information, and accumulation of unhealthy behaviour over time can eventually lead to chronic diseases or even premature death.

transportation options, including cycling and public transit, improves the environment and drives down obesity and other chronic illnesses. Outdoor and indoor air quality should be clean and safe to breathe. Children and adults alike should have access to safe and clean public spaces such as parks. Community should engage in emergency preparedness and have the tools and resources to be resilient against physical (infrastructure and human) and emotional damage. All these environmental health protection activities require participation of and collaboration among national, state/provincial, and local governments and civil society.

Impacts of environmental health hazards

Environmental health addresses all human health-related aspects of the natural environment and the built environment that may pose health risks to a population. It concerns air quality (including both ambient outdoor air and indoor air quality, which also comprises concerns about environmental tobacco smoke), water and sanitation, biosafety (chemicals, radiation), noise, occupational risks, agricultural and food practices, built environment, and climate change and its effects on health. The following sections will discuss health hazards that are associated with water and sanitation, air, living environment, food, toxic chemicals and waste, and energy.

Water

Water is essential for sustaining life and supporting good health. Safe drinking water, water access for personal hygiene and food preparation, and stagnant puddles of water outdoors are water-related issues that may affect human health (Chan and Ho, 2019). Inadequate or insufficient water quantity might lead to water-borne and water-washed (or hygiene contact-based) diseases (see Knowledge Box 6.2). It has been estimated that one human being requires 15 litres per day to fulfill basic personal and food hygiene needs (WHO, 2003; Sphere, 2018) and 50 litres per person per day for domestic purposes (United Nations Development Programme [UNDP], 2006).

However, access to water is not equal to all globally. Water stress and scarcity are a living reality for more than 2 billion people and this pattern is likely to remain with population growth and increase in global water usage (United Nations World Water Assessment Programme, 2015). Conservation and maintenance of water resources in urban areas is a major challenge for urban well-being. Historically, early civilizations were built in locations where there was access to water bodies and the cities flourished with stable access to the basic requirements for health, namely clean water and sanitation, food and nutrition, shelter and clothing, health services, and information (Bolton and Burkle, 2013). In modern world, although many major cities are still located along rivers, people have changed from direct usage of the water body to system-based dependency (Shaw and Thaitakoo, 2010) as urban populations have increased and technology has been improved. According to the WHO, in the twenty-first century, approximately one-third of the world's population live in countries with moderate to high water stress, with 2.1

Knowledge Box 6.2 Public Health Framework for Understanding Water

A safe, reliable, affordable, and easily accessible water supply is essential to sustain health and well-being of population. The WHO *Guidelines for Drinking-Water Quality* (WHO, 2017a) suggests a public health framework for assessing the adequacy of drinking-water supply in an area/context, which includes the following parameters:

Quality: The presence of regularly verified quality of water supply and water safety plan, with demonstrated compliance with regulations during periodic audits;

Quantity: The proportion of population with access to different levels of drinking-water supply (e.g. no, basic, intermediate, and optimal access) as a surrogate for health impacts in relation to the quantity of water used;

Reliability: The percentage of time in a given period during which drinking water is available;

Accessibility: The percentage of population with reasonable access to an improved drinking-water supply; and

Affordability: The cost of the water measured by the percentagae of income paid by domestic consumers as tariff.

billion people lacking access to safely managed drinking water services and 4.5 billion people lacking access to safely managed sanitation services (WHO and UNICEF, 2017).

In addition, water quality matters to protect health. **Biological** contamination (e.g. with pathogens such as microbes through faecal materials; see Chapter 5), **chemical** contamination (as a result of human activity), and **physical** contamination (e.g. taste, colour, and smell) may all compromise water quality and render water sources hazardous to consumption and well-being. Thus, water safety and quality are fundamental needs for healthy human development and well-being.

Ensuring access to safe water is one of the most effective instruments in promoting public health and reducing poverty. The WHO leads global efforts to prevent transmission of water-borne diseases by promoting health-based regulations to governments and working with partners to promote effective risk management practices to water suppliers, communities, and households (WHO, 2018b).

In addition, health implications of water pollution is not limited to drinking water sources. Non-drinking water, which is water that may not be used for drinking or food preparation, may affect plant and algae growth, and can reduce oxygen levels and harm aquatic life if polluted. Pollution may occur when gasoline, oil, road salts, or chemicals (e.g. lead) are leached into water from the soil (see Knowledge Box 6.3). The majority of the world's wastewater (80%) is dumped, mostly untreated, back into the environment, polluting rivers, lakes, and oceans (Denchak, 2018). Moreover, inadequate sanitation,

Knowledge Box 6.3 Lead Poisoning

Lead is a naturally occurring metal used to make common products like batteries and pipes. While it has beneficial uses, lead can be toxic. Generally, people can be exposed to lead by breathing contaminated air or dust, drinking contaminated water, or eating contaminated food. Children and pregnant women are at risk. Exposure to lead is particularly harmful to children because their bodies are still developing. Behaviours like putting hands and objects in their mouths leave infants and small children at increased risk of lead exposure. Children can be exposed by eating paint chips containing lead or eating contaminated soil. Lead can cross the placenta to the foetus and be passed through breast milk. Health risks of lead exposure to children and adults include slowed growth, lower IQ, learning difficulties, anaemia, reproductive problems, cardiovascular effects, and reduced kidney function.

To reduce potential exposure to lead, it is advisable to keep products containing lead out of the hands and mouths of children, wash children's hands and toys regularly, mop floors and wet-wipe window sills in routines (i.e. every 2–3 weeks), and to prevent or reduce access to lead-based paint that is peeling. Adults are most often exposed by work activities and hobbies (including rehabbing older homes, gardening in contaminated soil and making stained glass), or consuming food or water contaminated by lead.

Lead can contaminate drinking water via plumbing systems including the pipes and fixtures in people's homes, schools, and workplaces. Exposure risk is higher in older homes with corrosion of these pipes and fixtures that may allow lead to leach into the drinking water. In addition, the estimated economic benefit of reduced lead exposure for each year's cohort of 3.8 million 2-year-old children in the United States was estimated to be ranging from US$110 billion to US$319 billion.

Sources: Environmental Protection Agency (EPA, 2018a); Grosse, Matte, Schwartz, and Jackson (2002).

such as improper disposal of municipal sewage system and septic tank contents, or open defecation can easily contaminate this water.

To improve water and to safeguard health, there are four major categories of interventions, which target water supply, water quality, hygiene, and sanitation. Good indicators are also needed to monitor water to protect public health (Chan and Ho, 2019). For example, research is needed for the identification of appropriate microbial reference pathogens used to monitor water quality and reduce waterborne disease outbreaks, as the possible options are restricted by limited data on dose–response relationships of these pathogens.

Impact of climate change on water-related health risks, such as vector-borne diseases, constitutes another area where attention must be placed and further research is needed. As water is a multi-sectoral issue, tackling water and health issues requires a collaborative multi-sectoral approach. In urban areas, high population density, travel patterns, demographics and land use all contribute to a population's water-related health risk. As this health risk is constantly evolving, continuous monitoring, evaluation, and update of reference pathogens for each urban community should be conducted. Monitoring also incorporates the management and maintenance of the water supply system and its operations. Preventive and adaptive planning of the water supply system is needed to address increasingly stressed water sources, risks of disaster incidents, and impact of climate change as well as to ensure a low-cost and sustainable water management mechanism.

Sanitation

While water is essential for life, health, and human dignity and clean water is needed for drinking, cooking, and brushing teeth, **sanitation** is defined as the provision of facilities for safe disposal of human excreta (WHO, 2018a). Safe sanitation prevents infection and improves/maintains mental and social well-being. Hygiene promotion is a planned, systematic approach to enable people to take action to prevent and/or mitigate water-, sanitation-, and hygiene-related diseases (Sphere Project, 2011). Water, sanitation, and hygiene (WASH) initiatives aim to promote good personal and environmental hygiene in order to protect health.

Good hygiene practices are one of the most effective ways to reduce the spread of diseases (Boyce, Pittet, Healthcare Infection Control Practices Advisory Committee, and HICPAC/SHEA/APIC/IDSA Hand Hygiene Task Force, 2002). Although good personal hygiene practices, including bathing, washing clothing, washing hands, and using a toilet, are simple behavioural measures to protect health, there are major disparities of knowledge and attitude of hygiene practices across the world. In some developing areas, even with awareness, the lack of access to safe water, cleansing materials, and washing facilities may hamper the efforts to promote good hygiene practices. If water is not readily available, personal hygiene often is one of the first things to be surrendered (WHO, 2018b).

Well-organized sanitation system and safe wastewater treatment and reuse are also fundamental to protect public health. Global efforts are called to monitor the global burden of sanitation-related disease and access to safely managed sanitation and safely treated wastewater under the Sustainable Development Goals (SDGs) agenda. Factors that enable or hinder progress towards these targets should also be monitored. Implementation is supported by promoting risk assessment and management in normative guidelines and tools and collaborates among sectors in health initiatives such as: neglected tropical diseases; nutrition; infection prevention and control; and antimicrobial resistance to maximize health benefits of sanitation interventions (WHO, 2018a).

A safe sanitation system separates human excreta from human contacts at all steps of the sanitation process from toilet capture to containment through emptying, transport, treatment, and final disposal, as shown in Table 6.1 and Figure 6.4. Even with good water supply and quality control, sanitation and waste management are important dimensions

Table 6.1 Unsafe Sanitation and Service and the Health Risks

Unsafe toilet	Containment	Conveyance	Treatment	End use
Open defecation, inconsistent toilet use and poorly constructed pit toilets potentially causing faecal discharge into fields and providing vector breeding ground.	Poorly-constructed latrine pits or septic tanks causing leakage into groundwater and contamination of water sources.	Direct dumping into water bodies, drains, fields, groundwater, and open surfaces.	Insufficient pathogen removal from faecal sludge discharged into fields through fertilization or water bodies throughout runoff.	Discharge of untreated faecal sludge into environment causing pollution and disease risks.

to be addressed in order to protect community well-being. Inadequate **sanitation** and waste management practices can expose humans and animals to environmental health risks and cause diseases or even death in extreme contexts. Although most of the modern urban contexts have basic sanitation systems, disparity in urban infrastructure (such as poor infrastructure in slum areas) might provide only suboptimal sanitation standards. In informal settlements, pathogens associated with human biological waste (e.g. faeces) may contaminate water, food, and hands (WHO, 2018a). Ground and surface water pollution in developing contexts may further exacerbate poor sanitation.

An unsafe sanitation system includes open defecation or inconsistent use of a toilet, unsafe containment where septic tanks can overflow, unsafe transportation to a treatment facility, unsafe site treatment, or unsafe disposal, such as into a water body. The unsafe sanitation hazards can lead to hazardous events and disease exposure, as illustrated in Figure 6.4.

Disease outcome

Unsafe sanitation generates many health risks and poor health outcomes (see Table 6.2). Water-borne diseases are caused by bacteria or chemicals in water that can result in diarrhoea, fever, and vomiting. Diarrhoea is the leading cause of disease and death in children under 5 in low- and middle-income countries from unsafe WASH. The WHO (2018b) states that lack of access to safe WASH is estimated to cause 842,000 diarrhoeal deaths each year. In the absence of safe WASH, flies land on or breed in exposed human faeces, transporting faecal matter and pathogens to surfaces, food, and people, increasing the number of insect vector-borne diseases. Helminth-related infection typically transmits through human faeces and contaminated soil, crops, and water. Affected children may suffer from stunting, low birthweight, impaired cognitive function, pneumonia, and anaemia. In addition, unsafe access to WASH may cause anxiety, violence, and assault (see Knowledge Box 6.4). Clean water and improved sanitation may result in a 10% reduction of diarrhoeal illness (Prüss-Üstün, Bos, Gore, and Bartram, 2008).

Human host

Faeces/Urine

Sanitation hazards

Unsafe Toilet	**Containment**	**Conveyance**	**Treatment**	**End Use**
Open defecation, inconsistent use, or poorly constructed pit toilets causing discharge into fields	*Poorly-constructed latrine pits or septic tanks causing leakage into groundwater*	*Untreated excreta discharged into water bodies, drains, fields, groundwater, and open surfaces*	*Insufficient pathogen removal from faecal sludge discharged into fields through fertilization or water bodies throughout runoff*	*Discharge of untreated faecal sludge into environment*

Hazardous events

Files Water bodies/drains Fields Ground Water

Exposure

 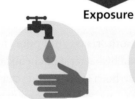 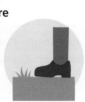

Crops/Food Water consumption/use Feet/skin Objects/Floors/surfaces

Figure 6.4 The health impact of unsafe sanitation

Reproduced with permission from World Health Organization World Health Organization. (2018). Guidelines on sanitation and health. Copyright © 2018 WHO. Available at: <http://apps.who.int/iris/bitstream/handle/10665/274939/9789241514705-eng.pdf?ua=1>

Table 6.2 The Direct Impacts of Unsafe Sanitation: Examples of Common Infections

Faecal-oral infections	**Helminth infections**	**Insect vector diseases**
– Diarrhoea	Hookworm	Dengue
– Cholera	Round worms	Japanese encephalitis
– Dysenteries	Schistosomiasis	

Source: (WHO, 2018a).

Knowledge Box 6.4 WASH, Sexual Assault, and Anxiety

The lack of safe access to WASH can have many adverse impacct on well-being. The task of collecting safe water often falls on women and children, causing them to have to walk long distances every day. Time and energy required for water collection may lead to the loss of other opportunities such as education or other employment. Less education can lead to fewer job opportunities and predispose people to a lower likelihood of economic success, furthering the poverty cycle (United Nations Population Fund, 2003). In addition, there is a greater risk of being sexually assaulted or exposed to violence and animal attack when traveling long distances to access WASH(WaterAid, The Water Supply and Sanitation Collaborative Council, and Domestos, 2013). Anxiety is found to be associated with unsafe sanitation from shame and embarrassment from open defecation and shared sanitation.

Waste management

Waste is generated every day by household, commercial, and industrial sectors. Although the definition of waste (material, substances, or product) might vary with judgement, culture, sources, and policy, waste is typically classified in the modern world by rules and regulations set up by government and authorities to facilitate its management. Waste might include, but not limited to: municipal solid waste, food waste, construction waste, chemical waste, clinical waste, waste cooking oils, and special wastes (see Figure 6.5). Typically, domestic and industrial wastes are the two main types of waste that are managed proactively by institutions and authorities.

Globally, the mining and construction industry produces the greatest quantity of waste by weight and high-income countries produce more waste per capita then low- or middle-income countries (Schrör, 2011). Composition of waste varies by region and organic waste is found to be of a larger proportion in the Pacific Region than in OECD (Organisation for Economic Co-operation and Development) countries. However, with economic and technology development, changes in practices and production patterns are likely to increase overall waste generation in the decades to come (UN-HABITAT, 2010).

Waste production affects environment, human health, and quality of life. Poorly managed waste can increase infectious disease risk as well as lead to contamination of drinking water and soil, emissions of air pollutants from incinerators, food contamination from waste chemicals, and gas migration and leachate discharges from a landfill. In addition, there is only a finite amount of land to use as landfills. Two most common methods of waste disposal are landfills and incinerators. Landfills compress solid waste with soil. Incinerators burn solid waste under controlled conditions to break down materials. Proper waste management can decrease the adverse impact of waste on human health and the environment.

Municipal Solid Waste	Municipal solid waste consists of plastic waste, paper waste, tins and metals, and ceramics and glass—all solid waste from household, commercial, and industrial sources.
Food Waste	Food waste is composed of waste produced during all processes of food production, processing, wholesale, resale, preparation, and disposal. Food is highly degradable, causing odour and hygiene problems.
Construction Waste	Construction waste results from construction, renovation, demolition, land excavation, and road works.
Chemical Waste	Chemical waste often poses a potential threat to public health and the environment. Chemical waste can be hazardous and explosive, corrosive, flammable, poisonous, or toxic. Chemical waste is often the by-products of manufacturing processes, discarded used materials or commercial products.
Clinical Waste	Clinical waste is generated from healthcare, laboratory, and research practices. Some healthcare waste is hazardous material that is infectious, toxic, or radioactive. Open burning and incineration of healthcare waste can result in the emissions of dioxins, furans, and particulate matter.
Waste Cooking Oils	Waste cooking oils are abandoned oils from any cooking process for human consumption.
Special Waste	Special waste includes animal carcasses, livestock waste, radioactive waste, grease trap waste, sewage sludge, and waterworks sludge.

Figure 6.5 Classification of waste

Source: Data from Environmental Protection Department of the Government of the Hong Kong Special Administrative Region. (n.d.-b). Waste. Available at: <https://www.epd.gov.hk/epd/english/environmentinhk/waste/waste_maincontent.html>

Plastic pollution

Plastic has been generated at an alarmingly increasing rate since the 1940s due to its versatile, cost-effective benefits such as easy sterilization, light weight, durability, and rapid disposability. However, as plastic is made to last long, such quality also creates major implications for health, environment, and sustainability (North and Halden, 2013). As plastic is not biodegradable and can only break down into smaller pieces, plastic pollution harms the environment, ocean, animal, and human health. Plastic ends up in the ocean, whether in its whole forms or smaller pieces, and will affect ocean lives. Plastic leaches toxic chemicals into groundwater, lakes, and rivers, attracting other toxins, and disrupting animal habitats (Hopewell, Dvorak, and Kosior, 2009). Animals can also get caught or entrapped in plastic, which leads to impaired movement and feeding, reduced

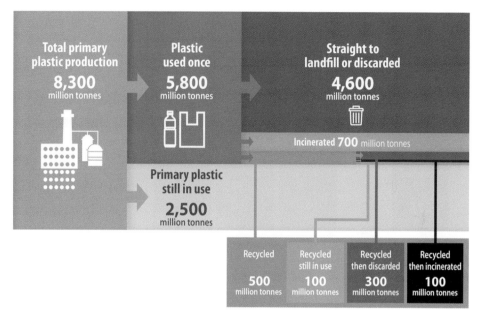

Figure 6.6 Global plastic production and its fate, 1950–2015
Reprinted with permission of AAAS from Geyer, Jambeck, Law Sci. Adv. 2017;3: e1700782. © The Authors, some rights reserved; exclusive licensee American Association for the Advancement of Science. Distributed under a Creative Commons Attribution NonCommercial License 4.0 (CC BY-NC) <http://creativecommons.org/licenses/by-nc/4.0/>

reproductive output, and death. Animals can mistake plastic for food and feed it to their young, who may choke to death on it (Thompson, Moore, vom Saal, and Swan, 2009). If marine animals consume plastic, they absorb their hazardous chemicals, displacing nutritious algae, also raising the risk of death. Plastic can then pass through the food chain, as other animals, such as humans, eat the contaminated fish and plankton. The exposure can then cause effects on human health as well (Andrady, 2011). Chemicals from plastics are detected in the blood and tissues of nearly all humans. Plastic can contain toxic chemicals like lead, cadmium, and mercury. Exposure to plastic in people's blood and tissue leads to cancer, birth defects, impaired immunity, endocrine disruption, etc. (Plastic Pollution Coalition, 2018). With the current trend in plastic waste production, it was estimated that oceans would contain more plastic than fish by weight by 2050 (Ellen MacArthur Foundation, World Economic Forum, and McKinsey Center for Business and Environment, 2016) (see Figure 6.7).

Recycling of plastic, whilst a good idea in theory, often presents practical challenges. Most of plastic ends up in landfills, with only 9% of plastic used once recycled and 6% of total primary plastic ever produced recycled (Geyer, Jambeck, and Law, 2017) (see Figure 6.6). Sorting plastics takes time, the recycle management cost is high, and the quality of recycling product is often low. As getting rid of plastic is difficult, the most sustainable solution is to control its supply.

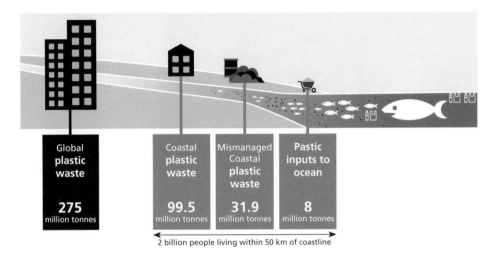

Figure 6.7 Plastic entering the world's oceans in 2010

Source: Data from Ritchie, H. and Roser, M. (2018). Plastic pollution [Online image]. Available at: <https://ourworldindata.org/plastic-pollution>

Principle of waste management

The principle of waste management may be based on the waste hierarchy that highlights the '4Rs' namely: 'reduce, reuse, recycle and refuse' (Wilson, Rodic, Modak, Soos, Rogero, et al., 2015). While the first three 'Rs' require changes in behavioural practices and systems to support the efforts (e.g. recycle systems), the last 'R', refuse, may pose environmental health challenges. Although the ideal waste management strategy aims to produce no waste at all, waste minimization is a goal that societies and communities might achieve over time rather than immediately. Reusing products can also support more efficient use of resources by saving energy, raw materials, and costs to consumers. To enable reuse products (e.g. drink and food containers), such products need to be designed and produced with materials that permit reusability. Recycling helps preserve natural resources, reduce energy consumption, and create economic activities that enable an active informal sector to flourish. In certain parts of the world, 50% of packaging might be recycled (Busby, 2016).

With the various approaches to reduce waste, one of the key paradigm shifts required is the heightening of the awareness of the environment or health cost associated with waste production for consumers. A number of waste subtypes cannot be reused and recycled and disposal is the only option to manage them. Landfills and incineration are typical approaches adopted in refuse (Busby, 2016). **Landfill** is a waste disposal approach that relies on natural decomposition, and the ability to maintain the integrity of landfill sites to avoid harmful by-products leaking into the neighbouring communities is essential to minimize harm to the community. Open dumps and poorly operated landfill sites in low-income communities often present major environmental hazards (quality of life affected through smell, sight, breeding sites for pests and diseases vectors) and evidence has been produced which associates landfill with low birth weight, congenital abnormalities, and non-specific health effects such as headaches and fatigue (Busby, 2016; Vrijheid, 2000).

Incineration might cause air pollution if not managed appropriately. The toxic gases released might be carcinogenic or tetarogenic as well as causing respiratory diseases following specific particulate exposure. It is not just nearby residents that are affected; workers in the waste management industry might also face a variety of health risks such as skin, gastrointestinal, and respiratory symptoms (Busby, 2016).

Globally, suboptimal waste management might affect living environment and contributed to the harmful effects of climate change. Health risks and impacts associated with waste include contamination of drinking water, soil, and food. Air pollution through gas emissions from combusted materials (e.g. plastic burning) and leakage of discharge from landfills as well as infectious diseases risks are common health risks associated with poor waste management. The by-product of incineration process may produce hazardous and toxic pollutants, which might be emitted to pollution levels. Acute toxicity, respiratory diseases, cancer, birth defects are some possible adverse health outcome associated with incinerators (Franchini, Rial, Buiatti, and Bianchi, 2004). Landfills may produce methane gas (CH_4); incinerators produce CO_2; and the waste management-related transportation for reuse and recycling may also incur potential environmental impact. The issue of suboptimal waste management due to lack of capacity (e.g. electronic waste) in developing countries and 'waste trafficking' (i.e. exporting hazardous waste for disposal in developing countries) reflect the issue of environmental justice, the effect of which might last for generations. Commercial and legal restrictions and environmental impact assessment when deciding on waste management practice will be two of the key areas supporting health protection in the decades to come.

Air pollution

One of the most important contributors of declining environmental health is the fine particulate matter (PM) pollution in urban air (Prüss-Üstün, Vickers, Haefliger, and Bertollini, 2011). Air pollution was found to increase premature deaths (WHO, 2018c, 2018g), hospital admissions (Chan, Goggins, Yue, and Lee, 2013), and emergency room visits due to premature death causes such as stroke, heart disease, chronic and acute lung cancer, and respiratory diseases (EPA, 2018b) (see Figure 6.8).

According to the WHO, urbanization, transportation, dust, agricultural practices, and suboptimal waste management cause outdoor air pollution (see Figure 6.9). While it is prevalent in both rural and urban areas, outdoor air pollution is usually magnified in urban areas due to the density and intensity of human activity. Outdoor air pollution is known to cause multiple health problems. Typical health outcomes include lung cancer, reduced lung function, respiratory infections, aggravated asthma, adverse birth outcomes, low birth weight, preterm birth, and small gestational age birth. New scientific evidence also shows impact on neurological development in children and can cause diabetes. Indoor (household) air pollution mainly comes from indoor smoking, waste burning, cooking, and using detergents, personal care products, kerosene and solid fuels

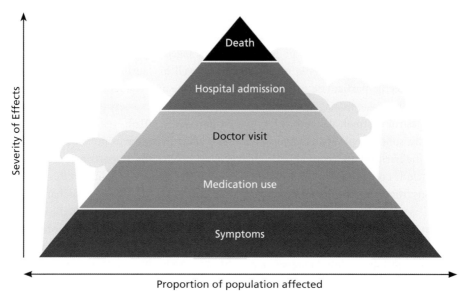

Severity of Effects

Death

Hospital admission

Doctor visit

Medication use

Symptoms

Proportion of population affected

Figure 6.8 Health outcome pyramid of air pollution

Source: Data from Environmental Protection Agency, United States. (2018b). How BenMAP-CE estimates the health and economic effects of air pollution [online]. Available at: <http//www.epa.gov/benmap/how-benmap-ce-estimates-health-and-economic-effects-air-pollution>

such as wood in polluting stoves, open fires, and lamps. Household air pollution can cause eye problems, respiratory illnesses, and cancer. Burden of disease from air pollution is already high but will continue to be in an increasing trend globally with the pace of socioeconomic development and current consumption patterns (ENVIS Centre on Control of Pollution Water, Air, Noise, 2016; WHO, 2018c) (see Figure 6.9; see also the next section).

Atmospheric pollutants

Many chemical entities can contribute towards polluting the ambient air. The air pollutants that cause the largest health implication and effect are particulate matter (PM), sulphur dioxide (SO_2), nitrogen oxides (NO_x), and ozone (O_3). The impact of these pollutants varies with cities and industries. For example, in Hong Kong, a city in southern China, the positive association between sulphur dioxide and mortality exhibited the strongest health impact on its population (Chan, Goggins, Kim, and Griffiths, 2012) (see Case Box 6.4, Table 6.3, Figures 6.10 and 6.11).

Housing environment

Indoor environments maintains optimal temperature, light, and noise level for physiological well-being and functioning. It protects dwellers from physical hazards (e.g. rain, wind, and extreme temperatures). It provides space, privacy, comfort, and security. With a significant proportion of time spend within their household, a healthy housing

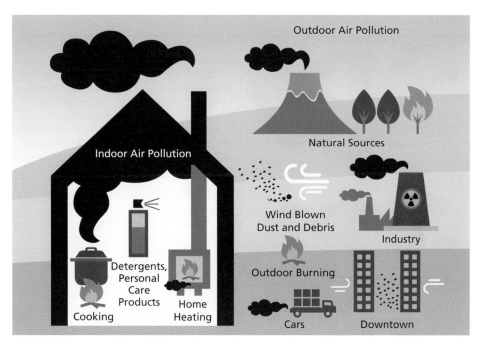

Figure 6.9 Sources of air pollution

environment may contribute to an individual's well-being. The maintenance of the indoor living environment is important for health and well-being (Milner and Hutchinson, 2016). Healthy housing also protects people from health risks such as infectious diseases. Well-thought-out building design and construction helps ensure physical safety and protects people from injury and thermal stress. However, construction materials might cause potential harm to human health (e.g. asbestos might cause lung cancer). Overcrowding, poor design, suboptimal maintenance, and informal settlements/slum development pose a potential high risk of collapse, accidents, and flooding.

Indoor air quality

As stated by the WHO (2018c), indoor/household air pollution is a major environmental health risk. By reducing indoor air pollution levels, countries can reduce stroke, heart disease, both chronic and acute lung cancer, and respiratory diseases. Every year, around 7 million deaths are due to exposure from both outdoor and household air pollution (WHO, 2018e). There are three types of indoor air quality issues:

1. Pollutants from indoor combustion of fuels: In developing countries, a significant portion of indoor air pollution comes from the burning of solid fuels for cooking, heating, and lighting, which causes allergy and respiratory and cardiovascular diseases (Gall, Carter, Earnest, and Stephens, 2013).

2. Chemical pollution: High amounts of radon also have been shown to rise through housing foundations and this can get trapped inside a house, which can lead to cancer

Table 6.3 Common Air Pollutants

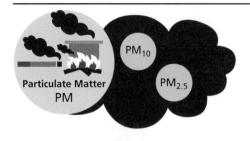	Particulate matter (PM) refers to particles such as dust, pollen, mould, organic compounds, and metals. In open air environment, PM frequently comes from dust from roads, agricultural processes, uncovered soil, or mining operations. In indoor environmental, it is mostly produced in cooking, burning, and smoking. Humans may easily inhale PM through the nose and mouth. PM is the most widely used indicator to assess the health effects from exposure to surrounding air pollution.
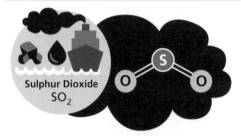	Sulphur dioxide is a gas generated by industrial activities such as power plants and fuel combustion. While invisible, it has a potent smell that can react with other substances to create harmful compounds.
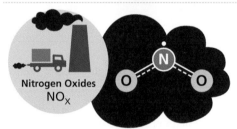	Nitrogen oxides are created from power generation, industrial, and traffic sources. These chemicals can combine with water in the air to turn into acid rain, damaging trees, crops, and buildings.
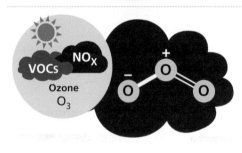	There are two types of ozone: naturally occurring ozone in the upper atmosphere and ground-level ozone. Ozone in the upper atmosphere protects life on the Earth from the sun's harmful ultraviolet rays. Ozone at the ground level is harmful to people and the environment. Ground-level ozone is created by chemical reactions between oxides of nitrogen (NO_x) and volatile organic compounds (VOC). In the environment, ozone can reduce photosynthesis, slow or harm plants' growth, contribute to loss of species diversity, and change habitat quality, water, and nutrient cycles, and variety of plants (EPA, 2018c).

Source: WHO (2018d).

(WHO, 2016a). Harmful impacts of indoor environments on human and environmental health include chemical substances such as benzene and carbon monoxide that decrease the amount of red blood cells in the human body (WHO Regional Office for Europe, 2010).

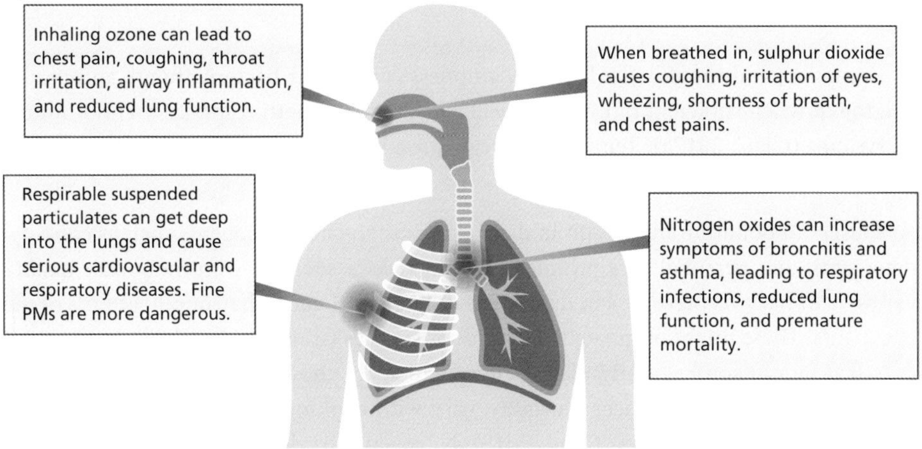

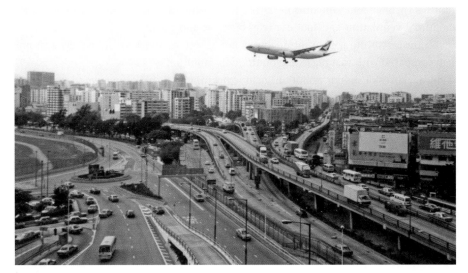

Inhaling ozone can lead to chest pain, coughing, throat irritation, airway inflammation, and reduced lung function.

When breathed in, sulphur dioxide causes coughing, irritation of eyes, wheezing, shortness of breath, and chest pains.

Respirable suspended particulates can get deep into the lungs and cause serious cardiovascular and respiratory diseases. Fine PMs are more dangerous.

Nitrogen oxides can increase symptoms of bronchitis and asthma, leading to respiratory infections, reduced lung function, and premature mortality.

Figure 6.10 Effects of air pollutants on human health

Figure 6.11 Relative sizes of particulate matters

Case Box 6.4 Air Pollution Measurement in Hong Kong

To protect human and environmental health, it is important to test and monitor the air in the places one lives and works. Hong Kong adopts two public monitoring indicators to alert people to the quality of air in the city and allow global comparison and monitoring. These include the Air Quality Index (AQI) and the Air Quality Health Index (AQHI). These indexes help monitor and guide achieving targets for WHO's Air Quality Guidelines and emission reduction targets. The AQHI is reported hourly at many stations across Hong Kong to help people take precautionary measures to protect their health and guide susceptible groups **short-term**. The monthly reported AQI supports community understanding of the health risks caused by **long-term** exposure to air pollutants.

3. Dampness and mould: The level of dampness can trigger bacteria, fungi, and mould growth when sufficient moisture is available and affect both respiratory and immune systems (CDC, 2017a). Temperature regulation is thus required to be maintained for heat and comfort (EPA, 2016).

Household pollution may result in daily exposure to chemical agents such as cooking, detergents, and personal care products. Health risks associated with indoor air quality varies, with hazards presented in different dwelling types and behavioural patterns of the occupants. These might originate from outdoor sources (traffic, industrial, construction) as well as indoor sources. Particulate matters, which are known to be associated with cardiopulmonary and lung cancer mortality, vary with cooking, ventilation, smoking, and waste management practices (Chan, 2018). Nitrogen dioxide (NO_2), carbon monoxide, radon, and environmental tobacco smoke (ETS) all increase health risks. Household air pollutants (HAP) is of particular health concern in low- and middle-income developing countries (Milner and Hutchinson, 2016) where indoor cooking and heating involves suboptimal ventilation and fuel use (e.g. biomass and burning of plastics and wastes). Notably, research into indoor air quality is not as well established and widely examined when compared with that regarding outdoor air pollution.

Typical causes of indoor pollution include burning fuels like dung, wood, and coal in inefficient stoves or open hearths, which produces a variety of health-damaging pollutants, such as particulate matter (PM), methane, carbon monoxide, polycyclic aromatic hydrocarbons (PAH), and volatile organic compounds (VOC). Particulate matter is a pollutant of special concern. Many studies have demonstrated a direct relationship between exposure to PM and negative health impacts. Smaller-diameter particles (PM2.5 or smaller) are generally more dangerous, as they can reach deep into the small airways of the body and deposit on the alveoli—the tiny sacs in the lungs where oxygen exchanges

Table 6.4 Health Risks Associated with Selected Common Air Pollutants and Their Sources

Pollutant	Sources	Health problems
Particular matter (PM)	Cooking, aerosol (e.g. burning of waste)	Cardiopulmonary and lung cancer mortality
Nitrogen dioxide (NO_2)	Cooking and heating appliances	Respiratory diseases
Carbon monoxide (CO)	Boilers, cooking, and heating appliances	Poisoning
Environmental tobacco smoke (ETS)	Cigarettes, cigars and smoking practices (primary and secondary/passive smokers)	Lung cancer, cardiovascular problems, carcinogenic, and tetarogenic
Allergens	Dust mites, moulds, air pollutants (chemical and cleaning product use)	Skin, eyes, gastrointestinal problems
Radon	Ground gas emission	Lung cancer and carcinogenic

Source: Milner and Hutchinson (2016).

with carbon dioxide in the blood. Ultrafine particles (one micron in diameter or less) can penetrate tissues and organs, posing an even greater risk of systemic health impacts. Exposure to smoke from cooking fires was estimated to have caused 3.8 million premature deaths each year, mostly in low- and middle-income countries (WHO, 2018f). Burning kerosene in simple wick lamps also produces significant emissions of fine particles and other pollutants. Case Box 6.5 illustrates household air pollution from solid fuel use (see also later section on outdoor air pollutants and particulate matter).

Exposure to indoor air pollutants can lead to a wide range of adverse health outcomes among both children and older people who tend to spend long duration indoor. Households with limited means or in poverty may have to rely on polluting fuels and devices and suffer a higher risk of exposure to pollutants and injuries such as burns, poisonings, and musculoskeletal injuries.

Case Box 6.5 Household Air Pollution from Solid Fuel Use: A Sustainability Challenge

Peter Ka-hung Chan

Affecting over 2.7 billion individuals worldwide, household air pollution from solid fuel (e.g. coal, wood) use is a classic example of complex sustainability challenges. Household air pollution is a major health threat to people relying on solid fuels for cooking, heating, or lighting, especially women and young children who are disproportionately exposed due to women's traditional gender role. Early-life exposure to solid fuel smoke is a leading cause of under-five mortality (due to pneumonia) (Gordon, Bruce, Grigg, Hibberd, Kurmi, et al., 2014). For adults, a recent prospective cohort study involving more than 270,000 adults in rural China observed that prolonged solid fuel use for cooking and heating were associated with 30–50% greater risk of cardiovascular death (Yu, Qiu, Chan, Lam, Kurmi, et al., 2018). Another report from the same cohort revealed that prolonged solid fuel use for cooking was associated with higher risks of a wide range of acute and chronic respiratory diseases, including chronic lower respiratory disease and acute lower respiratory infection (Chan, Kurmi, Bennett, Yang, Chen, et al., 2018).

The health impacts of household air pollution, together with time spent on fuel collection and cooking and loss of education opportunity, are major barriers to female empowerment and societal development, which are in turn linked to extensive health and social benefits (WHO, 2016b). This underlies the enormous potential of the United Nations SDG 7 to promote universal access to clean and affordable energy. Although there has been increasing effort made worldwide (most notably in India and China), most existing clean fuels promotion programmes are still in their pilot phase. Sustained effort and advocacy from researchers, public health practitioners, healthcare professionals, and policy-makers is crucial to drive this forward and alleviate this age-old sustainability challenge.

Living context

Living density matters to health in the indoor environment. People of extremes of age (young and old) living in crowded housing are more vulnerable to unintentional injury (such as falls) and inadequate physical activity level (Chan, Kim, Griffiths, Lau, and Yu, 2009). **Household pets** may present additional health risks (e.g. allergens, injury) in the urban household context (Chan, Gao, Li, and Lee, 2017). **Indoor temperature**, which is linked to thermal comfort and affects people with underlying health condition, is associated with adverse health outcomes (see Chapter 3). Suboptimal household dampness control may be associated with respiratory and asthma-related conditions in infants and children (Fisk, Lei-Gomez, and Mendell, 2007). Overcrowding in a suboptimal housing environment may also predispose at-risk individuals to stress and poor mental health outcomes.

Good quality housing, together with water and sanitation support, proper building codes, and standard maintenance, can support and maintain good health and well-being for individuals. In addition to protection from pollutants, important healthy housing considerations include the relationship between housing and amenities, water and sewage, public transport, education, work, and green space (Wilkinson, Smith, Joffe, and Haines, 2007; Milner and Hutchinson, 2016).

Outdoor air pollution

Outdoor air pollution is a major public health concern in the twenty-first century. Urbanization, technology advance, and industrial growth have increased energy requirements, transport use, and waste management. Outdoor air pollution mainly resulted from massive human activities in the urban area affects both urban and rural areas. Traffic-related emissions (petrol and diesel powered vehicles), energy-related emissions (burning of fossil fuels), and natural events (such as forest fires, volcano eruption and dust storms) can all generate high concentrations of pollutants and lead to major harm to the health and well-being of populations (e.g. people with chronic disease problems) (EPA, 2014; WHO, 2018e, 2018f).

Ambient (outdoor air) pollution is found to be a major cause of death and disease globally. It is estimated that 2% of premature deaths globally can be attributed to outdoor air pollution and high concentration of fine particulate matter in urban air is the most important cause. (Prüss-Üstün et al., 2011). Similarly, environmental exposures have been estimated to contribute to 4.9 million (8.7%) deaths and 86 million (5.7%) DALYs globally. The health effects range from increased out-patient service use, hospital admissions, and emergency room visits to increased risk of premature death. The estimated 4.2 million premature deaths globally are linked to ambient air pollution, which might have caused or exacerbated underlying heart disease, stroke, chronic obstructive pulmonary disease, lung cancer, and acute respiratory infections in children. In children and adults, both short- and long-term exposure to ambient air pollution were found to be linked to reduced lung function, respiratory infections, and aggravated asthma. Maternal exposure to ambient air pollution is associated with adverse birth outcomes, such as low birth weight, preterm birth, and small gestational age births. Emerging evidence also suggests ambient air pollution may cause diabetes and affect neurological development in children. Considering that the precise death and disability toll from many of the conditions mentioned here are not currently quantified in current estimates, with growing evidence, the burden of disease from ambient air pollution is expected to increase significantly. The health risks associated with particulate matters of 10 microns or less and 2.5 microns or less in diameter (PM10 and PM2.5) are especially well documented. These particulate matters are capable of penetrating deep into lung passageways and entering the bloodstream causing cardiovascular, cerebrovascular, and respiratory impacts, and it was classified as a cause of lung cancer by the WHO's International Agency for Research on Cancer (IARC) (Straif, Cohen, and Samet, 2013). It is used as the indicator to assess the health effects from exposure to ambient air pollution (see Case Box 6.6). Knowledge Box 6.5 discusses the limitation of facemask in protecting from health risks of small particulate matter.

Case Box 6.6 Air Pollution Is Destroying Human Health

Ambient air pollution is the leading contributor to the global disease burden. TheWHO estimated that fine particulate matter (PM2.5) alone contributed to 4.2 million deaths (7.5% of all-cause deaths) worldwide in 2016 (WHO, 2018g). Some 91% of those premature deaths occurred in low- and middle-income countries, and the greatest number in the WHO South-East Asia and Western Pacific regions (WHO, 2018g).

Previous research on the link between air pollution and health mostly focuses on short-term effects such as mortality, mainly for sensitive individuals or vulnerable populations. Scientists recently found that long-term exposure to air pollution may cause physiopathological changes in all individuals, resulting in a much more serious disease burden. For example, studies show that long-term exposure to PM2.5 air pollution may increase the level of inflammation and coagulation (Zhang, Chang, Lau, Chan, Chuang, et al., 2017; Zhang, Chan, Guo, Chang, Lin, et al., 2018) and the risk of hypertension and chronic kidney disease (Chan, Zhang, et al., 2018; Zhang, Guo, Lau, Chan, Chuang, et al., 2018), which ultimately cause cardiovascular morbidity and mortality. Long-term exposure to air pollution can also reduce pulmonary function and result in chronic obstructive pulmonary disease (Guo, Zhang, Lau, Lin, Chuang, et al., 2018) and mortality.

More than 90% of the world's population lives in a place where the air quality does not reach the standards recommended by the WHO. From 30 October to 1 November 2018, the First WHO Global Conference on Air Pollution and Health took place in Geneva and an aspirational goal was proposed to reduce the number of deaths from air pollution by two-thirds by 2030 (WHO, 2018g).

Knowledge Box 6.5 A Rethink of Health Protection Ability of Facemasks

Although facemask is regarded as an individual health protection measure against airborne/droplet-borne infection (e.g. common cold, influenza, and SARS), typical facemasks cannot prevent the inhalation of gaseous air pollutants carbon monoxide, nitrogen dioxide, ozone, and sulphur dioxide. This may be due to poor facial fit and some of these facemasks intend for filtering larger particles rather than small particles/pathogens (Cherrie, Apsley, Cowie, Steinle, Mueller, et al., 2018). Although most facemasks may only partially reduce the negative health effects of air pollution, there are workplace masks which are designed to protect against fine particle pollution under PM2.5. Other complementary avoidance behaviours such as staying indoors and personal hygiene measures should also be adopted to maximize the health protection effect (Zhang and Mu, 2017).

Urban environment

Built environment

The built environment refers to all human-made physical spaces such as buildings, furnishings, public spaces, and all infrastructure such as roads and utilities. Buildings can protect health and well-being; yet, those of poor quality may accelerate infectious disease transmission and pose hazards and disaster risks such as Natech (see Chapter 4), which are secondary disasters associated with reliance on lifeline infrastructures. Busy roads are likely to cause air pollution and increase risks of traffic accidents. Built environment can also be affected by factors such as access to air, water, transportation, and services. It also leads to exposure to chemical substances, humidity, extreme temperatures, and waste. Knowledge Box 6.6 discusses strategies related to mitigation and adaptation for air pollution, while Knowledge Box 6.7 discusses urbanization and climate change.

Knowledge Box 6.6 Interventions for Air Pollution Mitigation and Adaptation

Cooperation across sectors and at different levels--city, regional, and national--is crucial to address air pollution effectively. Policies and investments supporting cleaner transport and power generation, as well as energy-efficient housing and municipal waste management can reduce key sources of outdoor air pollution. These interventions would not only improve health but also reduce climate pollutants and serve as a catalyst for local economic development and the promotion of healthy urban lifestyles.

Knowledge Box 6.6 Interventions for Air Pollution Mitigation and Adaptation *(continued)*

At the policy level, relevant interventions include improving the transport system by prioritizing rapid urban transit, walking and cycling networks in cities, rail inter-urban freight and passenger travel shifting to cleaner, heavy-duty diesel vehicles and low-emissions vehicles and fuels (including fuels with reduced sulphur content), and implementing stricter vehicle emissions and efficiency standards. At the infrastructure level, building safe and affordable public transport systems and pedestrian- and cycle-friendly networks can encourage the use of bicycles and other clean transportation.

Making cities more compact and thus energy efficient, creating spaces for safe walking and cycling, investing in bus rapid transit or light rail, creating green spaces that help remove particulate matter and reduce the heat island effect, and improving urban waste management (including capture of methane gas emitted from waste sites as an alternative to incineration) are all feasible interventions at the urban planning level.

At the household level, potential interventions may include replacing traditional solid fuel with lower-emission cook stoves and/or cleaner fuels and improving the energy efficiency of homes and commercial buildings through insulation and passive design principles such as natural ventilation and lighting. Shifting to cleaner cook stoves requires a multi-pronged approach including: (i) the introduction of cleaner technologies and fuels for cooking, heating, and lighting as well as improved housing and ventilation design; (ii) supportive government policies and economic incentives; and (iii) education and awareness-raising to support needed changes in cultural habits around cooking and household energy management.

Better waste management such as promoting waste reduction, waste separation, recycling, reuse, and waste reprocessing can also contribute to reducing the generation of air pollutants. Improving methods of biological waste management such as anaerobic waste digestion to produce biogas are feasible as low-cost alternatives to the open incineration of solid waste. Where incineration is unavoidable, combustion technologies with strict emission controls are critical.

At the industrial level, relevant measures include improving brick kilns and coke ovens that emit large amounts of black carbon, adopting clean technologies that reduce industrial smokestack emissions, and increased recovery and use of gas released during fossil fuel production. In the field of agriculture, reducing the burning of agricultural fields, promoting healthy diets low in red and processed meat and rich in plant-based food, alternating wet/dry rice irrigation, and improving the management of agricultural waste and livestock manure (including the capture of methane gas emitted from waste sites as an alternative to incineration) can all contribute to cleaner air.

The power generation process should be enhanced to make it cleaner by transitioning away from fossil fuel combustion (oil, coal) for large-scale energy production and diesel generators for small-scale production, increasing the use of low-emissions fuels and renewable combustion-free power sources (like solar, wind, or hydropower), and increasing reliance on the co-generation heat and power and distributed energy generation (e.g. mini-grids and rooftop solar power generation). Investing in energy-efficient power generation is beneficial to improve domestic, industry, and municipal waste management, as well as helping to reduce agricultural waste incineration. Additional community air quality improvement approaches also include producing greener and more compact cities with energy-efficient buildings, as well as offering universal access to clean affordable fuels and technologies for cooking, heating, and lighting.

Sources: CDC (2018a, 2018b); WHO (2018d).

Transport/roads

Transport offers multiple social, economic, and health benefits. Not only does a transport system improve economic and employment opportunities, but it also facilitates better access to health education, more efficient food distribution, and enhanced socio-economic development. Nevertheless, a number of health risk might be associated with transport development. For example, infectious disease transmission (see Chapter 5) increase with human migration and travel. As mentioned earlier, traffic-related air pollution includes but is not limited to CO_2, PM, nitrogen oxides, volatile organic compounds, and carbon monoxide. Poorly designed transport systems may lead to road traffic accidents, physical inactivity, and noise pollution (see the following section). It is estimated that traffic-related fatalities may increase to 66% by 2020 (from 2000) with large disparities shown between countries (Koptis and Cropper, 2005; Tonne and Sccvronick, 2016). Road designs and policies should aim at improving safety (e.g. banning of drink driving) and protecting communities from the risk of serious and fatal accidents.

While the transportation industry has evolved to decrease travel time significantly, transportation development is also accompanied by negative environment effects. There

Knowledge Box 6.7 Urbanization and Climate Change

Urbanization is drastically increasing climate change effects on communities. As people migrate to cities, trees and plants are cut down as buildings rise, creating more pollution. These cities consume so much energy, and carbon dioxide and other greenhouse gases are produced through energy generation, vehicles, and industries. This can affect cloud condensation, rainfall, and weather patterns. Urbanization can result in the high heat capacity of buildings absorbing and storing more energy, blocking heat release back to space. The closeness of buildings also reduces wind speeds and inhibits cooling by convection (Hong Kong Observatory, 2016). An urban heat island occurs when a city experiences much warmer temperatures than nearby rural areas.

Table 6.5 Sources of Common Environmental Noise

Type of environmental noise source	Examples
Transportation	Aircrafts, trains, road vehicles, vessels
Industrial buildings	Factories: machineries, air-conditioning systems
Commercial buildings	Office buildings: air-conditioning systems restaurants: air-conditioning systems, kitchen ventilating systems
Construction sites	Site formation (e.g. excavation), piling, road work, demolition, renovation
Domestic buildings	Mahjong playing, hi-fi, musical instruments
Public places	Open markets, streets, parks
Products	Intruder alarms of buildings and motor vehicles

may be: (i) increased road construction/maintenance which generates more noise, traffic, and air pollutants; (ii) increased congestion depletes natural gas and emits air pollutants; and (iii) increased traffic noise. The biggest source of community noise is road traffic (WHO, n.d.-c), which is associated with many health effects such as ischaemic heart disease, sleep disturbance, cognitive impairment in children, annoyance, stress, and tinnitus. Traffic noise has also been known to affect respiratory and metabolic health, and in some cases, cause heart attacks (Recio, Linares, Banegas, and Diaz, 2016; Seidler, Wagner, Schubert, Dröge, Pons-Kühnemann, et al., 2016).

Noise pollution

Globally, outdoor noise pollution is mainly caused by machines, transport, and transportation systems. Road traffic is the biggest cause of community noise in most cities, and typically noise levels increase with higher traffic volumes and speeds (WHO, n.d.-c). Poor

Case Box 6.7 Noise Pollution: The Case of Hong Kong Kai Tak Airport

Hong Kong, a subtropical southern China city, is affected by noise problems due to its high urban density. Lack of physical space, suboptimal urban planning (e.g. putting highways next to people's homes), and its continuous urban development contribute to urban noise problems. Noise in the urban centre was drastically reduced in 1998 when the international airport moved from the previous location at Kai Tak to the new Chek Lap Kok. The town-centre located airport had previously caused a great deal of noise affecting 380,000 residents living around the airport. With its new location, it was estimated that about 200 people are severely affected by the noise in the new airport (EPD, 2016) (see Figure 6.12).

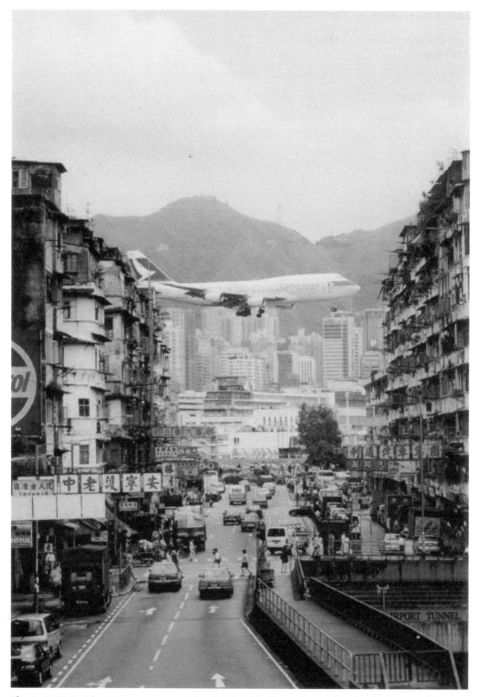

Figure 6.12 Residents in areas around the Old Kai Tak Airport located in the city centre of Hong Kong were troubled by noise from frequent flights just above their heads

Reproduced from Wikimediq Commons at: < https://commons.wikimedia.org/wiki/File:A_CX_Final_Approach_to_KaiTak.jpg) By Ywchow / Public Domain>. In public domain.

urban planning may give rise to noise pollution, and industry situated near residential developments can easily result in noise pollution in residential areas. Some of the main sources of noise in residential areas include loud music, transportation noise, lawn care maintenance, and construction. Noise pollution is also associated with the use of household electricity generators in many developing nations. Case Box 6.7 describes the case of noise pollution created by an airport in the middle of a city.

Human health impact caused by noise may range from hearing loss to coronary artery disease/hypertension. Environmental noise exposure is responsible for a range of health effects. Reported health impacts include increased risk of ischaemic heart disease, sleep disturbance, cognitive impairment among children, annoyance, stress-related mental health risks, and tinnitus. While road traffic is the most pervasive noise-related issue, children living in areas with high aircraft noise were also reported of delayed reading ages, poor attention levels, and high stress levels. In the workplace, noise-induced hearing loss is one of the most common occupational illness. In addition, noise also affects animal health by increasing the risk of death due to animals not being able to hear and thus avoid predators. It can also interfere with reproduction and navigation, and contribute to permanent hearing loss. In high-income European countries, it was estimated that environmental risk accounted for a loss of 1–1.6 million disability adjusted life years (DALYs)—a standardized measure of healthy years of life lost to illness, disability, or early death.

Reducing traffic volumes reduces noise exposures as well as air pollutants. Lower traffic values in neighbourhoods can generate economic and social co-benefits such as higher property values and increased levels of fitness and well-being due to pedestrian street activity and social interaction. Individuals measures may help reduce the harmful effects of noise pollution. Some of such examples include maintaining a level of around 35 decibels (dB) in bedrooms at night, and around 40 dB in houses during the day, choosing residential areas as far from heavy traffic as possible, and avoiding prolonged use of earphones, especially at elevated sound levels. If people must live or work around loud sounds, they can protect their ears with hearing protection (e.g., ear plugs or ear muffs). Mitigation policies may include restriction of activities and use of devices that generate noise in residential areas, occupational health protection rules and regulations, as well as noise control and monitoring mechanism.

Light pollution

Artificial light has benefited human productivity by allowing people to expand their activities beyond normal daylight hours. However, due to wealth and urbanization, the nights of the Earth surface is growing 20% brighter each year in certain regions. Artificial light sources like neon signs, light boards, large television screens, light shows, and lit-up buildings are becoming the norm in large cities. However, light is not always properly emitted from its source, causing it to reflect, spill, and glare. This wasteful light reflects upward into the night sky via suspended particulates in the atmosphere such as clouds, aerosol, and pollutants, effectively brightening the night sky and diminishing the ability to see the stars (Benn and Ellison, 1998). Light pollution affects not only human habitat

Case Box 6.8 Lights in Hong Kong

Hong Kong is famous for its night scene and evening lighting illumination. However, the city is also one of the most light-polluted cities in the world, with an average of 82 times brighter in Hong Kong at night than the global dark sky standard (Pun et al., 2014). Many advertising boards within the city have eight times greater luminous flux per unit area than normal. In the city, there are currently no laws controlling urban lighting but only voluntary charters that request businesses to turn off lights around midnight. Stricter legislation, enforcement, and control can help ease unnecessary light pollution while still maintaining safety. Meanwhile, the tourism industry in Hong Kong is worried that legislation for light pollution control might threaten business as the Victoria Harbour night skyline and bright signs is a huge tourist attraction. For instance, Hong Kong hosts 'A Symphony of Lights', a show using 44 buildings emitting novelty lighting every night. It generates light pollution to the night sky yet attracts millions of tourists.

but also the natural environment and ecosystem globally (Pun, So, Leung, and Wong, 2014). Light affects animals' migratory cycles as well as the survival of animals who thrive in the dark such as fireflies and owls. Environmentally, light consumes a lot of electricity and fossil fuels, generating carbon dioxide emissions, contributing to global warming (Lau, Ng, Tsang, and Vong, 2014).

While light at night makes streets safer and reduces accident as well as injury risks, excess light may damage people's eyes. Light may also suppress the production of melatonin, the hormone influencing tumour growth and circadian rhythms which dictate healthy sleeping patterns. In addition, light at night has been linked with an increased risk of diabetes, sleep disorders, cancer, insomnia, and obesity (Harvard Health Letter, 2015) (see Case Box 6.8).

Land pollution

Apiece of land is classified as 'contaminated' when it is deemed to be capable of causing adverse impacts on humans and the natural environment: where substances may cause immediate or future harm to the well-being of people, property, or protected species. This also includes the risk of how the land may cause significant pollution to surface waters (e.g. lakes and rivers) or groundwater, or may contain radioactive contamination. Contaminated land may previously have been used as a factory, mine, steel mill, refinery, or landfill site. Typical contaminated sites include land contaminated by improper handling or disposal of toxic and hazardous materials and wastes, sites where toxic materials may have been deposited as a result of natural disasters or acts of terror, and sites where improper handling or accidents resulted in release of toxic or hazardous industrial materials. Wastes generated by different industries can also contain contaminants such as heavy metals (such as arsenic, cadmium, and lead), oils and tars, chemical substances and preparations (like solvents), gases, asbestos, and radioactive substances (EPA, 2018e; London Borough of Bexley, n.d.).

Land contamination can result from a variety of intended, accidental, or naturally occurring activities and events (EPA, 2018c). Sources of contamination might include materials and activities associated with manufacturing, mineral extraction, abandonment of mines, national defence activities, waste disposal, accidental spills, illegal dumping, leaking underground storage tanks, hurricanes, floods, pesticide use, and fertilizer application. Contaminated sites vary with size and their significance depends on their activities or use (e.g. abandoned buildings in inner cities and large areas contaminated with toxic materials from past industrial or mining activities). Some contaminated sites pose limited risks to human health and the environment because the level of contamination and the chance of exposure to toxic or hazardous contaminants are low. Other contaminated sites are of greater concern because of the chemicals that may be present and their propensity to persist in or move through the environment, exposing humans or the environment to hazards. These sites must be carefully managed through containment or cleanup to prevent hazardous materials from causing harm to humans, wildlife, or ecological systems, both on- and off-site.

Some types of contaminated land are classed as 'special sites'. Examples of these include locations that seriously affect drinking water supplies, surface waters, or important groundwater sources; sites that have been, or are being, used for certain industrial activities, such as oil refining or making explosives; locations that are being or have been regulated using permits issued under the integrated pollution control or pollution prevention and control regimes; sites that are owned or occupied by ministries of defence; and locations that are contaminated by radioactive nuclear materials.

Chemical threats/chemical safety

Human beings are exposed to various chemical substances daily and through multiple physiological routes such as ingestion, inhalation, skin contact, and via the umbilical cord to the unborn child. Although most chemicals are harmless or even beneficial; others are a threat to human health and to the environment. Chemicals production and use continues to increase, particularly in the developing world, and, with it, the potential for chemical exposure. This is likely to result in greater negative effect on health if sound chemicals management is not ensured. The chemicals mentioned here are hazardous to human health, but exposure could potentially be reduced or removed through environmental management. They include pesticides, asbestos, various other household and occupational chemicals, ambient and household air pollution, secondhand tobacco smoke, lead, and arsenic. Estimates of health impacts are presented for a selection of chemicals with sufficient evidence for global quantification. The production and use of chemicals continues to grow worldwide, particularly in developing countries.

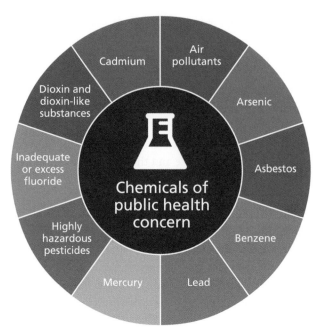

Figure 6.13 Chemicals of public health concern

It is important that the production and use of all chemicals, whether natural or manu-factured, are regulated for the safety of for both humans and the environment. According to the WHO, many chemicals used to human advantage to further the technology and improve the human existence can be hazardous to human health and the environment if not extracted, synthesized, produced, transported, or disposed of properly. Chemicals are all around us: in paints, plastics, cookware, public recreational spaces, cosmetics, build-ings, light bulbs, etc. (WHO, 2010). Figures 6.13 and 6.14 and Table 6.6 show and discuss chemicals of major public health concern. The following section discusses some common chemical substances (or groups of chemicals) that are of major public health concern listed by the WHO (2016c).

Arsenic

Arsenic is a natural component of the Earth's crust and is widely distributed throughout the environment in the air, water, and land. It is highly toxic in its inorganic form. The greatest threat to public health from arsenic originates from contaminated groundwater. Inorganic arsenic is naturally present at high levels in the groundwater of a number of countries including Argentina, Bangladesh, Chile, China, India, Mexico, and the United States. People may be exposed to elevated levels of inorganic arsenic-contaminated water through drinking, food preparation, food crops, irrigation, industrial processes, eating contaminated food, and smoking tobacco (WHO, 2018i). Long-term exposure to inor-ganic arsenic, again mainly through drinking water and food consumption, can lead to chronic arsenic poisoning. Skin lesions and skin cancer are the most characteristic effects.

Table 6.6 Chemical Substances of Public Health Concern

Lead	Lead is a naturally occurring metal that can be toxic. There is no known level of lead exposure that is deemed to be safe and it is harmful to both children and adults. Lead may be exposed through inhalation of particles released by industries or recycling, ingestion of contaminated soil or dust from decaying lead paint, contaminated food or water, and lead-containing products.
Arsenic	Arsenic can also be found distributed in water, food, and tobacco, leading to high levels of damage in water, unsafe food preparation, contaminated irrigation of food crops, and industrial processes. It is found naturally in the environment but is highly toxic in its inorganic form.
Mercury	Mercury, a naturally occurring metal, can be released into the environment from coal power plants, eating contaminated fish and shellfish, small-scale gold mining, blood pressure measuring devices, batteries, silver dental metal fillings, batteries, thermometers, skin lightening cosmetics, and lightbulbs.
Benzene	Benzene is a volatile chemical detected at high levels in indoor air from building materials, cigarette smoke, automobile exhaust, unflued oil heating, etc.
Asbestos	Asbestos, a carcinogenic (cancer-causing) mineral, is used as insulation due to its strength, poor heat conduction, and resistance to chemical attack in both homes and workplace.
Pesticides	Pesticides are used to control insects, rodents, and pests (Janssen, Solomon, and Schettler, 2011)

Asbestos

Asbestos is a group of naturally occurring fibrous minerals with current or historical commercial usefulness due to their extraordinary tensile strength, poor heat conduction, and relative resistance to chemical corrosion. Its chemical and physical properties have made asbestos a common temperature insulation material in buildings and as roofing shingles, water supply lines, and fire blankets, as well as clutches and brake linings, gaskets, and pads for automobiles. All forms of asbestos are harmful and carcinogenic to humans. Exposure to asbestos, including chrysotile, causes cancer of the lung, larynx, and ovaries, and also mesothelioma (a cancer of the pleural and peritoneal linings). Asbestos exposure is also responsible for other diseases such as asbestosis (fibrosis of the lungs) and plaques, thickening and effusion in the pleura.

Currently, about 125 million people in the world have been and are exposed to asbestos. Approximately half of the deaths from occupational cancer are estimated to be caused by asbestos. It is also estimated that several thousand deaths annually can be attributed to exposure to asbestos in the home. It has also been shown that co-exposure to tobacco smoke and asbestos fibres substantially increases the risk for lung cancer—and the heavier the smoking, the greater the risk.

The WHO, in collaboration with the International Labour Organization and other intergovernmental organizations and civil society, works with countries towards elimination of asbestos-related diseases by recognizing that the most efficient way to eliminate

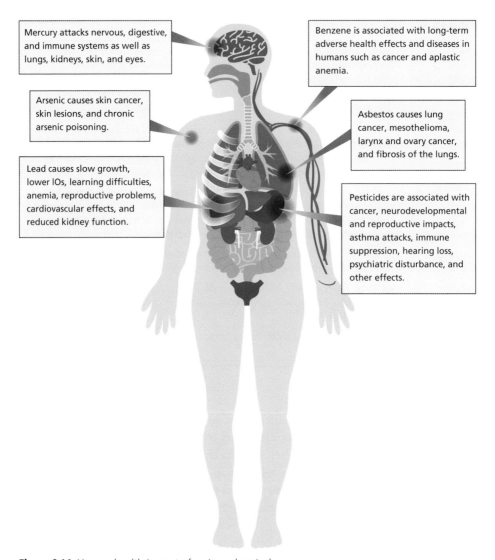

Mercury attacks nervous, digestive, and immune systems as well as lungs, kidneys, skin, and eyes.

Benzene is associated with long-term adverse health effects and diseases in humans such as cancer and aplastic anemia.

Arsenic causes skin cancer, skin lesions, and chronic arsenic poisoning.

Asbestos causes lung cancer, mesothelioma, larynx and ovary cancer, and fibrosis of the lungs.

Lead causes slow growth, lower IOs, learning difficulties, anemia, reproductive problems, cardiovascular effects, and reduced kidney function.

Pesticides are associated with cancer, neurodevelopmental and reproductive impacts, asthma attacks, immune suppression, hearing loss, psychiatric disturbance, and other effects.

Figure 6.14 Human health impact of various chemicals

asbestos-related diseases is to stop the use of all types of asbestos. It also provides information about solutions for replacing asbestos with safer substitutes, promotes the economic and technological mechanism development to stimulate asbestos replacement, and takes measures to prevent asbestos exposure during asbestos removal (abatement). The initiatives also advocate early diagnosis, treatment, and rehabilitation services for asbestos-related diseases, asbestos exposure registry development, medical surveillance for exposed workers, and awareness raising of waste containing asbestos to be treated as hazardous waste (WHO, 2018j).

Mercury

Mercury is a naturally occurring element found in air, water, and soil. Exposure to mercury—even small amounts—may cause serious health problems, and it is a threat to the development of the child *in utero* and in early life. Mercury may have toxic effects on the nervous, digestive, and immune systems, and on lungs, kidneys, skin, and eyes. Mercury is considered by the WHO as one of the top ten chemicals or groups of chemicals of major public health concern. People are mainly exposed to methylmercury, an organic compound, when they eat fish and shellfish containing the compound. Methylmercury is very different to ethylmercury. Ethylmercury is used as a preservative in some vaccines and does not pose a health risk (WHO, 2017b).

Mercury exists in various forms: elemental (or metallic) and inorganic (to which people may be exposed through their occupation), and organic (e.g. methylmercury, to which people may be exposed through diet). These forms of mercury differ in their degree of toxicity and in their effects on the nervous, digestive, and immune systems, and on lungs, kidneys, skin, and eyes.

Mercury occurs naturally in the Earth's crust. It is released into the environment as a result of volcanic activity, weathering of rocks, and human activity. Mercury may be released by coal-fired power stations, residential coal burning for heating and cooking, industrial processes, waste incinerators, as well as during the process of mining for mercury, gold, and other metals.

Once in the environment, mercury can be transformed by bacteria into methylmercury. Methylmercury typically bioaccumulates (bioaccumulation occurs when an organism contains higher concentrations of the substance than do the surroundings) in fish and shellfish. Methylmercury also biomagnifies. For example, large predatory fish are more likely to have high levels of mercury as a result of eating many smaller fish that have acquired mercury through ingestion of plankton. People may be exposed to mercury in any of its forms under different circumstances and exposure mainly occurs through consumption of fish and shellfish contaminated with methylmercury and through worker inhalation of elemental mercury vapours during industrial processes. Notably, as cooking does not eliminate mercury, food consumption is a typical exposure route for the general public. Case Box 6.9 describes the chemical incident in Minamata Bay of Japan in the twentieth century.

In modern world, humans are exposed to some level of mercury in their lifetime. Most people are exposed to low levels, often through chronic exposure (continuous or intermittent long-term contact). However, some people are exposed to acute high levels. An example of an acute exposure would be mercury exposure due to an industrial accident. To determine whether health effects occur and their severity, here are the factors to consider: the type of mercury concerned; the dose; the age or developmental stage of the exposed individual (the foetus is most susceptible); the duration of exposure; the route of exposure (inhalation, ingestion, or dermal contact).

Case Box 6.9 Minamata Disease

A notable example of mercury exposure that led to serious public health and medical implications happened in Minamata, Japan. Between 1932 and 1968, a factory discharged acetic acid waste liquid into Minamata Bay. The discharge included high concentrations of methylmercury. Minamata Bay was rich in fish and shellfish and marine products were the main economic livelihood for local residents and fishermen in the areas. For many years, the public was unaware of the marine contamination but noticed the increasing prevalence of strange diseases like brain damage, paralysis, incoherent speech, and delirium. Elemental and methylmercury are toxic to the central and peripheral nervous systems. The inhalation of mercury vapour can produce harmful effects on the nervous, digestive, and immune systems, lungs and kidneys, and may be fatal. The inorganic salts of mercury are corrosive to the skin, eyes, and gastrointestinal tract, and may induce kidney toxicity if ingested. Neurological and behavioural disorders may be observed after inhalation, ingestion, or dermal exposure of different mercury compounds. Symptoms include tremors, insomnia, memory loss, neuromuscular effects, headaches, and cognitive and motor dysfunction. Mild, subclinical signs of central nervous system toxicity can be seen in workers exposed to an elemental mercury level in the air of 20 μg/m^3 or more for several years. Kidney effects have been reported, ranging from increased protein in the urine to kidney failure. At least 50,000 people were affected to some extent and more than 2,000 cases of Minamata disease were certified. Minamata disease peaked in the 1950s.

In general, two population subgroups are more sensitive to the effects of mercury. Foetuses are most susceptible due to the detrimental developmental effects mercury may impose on human development. Methylmercury exposure in the womb can result from a mother's consumption of fish and shellfish. It can adversely affect a baby's growing brain and nervous system. Cognitive thinking, memory, attention, language, and fine motor and visual spatial skills may be severely affected among children who were exposed to methylmercury as foetuses. The second vulnerable group is people who are exposed to (chronic exposure) or consume high levels of mercury regularly (such as populations relying on subsistence fishing or people occupationally exposed). Among selected subsistence fishing populations, between 1.5/1,000 and 17/1,000 children showed cognitive impairment (mild mental retardation) caused by the consumption of fish containing mercury. These included at-risk populations living in Brazil, Canada, China, Columbia, and Greenland.

Prevention of the negative health impact of mercury
There are several ways to prevent adverse health effects of mercury. Clean energy promotion, banning use of mercury in gold mining, eliminating mercury mining, and phasing out non-essential mercury-containing products are some examples of population protection initiatives. In addition, as mercury is an element that cannot be destroyed,

mercury already in use should be recycled for other essential uses to avoid further need for further mercury mining. Mercury is contained in many products, including: batteries; measuring devices such as thermometers and barometers; electric switches and relays in equipment; lamps (including some types of light bulbs); dental amalgam (for dental fillings), skin-lightening products and other cosmetics; and pharmaceuticals. A range of actions are being taken to reduce mercury levels in these products, or to phase out mercury-containing products. For example, mercury-containing thermometers and sphygmomanometers are being actively replaced by alternative devices. Notably, mercury use in artisanal and small-scale gold mining is particularly hazardous, and health effects on vulnerable populations are significant. Thus, non-mercury (and non-cyanide) gold-extraction techniques need to be promoted and implemented, and where mercury is still used, safer work practices need to be employed to prevent exposure.

Energy generation

Electricity has changed the way humans live and conduct their activities since it became publicly accessible. Regulating light and temperature have increased economic productivity and expanded living environment possibilities. The ability to control temperature reduce heat stroke, hypothermia, and risks to chronic diseases. However, mankind has been using non-renewable energy resources such as the fossil fuels coal, petroleum, and natural gas for generating electricity. Coal and petroleum are known to cause harmful health and environmental effects at every step of electricity production process and use (Lockwood, Welker-Hood, Rauch, and Gottlieb, 2009). These processes have been maximized for cost effectiveness without considering the environmental health effects. Coal mining is physically dangerous, coal transportation adds pollution in the air, coal combustion releases mercury, particulate matter, nitrogen oxides, sulphur dioxides, and other gases, all significantly contributing to climate change. Natural gas is cleaner and cheaper than other fossil fuels. However, both oil and natural gas extraction can contaminate drinking and surface water as well as contribute to air pollution and climate change (Michaels, Simpson, and Wegner, 2010).

The use of other energy sources may reduce adverse environmental and human health impact. Alternative energy sources consist of solar, wind, and nuclear energy, hydropower, shale gas, and hydrogen fuel cells. While solar, wind, and hydropower have specific geographic requirement (e.g. close to water sources), nuclear power might be implemented with limited geographic requirement concerns. Energy generated by nuclear process generates electricity using uranium. However, uranium mining may contaminate air, water, and soil. Radioactive fission products, if released into air or water, will cause long-term catastrophic consequences to the ecological health of the context. There is also no safe way to dispose of nuclear waste. If buried underground, this waste will remain for hundreds of years and can potentially contaminate air and water. Shale gas is natural gas buried in shale rock formations and has increased the global energy supply. However, there remain concerns about water pollution from its extraction processes. Hydrogen fuel cell vehicles can reduce carbon emissions and fossil fuel consumptions. Nevertheless, this is an expensive technology and requires logistic infrastructure (e.g. fuel stations) to facilitate a scalable implementation.

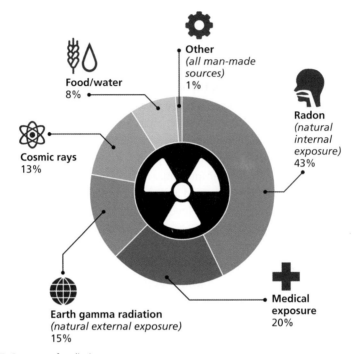

Figure 6.15 Sources of radiation exposure

Reproduced with permission from World Health Organization. (2004). Guidelines for drinking-water quality (3rd edn). Copyright © 2004 WHO. Available at: <https://www.who.int/water_sanitation_health/dwq/GDW9rev1and2.pdf>

Radiation

Radiation is a form of energy that is capable of travelling through space or a material medium. Ionizing radiation is a type of energy released by atoms in the form of electro-magnetic waves or particles (gamma, X-rays, neutrons, beta, alpha). Ionizing radiation is found in soil, water, vegetation, and human-made sources like X-rays and other medical devices (WHO, 2016d).

Radiological threats

Radiation exists naturally in the environment and, if harnessed safely, can serve as clean energy sources (see Figure 6.15). However, radiation can potentially pose health hazard as it can damage tissues or organs if humans/animals are exposed to excessive dose. Skin burns, acute radiation syndrome, or cancer may result from exposure to excess ionizing radiation (WHO, 2016d). Potential results of radiation explosure include death and in-jury (immediate deaths due to the radiation effects, longer-term deaths due to radiation-induced cancers, and injuries and chronic diseases due to radiation effects); contaminated land (which become unsuitable for agricultural use); contaminated water (leading to threats to the safety drinking water and adverse ecological impact, i.e. bio-accumulation of radioactivity in fish, resulting in concentrations significantly above guideline max-imum levels for consumption); contaminated flora and fauna (e.g. destroyed forest and farm animals dying from or suffering from thyroid diseases); extended affected area (i.e. spreading of radioactive substances by air and ocean current); and after-effects (e.g. residual radioactivity in the environment and prolonged recovery of the area, both ecologically and economically). Radiological threats cause acute and chronic impacts on human health, living organisms, and the environment and can cause disruption in the entire living ecology. Case Boxes 6.10 and 6.11 recount the radiation disasters occurred in Chernobyl of Ukraine in 1986 and Fukushima of Japan in 2011.

Ozone depletion

According to the WHO (n.d.-d), sunlight, which is a form of ultraviolet radiation, is one of the most important radiation sources for supporting human health in providing

---

Case Box 6.10 Chernobyl Disaster

On 26 April 1986, the nuclear power plant at Chernobyl in Ukraine exploded. Large amounts of radioactive materials were released into the atmosphere. The radioactive materials had caused many harmful effects on plants and animals within the proximity of the power plant, contaminating urban and agricultural areas, water, and forests. The nearest town to the power plant, Pripyat, was abandoned shortly afterwards.

The 1986 Chernobyl accident caused the deaths of 30 power plant employees and firemen within a few days or weeks (including 28 deaths due to radiation exposure). Immediately after the accident, two workers died due to the steam blast. Over the following weeks, 134 people were hospitalized with acute radiation sickness (ARS), of whom 28 firemen and employees died of the radiation effects in the following months and 14 died of radiation-induced cancer in the next decade. Among the wider population, as of 2011, there were more than 6,000 cases of thyroid cancer among people who were children or adolescents during the incident, of which 15 were fatal.

Cancer deaths caused by Chernobyl was estimated to reach about 4,000 among the 5 million persons residing in the contaminated areas. Four square kilometres of pine forest near the reactor died, animals in the worst-hit areas died or stopped reproducing, and domesticated horses and cattle left on an island in the Pripyat River a short distance from the power plant died as their thyroid glands were destroyed by high radiation doses.

The after-effects of Chernobyl nuclear incident are expected to unfold in the this century. Although the severity of the effects has declined gradually, since radioactive caesium-137 isotopes was taken up by fungi, which were in turn consumed by livestock, the long-term implications of the incident to the environment are still unfolding in the decades to come.

Sources: Chernobyl Forum (2005); World Health Organization (2005, 2011, April); Green Facts (2018); World Nuclear Association (2018, April).

Case Box 6.11 Fukushima Daiichi Nuclear Disaster: Environmental and Tertiary Impact on Evacuees

The Fukushima Daiichi nuclear accident happened following a major earthquake and its associated 15-metre tsunami disabled the power supply and cooling of three Fukushima Daiichi reactors, causing a nuclear accident on 11 March 2011. All three reactor cores largely melted within the first three days. There have been no immediate deaths or cases of radiation sickness from the nuclear accident, but over 100,000 people were evacuated from their homes to ensure their safety. The incident displaced 50,000 households after radioactive material leaked into the air, soil, and sea. Radiation checks led to bans on some shipments of vegetables and fish. On 11 April, experts from Kyoto University and Hiroshima University released a study of soil samples, revealing that up to 400 times the normal levels of radiation could remain in communities beyond a 30-kilometre radius from the Fukushima nuclear power plant site.

A Greenpeace Japan report conducted five years after the incident revealed that the environmental impacts of the Fukushima Daiichi nuclear disaster would last decades to centuries, due to man-made, long-lived radioactive elements being absorbed into the living tissues of plants and animals. The adverse impacts last not only locally but also spread globally by being recycled through food webs, and carried downstream to the Pacific Ocean by typhoons, snowmelt, and flooding. The environmental impacts are already becoming apparent, with studies showing high radiation concentrations in new leaves, and at least in the case of cedar, in pollen, and apparent increases in growth mutations of fir trees with rising radiation levels. Heritable mutations were found in pale-blue grass butterfly populations and DNA-damaged worms in highly contaminated areas. There were apparent reduced fertility in barn swallows, decreases in the abundance of 57 bird species with higher radiation levels over a 4-year study, high levels of caesium contamination in commercially important freshwater fish, and radiological contamination of one of the most important ecosystems—coastal estuaries (Greenpeace, 2016a, 2016b; World Nuclear Association, October 2018).

Tertiary Impact: Mental Health of Evacuees

The earthquake and tsunami that caused the nuclear disaster had meanwhile damaged or destroyed more than 1 million buildings, leading to a total of 470,000 people requiring evacuation, among whom the nuclear accident was responsible for 154,000 being evacuated (Reconstruction Agency, 2016).

Evacuation was the result of the damaged environment and the subsequent attempt to protect the residents in the affected area. However, mental health and change of socio-economic status of the evacuees should also be taken into consideration. In the former Soviet Union, many patients with negligible radioactive exposure after the Chernobyl disaster displayed extreme anxiety about radiation exposure. Relocation has also predisposed evacuees to develop many psychosomatic problems, including

---

Case Box 6.11 Fukushima Daiichi Nuclear Disaster *(continued)*

radiophobia along with an increase in fatalistic alcoholism. Life expectancy of the evacuees were found to have dropped from 65 to 58 years, not because of cancer, but because of depression, alcoholism, and suicide.

A survey by the Iitate local government obtained responses from approximately 1,743 evacuees within the evacuation zone (Pitta, 2015). The survey showed that many residents are experiencing growing frustration, instability, and an inability to return to their earlier lives. A relatively high percentage (66%) of respondents stated that their health and the health of their families had deteriorated after evacuating, while 39.9% reported feeling more irritated than they did normally before the disaster. Among all responses to questions related to evacuees' current family status, 33.3% of all sur-veyed families live apart from their children, while 50.1% live separate from other family members (including older parents) with whom they lived before the disaster. The survey also showed that 34.7% of the evacuees suffered salary cuts of 50% or more since the outbreak of the nuclear disaster. A total of 36.8% reported a lack of sleep, while 17.9% reported smoking or drinking more than before they evacuated (Shah and Rallapali, 2013).

Stress is often manifested in physical ailments, including behavioural changes such as poor dietary choices, lack of exercise, and sleep deprivation. Survivors, including some who lost homes, villages, and family members, were found likely to face mental health and physical challenges (Pitta, 2015). Significant portion of self-report stress was related to the lack of information and from relocation. A survey estimated that of some 300,000 evacuees, approximately 1,600 deaths were related to the evacuation conditions, such as living in temporary housing and hospital closures that had oc-curred as of August 2013, a number comparable to the 1,599 deaths directly caused by the earthquake and tsunami in the Prefecture (Pitta, 2015). The exact causes of these evacuation-related deaths were not specified because according to the municipalities, that would hinder relatives applying for compensation.

---

vitamin D. However, it is harmful if excessive doses are absorbed or ingested as it may cause acute and chronic health effects in the skin, eyes, and immune system. The ozone layer is a natural layer of gas in the stratosphere that helps protect living organisms from harmful ultraviolet radiation from the Sun. However, stratosphere can be destroyed and depleted by air pollution and man-made chemicals. When synthetic chemicals such as chlorofluorocarbons (CFCs) are exposed to ultraviolet radiation at low temperatures, they can damage the ozone layer. The depleted ozone layer will be unable to prevent ex-cessive ultraviolet (UV) radiation levels from reaching the ground surface of the Earth and cause skin cancer, eye cataracts, and immune deficiency disorders in humans. This will also affect plant and animal growth, therefore food chains, and biochemical cycles in terrestrial and aquatic ecosystems. Notably, ozone-depleting substances stay in the atmos-phere for many years and the ozone layer takes long time to recover. In recent decades,

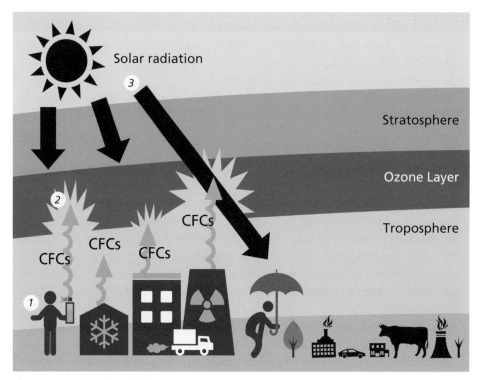

Figure 6.16 Ozone layer depletion

various restrictions on ozone-depleting substances have been imposed to allow the ozone layer to recover from environmental damage (European Commission, 2017; EPA, 2018c) (see Figure 6.16).

Resource depletion

Industrialization, science advancement and socio-economic development have greatly improved the quality of human life. However, along with such progress, human beings are consuming the Earth's resources at accelerating speed. As the global population continues to grow, various resource constraints will be more apparent. While alternatives to natural resources such as fossil fuels exist, not everything can be renewed. Improvement in energy use efficiency and new technologies will need to be developed to counteract the swiftness of natural resource depletion. Renewable energy resources and reusing and recycling resources are currently the frontier of scientific advancement.

Environmental health protection policies

Environmental health protection policies encompass activities and programme initiatives that aim to protect the public from avoidable health risks and minimize impacts on health where exposure cannot be avoided. Proactive and reactive actions to mitigate harm and benefit health from environmental determinants include local, regional, national, and international coordination and advice to maximize sanitation, safety, security, and quality.

Overall, environmental health protection policies may include the following approaches: legislations and policies (incorporating environmental/health standards) that protect the public from chemicals, poisons, and other environmental hazards; the training of a competent and resilient workforce with clearly defined workforce competency requirements and compliant procedures that are supported by specified minimum training standards; a high-quality inspection, regulation, and law enforcement capacity; responsive intervention services to protect against the acute and chronic exposure to chemicals and poisons; environmental services for zoonotic/vector-borne disease monitoring; and waste management including disposal/movement of hazardous waste. Other important health protection efforts include port health maintenance measures such as disinfection, sanitation, safe transportation of foodstuffs, and management of shipping waste.

Typical policies are prevention-focused such as legislation to ban harmful substances and practices, use of alternative chemicals, facility building and process, regulation enforcement, and development control via influencing rural/urban planning processes to minimize exposure potential. Relevant policies also include development or adaptation of protocols and guidance to manage public health risks from various environmental hazards (for example, chemical, biological, physical, radiation, and noise hazards), media (air, soil, water, and food), and living context (such as households, community settings, and road safety).

Preventing exposure to environmental hazards relies on partnership and participation of multiple stakeholders. Relevant human resources, sufficient surveillance capacity, and efficient response systems are important resources for investigating and responding to diseases, monitoring for hazards, and educating the public for health protection.

Constant efforts in capacity building and regular technology upgrade will be essential to enable appropriate measures and responses to be mounted in environmental incidents and crises. Operator controls, environmental sampling and monitoring, and effective alert systems should be implemented to reduce potential threats and risks for occurring or spreading.

Environmental health protection strategies and policies

With the constant changes in the human environment and the multidisciplinary nature of environmental health issues, regular updates and re-evaluation of public health risks associated with identified environmental health priorities are required. Environmental health training programmes should be tailored according to actual population risks, needs, and service needs. Skills and competences should include enquiry and incident response capabilities (comprising environmental public health field epidemiology investigation; sampling, monitoring, and analytical capabilities and expertise; risk assessment; data and risk interpretation; and risk management). Regular risk and crisis communication should be engaged for regular environmental hazard/health burden in defined areas/populations.;

Properly defined roles and hazard/scenario plans should be tested and reviewed via community participation in emergency preparedness, planning, and exercises. Actions and programmes should be implemented to reduce environmental inequities promote sustainable communities should be promoted by establishing relevant policies, legislation and human resources.

Robust health systems should have well-coordinated environmental health surveillance to enhance enquiry and incident response services. It should also have detailed service specification outlining multi-agency coordination and delivery standards. Examples include coordinated sampling and monitoring environmental hazards; continuous service quality improvement through regular audits. Risk assessment tools such as Health Impact Assessment should be developed to examine and monitor the well-being and quality of life of the population living in environment with specific hazard exposure. Environmental health assessment should be included in land use planning, housing development, community regeneration attempts, as well as climate change/sustainability agendas. Finally, communication strategies around identified priorities aimed at stakeholders including consumers, commercial interests (business relationship management), and policy-makers are also needed.

Environmental impact assessment (EIA)

Environmental impact assessments (EIA) can assist and facilitate decision-makers to examine environmental impacts of their project plan and implementation process. A typical EIA process involves identifying, assessing, evaluating, mitigating, planning, and managing the potential impact to the environment (see Case Box 6.12). Effective implementation of the EIA process will require the identification of programmes, policies, and projects that may have significant environmental effects on a community. EIA also allows early participation of the public and the affected community in the decision-making process.

Occupational health

In addition to community protection from environmental impacts, the protection of the well-being of the working population and protecting high-risk working population from occupation hazards are also important for the protection of public health. The WHO defines **occupational health** as all aspects of health and safety in the workplace with a strong focus on primary prevention of hazards (WHO, n.d.-e). According to the International Labour Organization, 2.02 million people die each year from work-related accidents or diseases. A further 317 million people suffer from work-related diseases, and there are an estimated 337 million fatal and non-fatal work-related accidents per year (International Labour Organization, n.d.). Case Box 6.13 discusses the occupational and environmental risk factors of lung cancer.

Many health risks and hazards exist in the workplace. These health issues may cause cancer, accidents, musculoskeletal diseases, respiratory diseases, hearing loss, circulatory diseases, stress-related disorders, communicable diseases, and etc. Indoor air pollutants, toxic chemicals such as lead and pesticides, carcinogens, noise, ergonomic stressors, and

Case Box 6.12 What Are the Stages of Environmental Impact Assessment? The Case of the United Kingdom

In the United Kingdom, the objective of conducting environmental impact assessment (EIA) is to protect the environment. The process ensures local planning authority, when deciding whether to grant planning permission for a project that is likely to have significant environment effect, takes the project's environmental implications into decision-making consideration. In general, there are five major stages of EIA.

Screening: The process is to determine if a proposed project falls within the remit of the relevant regulations and rules. It attempts to assess if the proposed project is likely to have significant effects on the environment and therefore requires an assessment.

Scoping: This stage is to review the extent and the scope of issues to be considered in the assessment. The applicant has to consult stakeholders or the local planning authority for their opinion on what information needs to be included (which is called a 'scoping opinion').

Preparing an environmental statement: If it is decided that an assessment of the proposed project/programme is required, public authorities have to make any relevant environmental information available to support the decision-making process. An environmental statement should include at least the information required to assess the likely significant environmental effects.

To ensure the completeness and quality of the environmental statement, the project party must ensure that the statement is prepared and made by competent experts. The environmental statement must be accompanied by a statement from the project party outlining the relevant expertise or qualifications of such experts.

Making a planning application and consultation: The environmental statement (and the application for development to which it relates) should be publicized by public notice. The statutory 'consultation bodies' and the public must be given an opportunity to give their views about the proposed development and the environmental statement.

Decision-making: The environmental statement, together with any other information that is relevant to the decision, and any comments and representations made on it, must be taken into account by the local planning authority and/or the Secretary of State in deciding whether or not to grant consent for the development. The public must be informed of the decision and explained of the main reasons for it, both through electronic media and by public notice.

Source: United Kingdom Ministry of Housing, Communities and Local Government (2019).

lack of proper equipment or training are common risk factors. As occupational health is affected by multiple determinants, protecting employee from unfavourable employee working conditions (such as working hours, salary, workplace policies concerning maternity leave, health promotion, and protection provisions) and work-related hazards (e.g. use of chemicals) are important considerations. Removing hazards at source, reducing

Case Box 6.13 Occupational and Environmental Risk Factors of Lung Cancer in Hong Kong

Shelly Lap-ah Tse

Lung cancer is the leading cancer incidence in Hong Kong as well as in other parts of the world. Many hazardous substances involved in employment in Hong Kong are confirmed or suspected occupational carcinogens, such as asbestos fibres, silica dust, and paints that are common in shipyard and car-repair work, and construction and renovation work. Results from a case-control study among 2,277 males (1,208 lung cancer cases versus 1,069 community controls) conducted from 2004–06 identified construction as the major hazardous industry associated with an increased risk of lung cancer (adjusted odds ratio = 1.37, 95% CI: 1.00–1.89). In terms of specific risk factors found in the workplace, silica dust, welding fumes, diesel exhaust, and man-made mineral fibres are the important occupational risk factors for lung cancer, and these four identified occupational risk factors contribute to an overall of 9.5% of excess lung cancer risk in Hong Kong general population (Tse, Yu, Qiu, Au, and Wang, 2012). We also identified second-hand smoke and burning incense resulting in indoor combustion and residential radon as the most important environmental risk factors of lung cancer in the Hong Kong male population (Tse, Yu, Qiu, Au, Yu, et al., 2009; Tse, Yu, Qiu, Au, and Wang, 2011). As lung cancer is the most fatal cancer worldwide including Hong Kong and China, prevention is thus key. Eliminating all the identified risk factors from occupational and environmental sources is challenging but plays an important role in cancer prevention.

contact between hazards and workers, and protecting workers in their employment are three key prevention and protection strategies.

Environmental health protection policy approach

Humans interact with the environment and these interactions may have implications on life expectancy and quality of life and may create health disparities. Maintaining a healthy environment may significantly improve quality of life and years of healthy life. Globally, 23% of all deaths and 26% of deaths among children under age 5 are due to preventable environmental factors. Exposure to hazardous substances in the air, water, soil, and food, natural and technological disasters, consequences of climate change, occupational hazards, and the built environment are some typical health risks that may influence human well-being and living environment (Prüss-Üstün et al., 2016). Creating healthy environments is a complex process and relies on continuous research and monitoring to understand the effects of exposure to environmental hazards on people's health. Countries have developed specific approaches that may address environmental health protection (see Case Box 6.14).

Case Box 6.14 Healthy People 2020 in the United States

Healthy People 2020 in the United States focus on six themes, which draw attention to elements of the environment and their links to health. Each theme highlights key components in environmental health, which include: outdoor air quality; surface and groundwater quality; toxic substances and hazardous wastes; homes and communities; infrastructure and surveillance; and global environmental health. The following describes some of these objectives.

Outdoor Air Quality

Poor outdoor air quality is associated with premature death, cancer, and long-term damage to respiratory and cardiovascular systems. Decreasing air pollution is an important step in creating a healthy environment and progress has been made to reduce unhealthy air emissions.

Surface and Groundwater

Contamination of surface and ground water by infectious agents or chemicals can cause mild to severe illness. Surface and groundwater quality concerns apply to both drinking water and recreational waters. Protecting water sources and minimizing exposure to contaminated water sources are important parts of environmental health actions and policies.

Toxic Substances and Hazardous Wastes

The health effects of toxic substances and hazardous wastes are not yet fully understood. Reducing exposure to toxic substances and hazardous wastes is fundamental to environmental health. Ongoing research aims to enhance understanding of how these exposures may impact health and policy efforts to reduce exposures continue.

Homes and Communities

People spend significant amount of their time at home, work, or school. Some of these environments may expose people to (i) indoor air pollution; (ii) inadequate heating and sanitation; (iii) structural problems; (iv) electrical and fire hazards; and (v) lead-based paint hazards. These hazards can impact health and safety. Maintaining healthy homes and communities is essential to environmental health.

Infrastructure and Surveillance

To protect environmental health, infrastructure maintenance, upgrading, and monitoring are important. Disease surveillance systems are essential to monitor system functioning and allow early detection of crisis.

Global Environmental Health

Environmental health hazards and crises transcend national boundaries. Global collaboration and partnerships need to be fostered to enhance capacity and maximize protection of population well-being.

Source: Office of Disease Prevention and Health Promotion, United States (n.d.).

International agreements and policies

For the past 50 years, more than 500 international agreements have attempted to enable health and environmental protection. Some examples include the Vienna Convention for the Protection of the Ozone Layer and the Montreal Protocol on Substances that Deplete the Ozone Layer, both of which aim to protect the globe's ozone layer. Another important agreements to protect the world's limited water supply are the Convention on the Protection and Use of Transboundary Watercourses and International Lakes, the 1989 Basil Convention on the Control of Transboundary Movements of Hazardous Wastes and Their Disposal, etc. For chemicals and hazardous wastes, the Minamata Convention on Mercury is an international agreement that aims to protect people and the environment from mercury (EPA, 2018d). It is working to phase out thermometers and blood pressure devices that contain mercury, promote oral health and so reduce dental amalgam use, implement strategies to protect small-scale gold miners and other vulnerable groups, and monitor mercury exposure and provide health advice.

There are also agreements and treaties related to oil pollution, hazardous waste dumping, prevention of marine pollution, and protection of endangered species and biodiversity to protect well-being of both humans and living environment. However, although these environmental goals, pledges, targets, protocols, and treaties are noble in nature, implementation of conventions, policies, and actions is not necessarily effective. National political commitments might affect success of these global efforts (see Case Box 6.15). In recent years, there appears to be 'treaty congestion' in which the number of international instruments has hindered implementation of these treaties (Anton, 2013).

Case Box 6.15 False Promises? Climate Action

Some famous climate action agreements resulted from the Framework Convention on Climate Change include the Kyoto Protocol and the Paris Agreement. The difference between the two treaties is that the Kyoto Protocol that sets carbon reduction targets is legally binding for developed countries, but not developing countries. The reduction targets were only 15% of total emissions worldwide, and many countries opted out of the Protocol since they could not achieve their targets and did not intend to pay the fines. The Paris Agreement does not group Member States according to their development status. All 195 nations have voluntary pledged to reduce emissions and self-declare how much they reduce.

Kyoto Protocol

The Kyoto Protocol is a multilateral agreement signed in 1997 aimed at reducing global warming by limiting greenhouse gas emissions, requiring developed countries to reduce the greenhouse gas emissions to 94.8% of their 1990 levels. These helped frame

Case Box 6.15 False Promises? Climate Action *(continued)*

the way for countries to develop their own policies and measurements. There were four methods the Protocol allowed to help achieve reduction targets:

- Emissions trading: a market-based approach to controlling pollution by providing economic incentives for achieving reduction in emissions. A central authority sells a limited number of permits to discharge specific quantities of a specific pollutant over a specific time. Countries can trade units if they run out.

- Net emission: amount of carbon dioxide taken up by forests being deducted from the total amount emitted.

- Clean development mechanism: any emissions reduced by developed countries to help developing countries reduce greenhouse gases being deductable from developing countries' emissions limits.

- Joint implementation: European Union Member States treated as a single unit so countries can work with others to help reduce emissions levels.

The Kyoto Protocol ultimately failed when its two largest carbon dioxide emitters, the United States and Canada, withdrew.

Paris Agreement

The Paris Agreement, designed to address the Kyoto Protocol's flaws, was signed in 2015 and is a universal legally binding global climate deal, trying to limit global warming to below 2 °C. Using a broader framework, 195 governments agreed to reduce emissions, ensure transparency in reporting, are accountable to each other, support developing countries, and strengthen societies' ability to deal with the impacts of climate change (United Nations Framework Convention on Climate Change [UNFCCC], 2018).

United States withdrawal from Paris Agreement

In 2017, President Trump pulled the United States out of the Paris Agreement, stating it would lead to a loss of millions of jobs and damage the economy. While the United States is no longer in the Paris Agreement, many think the Agreement will still succeed: people are beginning to grasp the dangers posed by climate change. The United States as a whole will not participate, but many states and companies have voiced their opinions and will independently reduce their emissions (White House, 2017).

Source: UNFCCC (2018).

Conclusion

The World Health Organization (WHO) defines environment, as it relates to health, as all the physical, chemical, and biological factors external to a person, and all the related behaviours that may influence human health outcomes. This chapter describes the key concepts and issues related to environmental health. Fundamentally, for environmental health protection, stakeholders must address various factors that increase health risks and the likelihood of exposure and disease.

References

Andrady, A. L. (2011). Microplastics in the marine environment. *Mar Pollut Bull 62*(8) 1596–605.

Anton, D. K. (2013). 'Treaty congestion' in international environmental law. In S. Alam, J. H. Bhuiyan, T. M. R. Chowdhury, and E. J. Techera (eds), *Routledge Handbook of International Environmental Law*. Abingdon: Routledge, pp. 651–66.

Bearer, C. F. (1995). Environmental health hazards: How children are different from adults. *Future Child 5*(2) 11–26.

Benn, C. R. and **Ellison, S. L.** (1998). Brightness of the night sky over La Palma. *New Astron Rev 42* 503–7.

Bolton, P. and Burkle, F. M. (2013). Emergency response. In C. Guest, W. Ricciardi, I. Kawachi, and I. Lang (eds), *Oxford Handbook of Public Health Practice* (3rd edn). Oxford: Oxford University Press.

Boyce, J. M., Pittet, D., Healthcare Infection Control Practices Advisory Committee, and HICPAC/ SHEA/APIC/IDSA Hand Hygiene Task Force (2002). Guideline for hand hygiene in health-care settings: Recommendations of the Healthcare Infection Control Practices Advisory Committee and the HICPAC/SHEA/APIC/IDSA Hand Hygiene Task Force. *Morb Mortal Wkly Rep 51*(RR-16) 1–45.

Busby, A. (2016). Waste. In E. Hutchinson and S. Kovats (Eds.), *Environment, Health and Sustainable Development* (2nd edn). London: Open University Press, McGraw-Hill Education.

Centers for Disease Control and Prevention (2017a). Basic facts: Molds in the environment. Available at: http://www.cdc.gov/mold/faqs.htm.

Centers for Disease Control and Prevention (2017b). *CDC Yellow Book 2018: Health Information for International Travel*. New York, NY: Oxford University Press.

Centers for Disease Control and Prevention (2017c). Children's Environmental Health. Available at: https://ephtracking.cdc.gov/showChildEHMain.action.

Centers for Disease Control and Prevention (2018a). Air quality. Available at: https://www.cdc.gov/air/default.htm.

Centers for Disease Control and Prevention (2018b). Air quality resources for professionals. Available at: https://www.cdc.gov/air/resources.htm.

Chan, E. Y. Y. (2018). *Building Bottom-Up Health and Disaster Risk Reduction Programmes*. Oxford: Oxford University Press.

Chan, E. Y. Y., Gao, Y., Li, L., and Lee, P.Y. (2017). Injuries caused by pets in Asian urban households: a cross-sectional telephone survey. *BMJ Open 7*(1):e012813.

Chan, E. Y. Y., Goggins, W. B., Kim, J. J., and **Griffiths, S. M.** (2012). A study of intracity variation of temperature-related mortality and socioeconomic status among the Chinese population in Hong Kong. *J Epidemiol Community Health 66*(4) 322–7.

Chan, E. Y. Y., Goggins, W. B., Yue, J. S. K., and **Lee, P.** (2013). Hospital admissions as a function of temperature, other weather phenomena and pollution levels in an urban setting in China. *Bull World Health Organ 91*(8) 576–84.

Chan, E. Y. Y. and Ho. J. Y. (2019). Urban water and health issues in Hong Kong. In B. Ray and R. Shaw (des), *Urban Drought*. Singapore: Springer.

Chan, E. Y. Y., Kim, J. H., Griffiths, S. M., Lau, J. T., and **Yu, I.** (2009). Does living density matter for nonfatal unintentional home injury in Asian urban settings? Evidence from Hong Kong. *J Urban Health 86*(6) 872–86. doi: 10.1007/s11524-009-9389-9

Chan, E. Y. Y., Wang, Z., Mark, C. K. M., and Liu, S. D. (2015). Industrial accidents in China: risk reduction and response. *Lancet* [Internet] *386*(10002) 1421–1422. doi:10.1016/S0140-6736(15)00424-9

Chan, K. H., Kurmi, O., Bennett, D., Yang, L., Chen, Y., Tan, et al. (2018). Solid fuel use and risks of respiratory diseases: A cohort study of 280,000 Chinese never-smokers. *Am J Respir Crit Care Med* *199*(3) 352–361. doi:10.1164/rccm.201803-0432OC

Chan, T. C., Zhang, Z., Lin, B. C., Lin, C., Deng, H. B., et al. (2018). Long-term exposure to ambient fine particulate matter and chronic kidney disease: A cohort study. *Environ Health Perspec 126* (10) 107002.

Chernobyl Forum (2005). Chernobyl's legacy: Health, environmental and socio-economic impacts and recommendations to the Governments of Belarus, the Russian Federation and Ukraine. International Atomic Energy Agency. Available at: https://web.archive.org/web/20100215212227/http://www.iaea.org/Publications/Booklets/Chernobyl/chernobyl.pdf.

Cherrie, J. W., Apsley, A., Cowie, H., Steinle, S., Mueller, W., et al. (2018). Effectiveness of face masks used to protect Beijing residents against particulate air pollution. *Occup Environ Med 75* 446–52.

Denchak, M. (2018). Water pollution: Everything you need to know. Available at: https://www.nrdc.org/stories/water-pollution-everything-you-need-know.

Ellen MacArthur Foundation, World Economic Forum, and McKinsey Center for Business and Environment (2016). The new plastics economy—Rethinking the future of plastics. Available at: http://www3.weforum.org/docs/WEF_The_New_Plastics_Economy.pdf.

Environmental Protection Agency (2014). Air quality index: A guide to air quality and your health. Available at: https://www3.epa.gov/airnow/aqi_brochure_02_14.pdf.

Environmental Protection Agency (2016). Heat island impacts. Available at: https://www.epa.gov/heat-islands/heat-island-impacts.

Environmental Protection Agency (2018a). Learn about lead. Available at: https://www.epa.gov/lead/learn-about-lead.

Environmental Protection Agency (2018b). How BenMAP-CE estimates the health and economic effects of air pollution. Available at: http://www.epa.gov/benmap/how-benmap-ce-estimates-health-and-economic-effects-air-pollution.

Environmental Protection Agency (2018c). Ground-level ozone basics. Available at: https://www.epa.gov/ozone-pollution.

Environmental Protection Agency (2018d). Minamata convention on mercury. Available at: http://www.epa.gov/international-cooperation/minamata-convention-mercury.

Environmental Protection Agency (2018e). Report on the environment: Contaminated land. Available at: https://www.epa.gov/report-environment/contaminated-land.

Environmental Protection Department of the Government of the Hong Kong Special Administrative Region (n.d.-b). Waste. Available at: https://www.epd.gov.hk/epd/english/environmentinhk/waste/waste_maincontent.html.

Environmental Protection Department of the Government of the Hong Kong Special Administrative Region (2016). *Noise*. Available at: http://www.epd.gov.hk/epd/english/environmentinhk/noise/noise_maincontent.html.

ENVIS Centre on Control of Pollution Water, Air, Noise (2016). Air pollution & control. Available at: http://www.cpcbenvis.nic.in/air_pollution_control.html.

European Commission (2017). Protection of the ozone layer. Available at: http://www.c.europa.eu/clima/policies/ozone_en.

Fisk, W. J., Lei-Gomez, Q., and Mendell, M. J. (2007). Meta-analysis of the associations of respiratory health effects with dampness and mould in home. *Indoor Air 17*(4) 284–96.

Franchin, M., Rial, M., Buiatti, E., and Biachi, F. (2004). Health effects of exposure to waste incinerator emissions: A review of epidemiological studies. *Annali dell'lstituto Superiore di Sanita 40*(1) 101–15.

Gall, E. T., Carter, E. M., Earnest, C. M., and Stephens, B. (2013). Indoor air pollution in developing countries: Research and implementation needs for improvements in global public health. *Am J Public Health 103*(4) e67–72.

Geyer, R., Jambeck, J., and Law, K. L. (2017). Production, use, and fate of all plastics ever made. *Sci Adv 3*(7) e1700782.

Gordon, S. B., Bruce, N. G., Grigg, J., Hibberd, P. L., Kurmi, O. P., et al. (2014). Respiratory risks from household air pollution in low and middle income countries. *Lancet Respir Med 2*(10) 823–60. doi:10.1016/s2213-2600(14)70168-7.

Green Facts (2018). Chernobyl nuclear accident. Available at: http://www.greenfacts.org/en/chernobyl/l-2/3-chernobyl-environment.htm.

Greenpeace (2016a). Fukushima nuclear disaster will impact forests, rivers and estuaries for hundreds of years, warns Greenpeace report. Available at: http://www.greenpeace.org/archive-international/en/press/releases/2016/Fukushima-nuclear-disaster-will-impact-forests-rivers-and-estuaries-for-hundreds-of-years-warns-Greenpeace-report-/.

Greenpeace (2016b). Radiation reloaded. Available at: https://www.greenpeace.org/archive-japan/ja/library/publication/20160304_report/.

Grosse, S. D., Matte, T. D., Schwartz, J., and Jackson, R. J. (2002). Economic gains resulting from the reduction in children's exposure to lead in the United States. *Environ Health Perspect 110*(6) 563–9. doi: 10.1289/ehp.02110563.

Guo, C., Zhang, Z., Lau, A. K. H., Lin, C. Q., Chuang, Y. C., et al. (2018). Effect of long-term exposure to fine particulate matter on lung function decline and risk of chronic obstructive pulmonary disease in Taiwan: A longitudinal, cohort study. *Lancet Planetary Health 2*(3): e114–e125.

Harvard Health Letter (2015). Blue light has a dark side. Available at: http://www.health.harvard.edu/staying-healthy/blue-light-has-a-dark-side.

Hong Kong Observatory (2016). Urbanization effect. Available at: https://www.hko.gov.hk/climate_change/urbanization_e.htm.

Hopewell, J., Dvorak, R., and Kosior, E. (2009). Plastics recycling: Challenges and opportunities. *Philos Trans R Soc B Biol Sci 364*(1526) 2115–26.

Integrated Environmental Health Impact Assessment System (n.d.-a). The causal chain. Available at: http://www.integrated-assessment.eu/eu/indexeba5.html?q=guidebook/causal_chain.

Integrated Environmental Health Impact Assessment System (n.d.-b). The DPSEEA framework. Available at: http://www.integrated-assessment.eu/eu/index7544.html?q=guidebook/dpseea_framework.

International Labour Organization (n.d.). International labour standards on occupational safety and health. Available at: https://www.ilo.org/global/standards/subjects-covered-by-international-labour-standards/occupational-safety-and-health/lang--en/index.htm.

Janssen, S., Solomon, G., and Schettler, T. (2011). Toxicant and disease database. Available at: https://www.healthandenvironment.org/our-work/toxicant-and-disease-database/.

Kjellén, M. (2001). Health and environment. Available at: https://www.sida.se/contentassets/f878f9d4943e4e1c97f6d6f62edff9d2/20012-health-and-environment.-issue-paper_641.pdf.

Kopits, E. and Cropper, M. (2005). Traffic fatalities and economic growth. *Accid Anal Prev 37*(1) 169–78.

Lau, S. Y., Ng, K. L., Tsang, H. T., and Vong, Y. C. C. (2014). Light pollution in Hong Kong (Outstanding Academic Papers by Students (OAPS)). Available at: http://lbms03.cityu.edu.hk/oaps/ef2014-1205-lsy694.pdf.

Lockwood, A. H., Welker-Hood, K., Rauch, M., and Gottlieb, B. (2009) Coal's assault on human health: A report from physicians for social responsibility. Available at: https://www.psr.org/wp-content/uploads/2018/05/coals-assault-on-human-health.pdf.

London Borough of Bexley (n.d.). Contaminated Land. Available at: https://www.bexley.gov.uk/services/environmental-issues/contaminated-land.

Martens P. and McMichael A. J. (eds). (2009). *Environmental Change, Climate and Health: Issues and Research Methods*. Cambridge: Cambridge University Press.

Mcgarry, S. L., Balsari, S., Muqueeth, S., and Leaning, J. (2017). Preventing the preventable: The 2015 Tianjin explosions. Available at: http://www.hkjcdpri.org.hk/download/casestudies/Tianjin_CASE.pdf.

Michaels, C., Simpson, J. L., and Wegner, W. (2010). Fractured communities: Case studies of the environmental impacts of industrial gas drilling. Available at: https://www.riverkeeper.org/wp-content/uploads/2010/09/Fractured-Communities-FINAL-September-2010.pdf.

Milner, J. and Hutchinson, E. (2016). Housing and indoor environment. In E. Hutchinson and S. Kovats (eds), *Environment, Health and Sustainable Development* (2nd edn). London: Open University Press, McGraw-Hill Education.

Moeller, D. W. (2005). *Environmental Health* (3rd edn). Cambridge: Cambridge University Press.

National Environmental Health Association (2016). Investing in an effective environmental health system. Available at: https://www.neha.org/sites/default/files/about/Investing%20in%20an%20Effective%20Environmental%20Health%20System_FINAL.pdf.

Nishijo, M., Nakagawa, H., Suwazono, Y., Nogawa, K., and Kido, T. (2017). Causes of death in patients with Itai-itai disease suffering from severe chronic cadmium poisoning: A nested case–control analysis of a follow-up study in Japan. *Br Med J Open 7*(7) e015694. doi: 10.1136/bmjopen-2016-015694.

North, E. J. and Halden, R. U. (2013). Plastics and environmental health: The road ahead. *Rev Environ Health 28*(1) 1–8.

Office of Disease Prevention and Health Promotion (n.d.). Healthy People 2020: Environmental health: Objectives. Available at: https://www.healthypeople.gov/2020/topics-objectives/topic/environmental-health/objectives.

Pampel, F. C., Krueger, P. M., and Denney, J. T. (2010). Socioeconomic disparities in health behaviors. *Ann Rev Sociol 36* 349–70.

Pitta, T. (2015). *Catastrophe: A Guide to World's Worst Industrial Disasters*. New Delhi: Vij Books India Pvt Ltd.

Plastic Pollution Coalition (2018). Why is plastic harmful [online]? Available at: https://plasticpollutioncoalition.zendesk.com/hc/en-us/articles/222813127-Why-is-plastic-harmful-.

Prüss-Üstün, A., Bos, R., Gore, F., and Bartram, J. (2008). Safer water, better health: Costs, benefits and sustainability of interventions to protect and promote health. Available at: http://apps.who.int/iris/bitstream/handle/10665/43840/9789241596435_eng.pdf?sequence=1.

Prüss-Üstün, A., Vickers, C., Haefliger, P., and Bertollini, R. (2011). Knowns and unknowns on burden of disease due to chemicals: a systematic review. *Environ Health 10*(9). doi: 10.1186/1476-069x-10-9.

Prüss-Üstün, A., Wolf, A., Corvalán, C., Bos, R., and Neira, M. (2016). Preventing disease through healthy environments: A global assessment of the burden of disease from environmental risks. Available at: http://apps.who.int/iris/bitstream/handle/10665/204585/9789241565196_eng.pdf?sequence=1.

Pun, C. S. J., So, C. W., Leung, W. Y., and Wong, C. F. (2014). Contributions of artificial lighting sources on light pollution in Hong Kong measured through a night sky brightness monitoring network. *J Quant Spectrosc Ra 139* 90–108. doi: 10.1016/j.jqsrt.2013.12.014.

Recio, A. Linares, C., Banegas, J. R., and Diaz, J. (2016). Road traffic noise effects on cardiovascular, respiratory, and metabolic health: An integrative model of biological mechanisms. *Environ Res 146* 359–70.

Reconstruction Agency (2016). Great East Japan Earthquake. Available at: http://www.reconstruction. go.jp/english/topics/GEJE/index.html

Ritchie, H. and Roser, M. (2018). Plastic pollution [Online image]. Available at: https://ourworldindata. org/plastic-pollution.

Schrör, H. (2011). Generation and treatment of waste in Europe 2008: Steady reduction in waste going to landfills. Available at: http://edz.bib.uni-mannheim.de/edz/pdf/statinf/11/KS-SF-11-044-EN.PDF.

Schweihofer, J. and Wells, S. (2013). Biological, chemical and physical hazards assessed with HACCP. Available at: https://www.canr.msu.edu/news/biological_chemical_and_physical_hazards_assessed_with_haccp.

Seidler, A., Wagner, M., Schubert, M., Dröge, P., Pons-Kühnemann, J., et al. (2016). Myocardial infarction risk due to aircraft, road, and rail traffic noise. *Deutsches Ärzteblatt International 113*(24) 407–14.

Shah, H. N. and Rallapali, R. (2013). Fukushima Daiichi - 2011: Nuclear disaster: Lessons learned: Where we stand in India. *Int J Health Syst Disaster Manag 1*(3).

Shaw, R. and Thaitakoo, D. (2010). Water communities: Introduction and overview. In R. Shaw and D. Thaitakoo (Eds). *Water Communities* (Community, Environment and Disaster Risk Management series Vol. 2, 1–13). Bingley, England: Emerald Publishing.

Smith, K. R., Corvalan, C. F., and Kjellstorm, T. (1999). How much global ill health is attributable to environmental factors? *Epidemiology 10*(5) 573–84.

Sphere (2011). The Sphere Project: Humanitarian charter and minimum standards in humanitarian response (3rd edn). Available at: https://www.spherestandards.org/wp-content/uploads/2018/06/Sphere_Handbook_2011_English.pdf.

Sphere (2018). The Sphere Handbook: Humanitarian charter and minimum standards in humanitarian response (4th edn). Available at: https://www.spherestandards.org/.

Straif, K., Cohen, A., and Samet, J. (Eds). (2013). *Air Pollution and Cancer* (IARC Scientific Publications No. 161). Lyon, France: International Agency for Research on Cancer, World Health Organization.

Thompson, R. C., Moore, C. J., vom Saal, F. S., and Swan, S. H. (2009). Plastics, the environment and human health: current consensus and future trends. *Philos Trans R Soc B Biol Sci 364*(1526) 2153–66.

Tonne, C. and Scovronick, N. (2016). Outdoor air pollution and road transport. In E. Hutchinson and S. Kovats (eds), *Environment, Health and Sustainable Development* (2nd edn). London: Open University Press, McGraw-Hill Education.

Tse, L. A., Yu, T. S. I., Qiu, H., Au, J. S., and Wang, X. R. (2011). A case-referent study of lung cancer and incense smoke, smoking, and residential radon in Chinese men. *Environ Health Perspect 119*(11) 1641–6.

Tse, L. A., Yu, T. S. I., Qiu, H., Au, J. S., and Wang, X. R. (2012). Occupational risks and lung cancer burden for Chinese men: A population-based case-referent study. *Cancer Causes Control 23*(1) 121–31.

Tse, L. A., Yu, T. S. I., Qiu, H., Au, J. S., Yu, K. S., et al. (2009). Environmental tobacco smoke and lung cancer among Chinese nonsmoking males: Might adenocarcinoma be the culprit? *Am J Epidemiol, 169*(5) 533–41.

United Kingdom Ministry of Housing, Communities & Local Government (2019). Guidance: Environmental Impact Assessment. Available at: https://www.gov.uk/guidance/environmental-impact-assessment.

United Nations Framework Convention on Climate Change (2018). The Paris Agreement. Available at: https://unfccc.int/process-and-meetings/the-paris-agreement/the-paris-agreement.

UN-HABITAT (2010). *Solid Waste Management in World's Cities: Water and Sanitation in the World's Cities 2010*. London: Earthscan.

United Nations Development Programme (2006). Human development report 2006: Beyond scarcity: Power, poverty and the global water crisis. Available at: http://www.undp.org/content/dam/undp/library/corporate/HDR/2006%20Global%20HDR/HDR-2006-Beyond%20scarcity-Power-poverty-and-the-global-water-crisis.pdf.

United Nations Population Fund (2003). Population and poverty: Achieving equity, equality and sustainability. Available at: https://www.unfpa.org/sites/default/files/pub-pdf/population_poverty.pdf.

United Nations World Assessment Programme (2015). The United Nations world water development report 2015: Water for a sustainable world. Available at: http://www.unesco.org/new/fileadmin/MULTIMEDIA/HQ/SC/images/WWDR2015_03.pdf.

University of Washington (2005). What is environmental health? A student introduction. Available at: https://depts.washington.edu/ceeh/downloads/Intro_to_EH_slideset.pdf.

von Schirnding, Y. (2002). Health in sustainable development planning: The role of indicators. Available at: http://apps.who.int/iris/bitstream/handle/10665/67391/WHO_HDE_HID_02.11.pdf?sequence=1&isAllowed=y.

Vrijheid, M. (2000). Health effects of residence near hazardous waste landfill sites: A review of epidemiologic literature. *Environ Health Perspect 108*(suppl.1) 101–12.

WaterAid, The Water Supply and Sanitation Collaborative Council, and Domestos (2013). We can't wait: A report on sanitation and hygiene for women and girls. Available at: https://www.unilever.com/Images/we-can-t-wait---a-report-on-sanitation-and-hygiene-for-women-and-girls--november-2013_tcm244-425178_1_en.pdf.

White House (2017). Statement by President Trump on the Paris Climate Accord. Available at: http://www.whitehouse.gov/briefings-statements/statement-president-trump-paris-climate-accord/.

Wilkinson, P., Smith, K. R., Joffe, M., and Haines, A. (2007). A global perspective on energy: Health effects and injustices. *Lancet 370* 965–78.

Wilson, D. C., Rodic, L., Modak, P., Soos, R., Rogero, A. C., et al. (2015). Global waste management outlook. Available at: http://www.greenreport.it/wp-content/uploads/2015/09/Global-Waste-Management-Outlook-2015.pdf.

World Health Organization (n.d.-a). Environmental health. Available at: http://www.searo.who.int/topics/environmental_health/en/.

World Health Organization (n.d.-b). PHE infographics: Protecting the children from the environment. Available at: http://www.who.int/phe/infographics/protecting-children-from-the-environment/en/.

World Health Organization (n.d.-c). Noise. Available at: http://www.who.int/sustainable-development/transport/health-risks/noise/en/.

World Health Organization (n.d.-d). Environmental radiation. Available at: http://www.who.int/ionizing_radiation/env/en/.

World Health Organization (n.d.-e). Occupational health. Available at: https://www.who.int/topics/occupational_health/en/.

World Health Organization (2003). Domestic water quantity, service level and health. Available at: https://www.who.int/water_sanitation_health/publications/wsh0302/en/.

World Health Organization (2004). Guidelines for drinking-water quality (3rd edn). Available at: https://www.who.int/water_sanitation_health/dwq/GDW9rev1and2.pdf.

World Health Organization (2005). Chernobyl: The true scale of the accident. Available at: https://www.who.int/mediacentre/news/releases/2005/pr38/en/.

World Health Organization (2010). Ten chemicals of major public health concern. Available at: http://www.who.int/ipcs/assessment/public_health/chemicals_phc/en/.

World Health Organization (April 2011). Chernobyl at 25th anniversary: Frequently asked questions. Available at: https://www.who.int/ionizing_radiation/chernobyl/20110423_FAQs_Chernobyl.pdf.

World Health Organization (2016a). Radon and health. Available at: http://www.who.int/mediacentre/factsheets/fs291/en/.

World Health Organization (2016b). Burning opportunity: Clean household energy for health, sustainable development, and wellbeing of women and children. Available at: http://apps.who.int/iris/bitstream/handle/10665/204717/9789241565233_eng.pdf?sequence=1.

World Health Organization (2016c). The public health impact of chemicals: Knowns and unknowns. Available at: http://apps.who.int/iris/bitstream/handle/10665/206553/WHO_FWC_PHE_EPE_16.01_eng.pdf?sequence=1.

World Health Organization (2016d). Ionizing radiation, health effects and protective measures. Available at: https://www.who.int/news-room/fact-sheets/detail/ionizing-radiation-health-effects-and-protective-measures.

World Health Organization (2017a). Guidelines for drinking-water quality (4th edn, incorporating the 1st addendum). Available at: https://apps.who.int/iris/bitstream/handle/10665/254637/9789241549950-eng.pdf;jsessionid=CB4858822EC2419ED04E59FD4106111B?sequence=1.

World Health Organization (2017b). Mercury and health. Available at: https://www.who.int/news-room/fact-sheets/detail/mercury-and-health.

World Health Organization (2018a). Guidelines on sanitation and health. Available at: http://apps.who.int/iris/bitstream/handle/10665/274939/9789241514705-eng.pdf?ua=1.

World Health Organization (2018b). Drinking-water. Available at: https://www.who.int/en/news-room/fact-sheets/detail/drinking-water.

World Health Organization (2018c). Air pollution: Air pollution and health. Available at: http://www.who.int/airpollution/en/.

World Health Organization (2018d). Ambient air pollution: Pollutants. Available at: http://www.who.int/airpollution/ambient/pollutants/en/.

World Health Organization (2018e). 9 out of 10 people worldwide breathe polluted air, but more countries are taking action. Available at: https://www.who.int/news-room/detail/02-05-2018-9-out-of-10-people-worldwide-breathe-polluted-air-but-more-countries-are-taking-action.

World Health Organization (2018f). Household air pollution: Health impacts. Available at: https://www.who.int/airpollution/household/health-impacts/en/.

World Health Organization (2018g). Public health, environmental and social determinants of health (PHE): PHE infographics: Air pollution. Available at: https://www.who.int/phe/infographics/air-pollution/en/.

World Health Organization (2018h). Ambient (outdoor) air quality and health. Available at: http://www.who.int/en/news-room/fact-sheets/detail/ambient-(outdoor)-air-quality-and-health.

World Health Organization (2018i). Arsenic. Available at: https://www.who.int/en/news-room/fact-sheets/detail/arsenic.

World Health Organization (2018j). Asbestos: Elimination of asbestos-related diseases. Available at: https://www.who.int/news-room/fact-sheets/detail/asbestos-elimination-of-asbestos-related-diseases.

World Health Organization Regional Office for Europe (2009). Night noise guidelines for Europe. Available at: http://www.euro.who.int/__data/assets/pdf_file/0017/43316/E92845.pdf.

World Health Organization Regional Office for Europe (2010). WHO guidelines for indoor air quality: Selected pollutants. Available at: http://www.euro.who.int/__data/assets/pdf_file/0009/128169/e94535.pdf.

World Health Organization and United Nations Children's Fund (2017). Progress on drinking water, sanitation and hygiene: 2017 update and SDG baselines. Available at: https://www.who.int/mediacentre/news/releases/2017/launch-version-report-jmp-water-sanitation-hygiene.pdf.

World Nuclear Association (April 2018). Chernobyl accident 1986. Available at: http://www.world-nuclear.org/information-library/safety-and-security/safety-of-plants/chernobyl-accident.aspx.

World Nuclear Association (October 2018). Fukushima Daiichi accident. Available at: http://www.world-nuclear.org/information-library/safety-and-security/safety-of-plants/fukushima-accident.aspx.

Yu, K., Qiu, G., Chan, K. H., Lam, K. H., Kurmi, O. P., et al. (2018). Association of solid fuel use with risk of cardiovascular and all-cause mortality in rural China. *JAMA 319*(13) 1351–61. doi:10.1001/jama.2018.2151.

Zhang, Z., Chang, L. Y., Lau, A. K. H., Chan, T. C., Chuang, Y. C., et al. (2017). Satellite-based estimates of long-term exposure to fine particulate matter are associated with C-reactive protein in 30034 Taiwanese adults. *Int J Epidemiol 46* 1126–36.

Zhang, Z., Chan, T. C., Guo, C., Chang, L. Y., Lin, C., et al. (2018). Long-term exposure to ambient particulate matter ($PM_{2.5}$) is associated with platelet counts in adults. *Environ Pollut 240* 432–9.

Zhang, Z., Guo, C., Lau, A. K. H., Chan, T. C., Chuang, Y. C., et al. (2018). Long-term exposure to fine particulate matter, blood pressure, and incident hypertension in Taiwanese adults. *Environ Health Perspect 126*(1) 017008.

Zhang, J. and **Mu Q.** (2017). Air pollution and defensive expenditures: Evidence from particulate-filtering facemasks. *J Environ Econ Manag 92* 517–36. doi:10.1016/j.jeem.2017.07.006.

Chapter 7

Planetary Health and Sustainability

Human environment has undergone substantial changes during the past few decades and as a result, health risks change with context and time. The ability to protect health of a population might be subject to the understanding of health risks and approaches to manage and safeguard the well-being of the potentially at-risk community. Although the previous chapters have highlighted various traditional health protection subject domains that help examine human health protections, the mostly human-focused conceptual frameworks might be inadequate to address the current health risks. Globalization of trade, travel, and culture is likely to bring bi-directional impacts on health. Increased trade and international exchange of products may improve material access and services, but may also bring harm to health and the environment. Travel and human migration enrich human experiences but exacerbate health threats such as the rapid dissemination of communicable diseases. Increased frequency of incidents of food safety in agricultural and livestock management as a result of technology use and ineffective regulation of the safety of food production (e.g. use of chemical substances and additives) has led to a number of serious human health outcomes.

This chapter will discuss a few concepts that attempt to expand the current health protection concepts and bridge traditional public health subject disciplines to include multidisciplinary actors and other related frameworks. Specifically, the concepts of "One Health", "planetary health", and "sustainable development" may support the conceptualization of human well-being together with other living organisms and its living ecosystem. It also explains how health protection might be linked to some important global policies such as Sustainable Development Goals and the New Urban Agenda. These ideas may help inform health protection practices and policy development to protect human health in the decades to come.

Survival of living creatures on Earth depends on and is affected by the complex interaction within its biosphere. With industrialization, urbanization, climate change, and globalization, the complex geophysical and ecological systems have changed drastically in recent decades. Predicting future living context based on historical patterns and trends may no longer be accurate for understanding health risks and hazards.

Global environmental changes

With the exponential increase in population, demands on energy supply, emission-intense economic activities, and rates of harmful waste generation, it is uncertain if the carrying capacity of Earth may be able to support future consumption patterns. Global

Essentials for Health Protection. Emily Ying Yang Chan, Oxford University Press (2020).
© Oxford University Press
DOI: 10.1093/oso/9780198835479.001.0001

environmental changes (GECs) are a range of ecological changes occurring in living environment, which are associated with both natural and man-made factors (McMichael, 2005). Some key GECs include: (i) human-induced changes in atmosphere such as greenhouse gas accumulation, which lead to climate change (see Chapter 3), and stratosphere ozone depletion (see Chapter 6); (ii) changes in global elemental cycles (e.g. carbon, nitrogen, phosphorus, and sulphur); (iii) changes in the hydrological cycle that might affect fresh water supply; (iv) changes in food production ecosystems that alter land use, soil fertility, agricultural and livestock production, coastal and marine ecosystem (e.g. due to over-fishing), etc.; (v) desertification; (vi) loss of biodiversity; (vii) pollution by persistent organic pollutants (POP); and (viii) urbanization that exacerbate pollution, waste production, and pressure on micro-ecosystems. All these GECs will have exerted their influences on the health and well-being of the living community.

Depending on hazards (e.g. microbiological and toxicological), some of these environmental changes not only affect immediate well-being, but also they might have catastrophic long-term impacts on human health. For instance, the use of hormones, antibiotics, and additives in livestock and agriculture for food production might have long-term effects to health outcomes that have yet to be exhibited. The health impact might be direct through consumption (e.g. poisonous and leading to various levels of direct physiological process) or indirect (e.g. socio-economically, causing loss of livelihood due to the disappearance of living ecosystems).

Contaminations of soil and water are important global environmental changes that affect sustainability and health in the twenty-first century. **Soil pollution** might result from contamination by urban and industrial wastes. Poor waste management (e.g. illegal disposal and lax disposal policies), unintended contamination (e.g. application of persistent organic pollutants such as DDT and TCDD dioxins, which are carcinogenic), and industry-polluted grounds (i.e. 'brownfields') are examples of land pollution that threaten the health and well-being of humans and animals. In addition, contamination of freshwater, surface water, and groundwater sources (as described in Chapter 6) also affect human well-being. Chemical, biological, and thermal discharges from sewage disposal can pollute ocean life forms. Suboptimal management of agricultural (e.g. pesticides and fertilizers) and industrial wastes will also pollute lakes, rivers, and oceans. Contaminated ocean can become breeding grounds for infectious diseases (e.g. cholera, hepatitis, and salmonella), which exact severe human health toll. Contamination of beaches by sewage overflows can cause disease outbreaks (Dorfman and Rosselot, 2011). Thermal discharges (i.e. heated water) from power stations also affect ecosystems and well-being of living organisms.

Human activities have also led to **land degradation, deforestation**, and **changes to the oceans**. The conversion of forest for agricultural, transport, mining, and urban uses changes a habitat's ecological system for both human and living creatures. Mismatch of land use can cause land degradation and challenge food production. Desertification can also lead to the loss of habitat and livelihood. Especially in developing nations, such impacts may lead to major nutritional and food insecurity and subsequently, health crisis.

Human consumption patterns have led to various forms of land pollution (e.g. metal pollution of river from mining, forest fires for clearing forests that lead to air pollution, and freshwater contamination), communicable disease transmission (e.g. malaria due to proliferation of mosquitoes as a result of favourable context of stagnant water, temperature, and humidity for increased transmission of vector-borne diseases), and the loss of biodiversity (see Case Box 7.3). Numerous potential medicinal resources (e.g. taxol for the treatment for breast and ovarian cancers, vinblastine and vincristine for leukaemia and lymphoma, and prostratin for HIV/AIDS management) that are derived from forests may be lost due to the destruction of these forests.

Marine resources are being depleted as a result of overconsumption by commercial fishing operations. Climate change-related ocean warming leads to harmful algal bloom (HAB) outbreaks that cause fish and shellfish poisoning. In addition, **climate change** threatens the availability of freshwater and food supply, natural disaster increase, the proliferation of infectious diseases, sea-level rise, alternation of precipitation patterns, and increased frequency of extreme climate events. These phenomena often impinge particularly harshly upon the least developed countries (see Chapter 3 on climate change).

One Health

In recent decades, a number of global public health incidents have revealed the emergence of a plethora of the health risks converging on human, animal, and environmental health. Many lethal human diseases such as bovine spongiform encephalopathy (BSE), severe acute respiratory syndrome (SARS), H5N1 influenza, Ebola, West Nile virus infection, Middle East respiratory syndrome (MERS), and Zika virus infection demonstrate the intimate links and relationship between human and other animals (see Chapter 5). Case Box 7.1 discusses the increasing incidence of zoonotic diseases.

Although One Health is not a new concept, it has only started to receive more attention in recent years. The concept of zoonotic diseases (i.e. diseases that are transmitted

Case Box 7.1 Zoonotic Diseases

Zoonotic diseases are infectious diseases that can be shared between animals and humans. They are examples to illustrate how human health may be associated with animal health and the environment. Some notable examples include rabies, salmonella infection, West Nile virus fever, and Q fever (*Coxiella burnetti*). Animals also share humans' susceptibility to some diseases and environmental hazards. Monitoring animal well-being may thus provide early warning signals and reminders of potential related human illness. For example, West Nile virus-related avian deaths often occur before people get sick with West Nile virus fever.

from animals to humans), and social and environmental determinants of health are well recognized within the public health community (Frankson, Hueston, Christian, Olson, Lee, et al., 2016). Most research and clinical disease management for zoonotic diseases still adopts an approach which takes a human health management perspective. Education of health and medical professionals remains segregated between human health (human medicine, nursing, and public health), animal health (veterinary medicine and agriculture), and environmental health (ecology).

The One Health framework highlights that the health of humans is connected to the health of animals and the environment. As estimated, six out of every ten infectious diseases in humans are spread from animals (United States Centers for Disease Control and Prevention [US CDC], 2017, see Chapter 5). Globally, nearly 75% of all emerging human infectious diseases in the past three decades originated in animals. Many factors might be related to this epidemiological pattern, but One Health argues that the changes in **the interactions between people, animals, and the environment** have exacerbated health risks and disease manifestation in living world. Not only have these changes made disease control challenging but also the changing pattern of modern living, consumption, and production have led to the emergence and re-emergence of many diseases. Table 7.1 shows how human, animal, and environmental conditions affect each other.

Although critics of One Health argue that the concept is incomplete because it only focuses on animal and human health with only marginal interest in other living environments (e.g. plants and environment context), the framework creates interdisciplinary platforms that venture beyond human health. Its approach helps fill knowledge gaps by bridging the relationship among human, animal, and environmental communities.

Table 7.1 Human, Animal, and Environmental Interactions That Might Affect 'One Health'

Factor (Cause)	Change (Effect)
Human populations are growing and expanding into new geographic areas.	As a result, people live in closer contact with livestock and wild animals, which provides more opportunities for diseases to pass between animals and people.
The Earth has experienced changes in climate and natural resource use (e.g. land, water, forest, etc.).	Disruptions in environmental conditions and habitats provide new opportunities for diseases to pass to animals and eco-living system.
International travel and trade have increased.	As a result, diseases transmit more quickly and unexpectedly across the globe. Consumer food choice expands and diversifies. New food demand may put pressure on certain animal species (e.g. fish). Diseases also transmit among human and animal communities more readily.

Source: Adapted from US CDC (2018).

Conversely, human–animal interactions and bonds can have beneficial impacts on the health of both people and animals (Atlas and Maloy, 2014).

Effective One Health protection strategies are collaborative, multi-sectoral, and transdisciplinary. Physicians, veterinarians, ecologists, and many others to monitor and control public health threats and to learn about how diseases spread among people, animals, and the environment. Collaborative efforts of multidisciplinary experts such as physicians and veterinarians may be able to work across and beyond the current compartmentalized frameworks of animal, human, and environmental health. Health of people and animals, including pets, livestock, and wildlife, can all be improved. One Health argues that health and well-being may be improved through the prevention of risks and the mitigation of effects of crises that originate at the interface between humans, animals, and their various environments. The One Health framework helps to design and implement programmes, policies, legislation, and research that analyses the health of humans, animals, and the general environment as one entity and recognizes that their well-being determinants are mutually inclusive and relevant. Training, education, research, and policy formulation using a One Health approach may enable better information sharing in disease prevention, detection, and diagnosis. One Health research also encourages new therapies and approaches to treatment, which will benefit both human and animal health.

In addition to the control of zoonotic disease, the One Health approach is particularly relevant also to the control and the management of human health risks in areas such as food safety and combatting antibiotic resistance (when bacteria change after being exposed to antibiotics and become more difficult to treat). Many of the same microbes infect both animals and humans as they share eco-systems. Efforts by one sector alone cannot prevent or eliminate the problem. Information on influenza viruses circulating in animals is crucial to the selection of viruses for human vaccines for potential influenza pandemics. Rabies in humans is effectively prevented only by targeting the animal source of the virus (e.g. by vaccinating dogs). Drug-resistant microbes can be transmitted between animals and humans through direct contact between animals and humans or through contaminated food and so to contain it effectively, a well-coordinated approach in humans and in animals is required (Frankson et al., 2016).

Health protection and education initiatives might be more effective if the One Health approach is adopted. Case Box 7.2 discusses how technology-based health education initiatives based on the One Health concept might address a wide range of health issues (see Chapter 8 on technological transition). In addition, the One Health concept is also part of the sustainability discussion as it focuses on the interconnectedness of human, animal, and ecological health (Zinsstag, Schelling, Waltner-Toews, and Tanner, 2011).

Planetary health

Planetary health extends the traditional definition of health that focuses on individuals and populations to include the health and sustainability of human civilization and its supporting natural and man-made systems. During the past few centuries, human

Case Box 7.2 'Technological Interventions' for Promoting 'One Health Approach' to Enhance Rural Health Resilience

Carol Ka-po Wong and Emily Ying Yang Chan

Information and communications technology (ICT) may play a crucial role in supporting mHealth education training in the community. A mobile application that aims to enhance knowledge and promote self-help in health protection for health emergency disaster risk management (H-EDRM) in rural communities of China has been developed by the CCOUC since 2018. With this mobile app, community dwellers and key stakeholders (e.g. village doctors and teachers) living in remote communities can access health-related information and acquire training material through an health intervention app that contains health educational videos and mini-games.

The 'One Health' approach is used in health education content development to build a holistic health protection programme that addresses context reality and knowledge needs in rural area where humans and animals are living in close proximity. With modern changes and challenges in living standards, pathogens, pollutants, food safety, and waste management, multidisciplinary-based training materials will be needed to help at-risk population cope with all the human-induced disruptions to the environment. Cultural and language contexts, religion- and ethnicity-specific practices (such as spoken dialects, diet preference, and housing structures among different ethnic minority groups in China), as well as ease of use and data connectivity are also key consideration during the development of this mHealth tool.

Although the long-term utilization pattern and behavioural impact of such mobile tools in health protection are yet to be determined, technological advancement has heralded a major transformation in the health education, especially in rural and remote communities that traditionally might face barriers in access to information and materials, as well as constraints in technical capacity.

Sources: WHO (2011); Marcolino, Oliveira, D'Agostino, Ribeiro, Alkmim et al. (2018).

over-consumption patterns have led to natural system degradation, climate change, biodiversity loss, land degradation, water scarcity, and the deterioration of multiple other related systems essential to maintaining life (see Case Box 7.3 on biodiversity).

The field of **planetary health** highlights how human actions (e.g. pollution, exploitation of resources) and global environmental changes (e.g. loss of biodiversity and invasive plant and animal proliferation) are inter-related and interdependent for the sustainability of the Earth and its living creatures. From the perspective of planetary health, sustainability refers to the idea that the ecology system on the Earth is finite and the challenge to address its needs ever-increasing and expanding. The assumption is based on the current level of technology available and the ability of mankind to organize itself to address potential threats to its collective and individual well-being. The framework attempts to

Case Box 7.3 Biodiversity

Biological diversity, or 'biodiversity', refers to the variability among living organisms (both within and between species) and the ecological systems they comprise (United Nations, 1992). As a central determinant of ecosystem integrity, biodiversity is important for maintaining the structure of ecosystem services, including provision of food and water, clean air, disease and pest control, and both traditional and modern medicines. Biodiversity is linked both directly and indirectly to human health, with interactions occurring at the individual, community, landscape, and global scales. Human health is dependent on its environment and human activities have resulted in significant cause biodiversity losses across Asia.

Land clearing driven by rapid population growth, urbanization, industrialization, and associated demands for, and over-exploitation of, natural resources is a key driver of habitat destruction (World Health Organization [WHO], 2015). In South-East Asia, land clearing is driven particularly by high demands for palm oil, rubber, and wood pulp; charcoal production is another contributor, highlighting the urgent need for equitable access to clean fuel technologies. Other drivers of biodiversity loss include water-management strategies (e.g. construction of dams, reservoirs, and hydropower facilities), pollution, illegal trade of plants and wildlife, invasive species, unsustainable fishing practices, mining, and other resource extraction processes, fires, and climate change (WHO and Secretariat of the Convention on Biological Diversity, 2015). These issues are compounded by inadequate regulations, and by ineffective monitoring and enforcement of protective mechanisms. Given the integral role of biodiversity to ecosystem function, biodiversity loss is regarded as a potential 'tipping point' or fundamental threat to Earth's life support systems, though thresholds for such losses have not yet been defined.

evaluate how human actions might both disrupt and promote the well-being and preservation of ecosystems.

In 2014, academics called for a united movement to examine and promote planetary health (Horton, Beaglehole, Bonita, Raeburn, McKee, et al., 2014). Specifically, Horton and colleagues (2014) highlighted three challenges that must be overcome to achieve and planetary health. These challenges include the conceptual/empathy failures (e.g. over-fixation on GDP as measurement of human progress, overemphasis on present gains at the cost of future environmental and health, etc.); knowledge failures (limited available information and interdisciplinary research); and implementation failures (governmental and institutional inaction or delay). For example, although evidence for causality between environmental change through deforestation and many disease outbreaks is inconclusive, loss of forest land has put people and wildlife into closer contact and enhanced transmission risks of zoonotic diseases. Moreover, arguments for sustainability highlight the responsibility the current generation has to its descendants to do no further harm to the planet and to create the systems which will allow future generations to thrive and prosper—mentally, physically, and materially.

Planetary health is a new scientific discipline that is gaining momentum of academic interests and advocates. This subject demands new coalitions and partnerships to support knowledgement advance, governance, and potential implementation across different disciplines to meet the pervasive knowledge failures. It requires creativity and imagination among scientists and practitioners working in health to redefine the meaning of human progress, rethinking the possibilities for human cooperation, and revitalizing the prospects for the health of human civilizations. Case Box 7.4 explains how planetary

---

Case Box 7.4 Rockefeller Foundation–*Lancet* Commission on Planetary Health

The Lancet Commission on Planetary Health has examined and explored the scope and the concept of planetary health (Horton et al., 2014). The Commission argued that a more united global agenda should be formulated to advocate for the alignment of planetary and human health targets. It recommends the addressing of

1. growing **food** demands through integrated strategies, such as

    a. sustainable **agriculture and fisheries**,

    b. diversification of **crops**,

    c. efficient **water use**,

    d. reduction of **food waste**, and

    e. promotion of healthy, low-environmental impact **diets**.

2. reducing **greenhouse gas** emissions and other **pollutants**,

3. developing a sound management of **chemicals**,

4. building **sustainable cities**,

5. improving access to modern **family planning**; and

6. **integrating environmental care with health systems**.

Potential synergies should be found among the various manifestos that concern health to maximize their impact on health protection. The Global Action Plan for the Prevention and Control of NCDs, the Sustainable Development Goals, and efforts to close the nutrition divide manifest in the triple burden of malnutrition are all interlinked since issues highlighted in these agreements are occurring simultaneously within Earth's critical and non-negotiable planetary boundaries. The discussion has called for improved governance to aid the integration of social, economic, and environmental policies as well as the creation, synthesis, and application of interdisciplinary knowledge to strengthen the health of the planet. The Commission also calls for the redefinition of prosperity to incorporate improved health and quality of life for all, together with respect for the integrity of natural systems. The goal is to allow societies to address the drivers of environmental change by promoting sustainable and equitable patterns of consumption and reducing population growth.

health might be defined by the Rockefeller Foundation–Lancet Commission on Planetary Health established in 2014.

Mitigation policies need to include health and ecosystem externalities through appropriate and progressive pricing mechanisms. Policies will be needed to protect transboundary resources such as freshwater, tackle food waste, encourage regional investment in urban active transport infrastructure, etc. Strong inter-sectoral governance will help policy-makers understand how economic, social, and environmental policies jointly impact on health, and vice versa. Trade-related laws and policies, combined with domestic tax regimes and regulation, can serve to maintain access to high-quality, affordable health technologies, and reduce the demand for alcohol, tobacco, refined sugars, and ultra-processed food.

From One Health to planetary health

One Health and planetary health are two related health concepts that attempt to describe and examine the relationship among human, animal, and ecosystem. Although they have a lot in common, some important differences between them exist. Planetary health concerns about the health of human civilization and the state of natural systems on which it depends. It extends beyond individuals and populations and includes the health and sustainability of human civilization. Although humans are healthier than their ancestors, environment degradation, climate change, biodiversity loss, land degradation, and water scarcity are examples of ecological change that affect long-term health and well-being of humans. Planetary health can strengthen the theoretical framework to analyse the environment challenges that involve: (i) conceptual/empathy failures; (ii) knowledge failures; and (iii) implementation failures. Planetary health calls for all levels of society to take action and collaborate to safeguard human health through nurturing the health of Earth, with win–win policies such as protecting freshwater resources, reducing food waste, and investing in scalable plans and financing models for implementing renewable energies.

Comparison of the two frameworks

One Health and planetary health are important interdisciplinary concepts to promote the synergy between humans, animals, and environments. However, definitions of the two concepts differ. One Health focuses more on biomedical sciences, human, and veterinary medicine, while planetary health primarily focuses on human health, natural resource systems, sustainability, and biodiversity (Lerner and Berg, 2017).

Sustainability, development policy, and human health

Sustainability and health

Public health is intricately linked with the living environment. In the modern world, the living environment includes both the natural and built contexts. **Sustainability** emphasizes the need to support and provide for current human needs without compromising the ability of future generations to meet their needs (World Commission on Environment and Development, 1987). **Carrying capacity** is the maximum human population that the planet might be able to sustain. Standard of living, population density, and natural resources (i.e. land and water resources that might support human and living creatures' survival) are all important considerations when evaluating carrying capacity. **Ecological footprint** measures the burden of human consumption has imposed in the biosphere. Population size, resources use, and consumption patterns affect environmental capacity of sustaining current lifestyles. Theoretically, people living in high-income countries with more intense resource-based living would tend to have larger ecology footprints when compared with their low-income countries counterparts. **Sustainability development** describes the interaction between the economy, social equity, and the environment (Goodland, 1995). Sustainability of the planet ecosystem is essential to sustain human life. Changes in climate change, depletion of the ozone layer, reduction of biodiversity, degradation of ecosystems, and the spread of persistent organic pollutants present long-term health consequences on humankind.

Sustainable development and public health are thus closely associated because an unsustainable environment adversely affects the well-being of individuals. For example, well-being (e.g. quality of life) and chronic disease status, such as cardiovascular, obesity, and cancer risks, are found to be strongly associated with environmental (e.g. urban living context, sedentary lifestyle, and pollution level) and behavioural (e.g. food consumption patterns) factors.

Global environmental hazards are often also human health threats. However, as described in Chapter 6, environmental hazards do not affect populations equally. Certain demographic subgroups, due to their underlying physiological vulnerabilities (e.g. extremes of age), activities (e.g. outdoor workers) and social context (e.g. living in polluted areas or with material deprivation) are more vulnerable to environmental risk than others. Despite technology and health advances, poor health continues to be a constraint on development efforts. Development process may create conditions that causes economic, political, and social upheaval, environmental degradation, and increasing inequities. As a result, human health suffers (WHO, 2002).

Urbanization, health, and sustainability

As of 2018, over 55% of global population are urban dwellers (United Nations Department of Economics and Social Affairs [UNDESA], 2018). The urban population is further projected to rise to 68% of the world's population by 2050. Among the urban areas, 33 megacities globally are inhabited by 10 million people and the population size is still growing. In these cities, urban growth can outstrip the resource capacity of governments to provide even basic health services. It challenges many current assumptions that the urban infrastructure and system might have the capacity to protect communities from potential health risks with better concentration of resources. Older cities with suboptimal infrastructure might have poorer sewage and disposal systems, which render their residents more likely to suffer from public health risks and disease outbreaks. Urban planning and management thus require continuous improvements to keep up with the living and survival demands in urban settings (Baker, 2012). In addition, already more than 1 billion people in urban areas are exposed to health-threatening levels of air pollution.

Underlying health problems of residents may be exacerbated by pollution, noise, crowding, inadequate water and sanitation, improper waste disposal, chemical contamination, poisonings, and physical hazards associated with the growth of densely populated cities. Air pollution, both ambient and indoor (including the work environment), will continue to be a major contributor to respiratory and other ill-health conditions. Suboptimal urban settlements and overcrowded housing are more prone to infectious disease transmission, illicit drugs, and violence (see Case Box 7.5). Urban growth will also lead to greater dependence on transport systems which, if automobile-based, generate further risks of pollution and injuries. Case Box 7.6 describes the latest global policy on sustainable urban development.

Among the urban vulnerable population, those dwelling in informal settlements and slum areas in a city are at a higher risk of adverse outcomes in disasters. Without adequate basic services, hazards that would have minor impact in formal settlements, such as a small fire or heavy rainfall, may develop into a major crisis or disaster in overcrowded living conditions (Baker, 2012). Thus, environmental sustainability and its associated

Case Box 7.5 Housing and Health

Sharon Chow

Housing is one of the main determinants that affects human health (Bonnefoy, 2007). Physical structure can present a number of potential hazards to health. Temperature, dampness, pollutant concentrations, injury risks, and hygiene conditions may render its residents vulnerable to major health problems. In addition to indoor and outdoor environment, the social aspects of housing (e.g. living density and economic burden from mortgage) are all housing-related factors that may also influence the physical, social, and mental well-beings of inhabitants.

Urbanization, population ageing, climate change, and epidemiological disease burden may affect resilience of population health (WHO, 2002). Housing is an intervention point for primary prevention and intersectoral public health programmes.

In rural China, a diversity of vernacular houses is built with different local natural materials, using different methods and styles harnessing a wealth of local wisdom and traditional culture. These structures and building materials have proven to respond well to local climate, geography, and socio-cultural needs. With proper technical advances that may help overcome limitations and drawbacks regarding construction and structural safety, a rethink of the best way to re-adapt these traditional wisdoms to construct updated and modern housing options may offer as solution to housing important for indigenous rural and even transitional communities.

Case Box 7.6 The New Urban Agenda

The New Urban Agenda was adopted in October 2016 at the United Nations Conference on Housing and Sustainable Urban Development (Habitat III) in Quito, Ecuador. The policy framework document that set the global agenda for sustainable and inclusive urbanization for the subsequent 20 years was agreed by the heads of states, local government leaders, government ministers, the private sector, civil society, experts, and community members. The New Urban Agenda document incorporates both the *Quito Declaration on Sustainable Cities and Human Settlements for All* and the *Quito Implementation Plan for the New Urban Agenda*. It aims to highlight five pillars of implementation: national urban policies; urban legislation and regulations; urban planning and design; local economy and municipal finance; and local implementation (United Nations, 2016).

health-related impacts are likely to be unevenly distributed in a community. Protection of human health from the potential impacts of global environmental threats requires an improved understanding of the disease-inducing mechanisms involved and the vulnerability of populations.

Sustainable Development Goals (2015–30)

The Sustainable Development Goals (SDGs) were adopted in September 2015 at the United Nations Sustainable Development Summit, succeed the Millennium Development Goals (MDGs). The MDGs were a global effort mounted between 2000 and 2015 to combat poverty, hunger, and ill-health. World leaders and heads of state set an ambitious universal agenda of 17 Sustainable Development Goals with 169 targets that guide global and national action between 2015 and 2030. Expanding beyond the eight original MDGs, the SDGs seek to address and balance the three dimensions of sustainable development: economic growth, social inclusion, and environmental protection, also known as prosperity, people and the planet. With the SDGs, the goals have been expanded to include the planet, people, prosperity, peace, and partnership (see Case Box 7.7).

Recognizing that different countries face specific obstacles to achieving sustainable development, the 2030 Agenda for Sustainable Development maintains that the primary responsibility for achieving the SDGs in national development lies within each country, while a global partnership can enhance implementation (United Nations General Assembly, 2015). Periodic reviews and follow-ups will be held from national to global levels, and indicator data will be collected to track the progress of attaining these SDGs. Case Box 7.8 discusses how health is included in the discussion of SDGs in SDG Goal 3.

In addition to the health focus of SDG 3, all the other SDGs have health implications. For example, SDG 1 targets poverty, a health determinant that has long been recognized to be closely linked to material access, health maintenance, and health protection efforts.

Case Box 7.7 The Sustainable Development Goals (SDGs) (see Figure 7.1)

There are 17 sustainable development goals highlighted by the United Nations (n.d.-b). These are:

Goal 1. End poverty in all its forms everywhere

Goal 2. End hunger, achieve food security and improved nutrition, and promote sustainable agriculture

Goal 3. Ensure healthy lives and promote well-being for all at all ages

Goal 4. Ensure inclusive and equitable quality education and promote lifelong learning opportunities for all

Goal 5. Achieve gender equality and empower all women and girls

Goal 6. Ensure availability and sustainable management of water and sanitation for all

Goal 7. Ensure access to affordable, reliable, sustainable, and modern energy for all

Goal 8. Promote sustained, inclusive, and sustainable economic growth, full and productive employment, and decent work for all

Goal 9. Build resilient infrastructure, promote inclusive and sustainable industrialization, and foster innovation

Goal 10. Reduce inequality within and among countries

Goal 11. Make cities and human settlements inclusive, safe, resilient, and sustainable

Goal 12. Ensure sustainable consumption and production patterns

Goal 13. Take urgent action to combat climate change and its impacts*

Health protection for the poor requires more consideration and support because those living in poverty tend to have access to fewer resources, are living under more suboptimal conditions, with greater pre-existing health risks due to the limited access to medical services. SDG 2 focuses on nutrition and food security. Adequate and appropriate nutrition is essential to human health and well-being. Malnutrition, includes both undernutrition and over-nutrition, may result from an inadequate as well as excessive consumption of macronutrients or micronutrients. Those who are malnourished are more likely to be vulnerable and require more support. SDG 4 emphasizes the importance of education. Education enables every individual to acquire health literacy and the capacity to engage in self-care and health protection at the individual and community level. SDG 5 promotes gender equality as gender is often a determinant of a person's duties, power, and ability to access and control resources (Inter-Agency Standing Committee [IASC], 2017). Existing gender inequalities are usually further exacerbated in the capacity to engage in health protection actions. For example, women and men experience different vulnerabilities and needs during and after a disaster, which are not only a result of biological and physiological differences but also socio-economic and power differences. Better gender equality will help reduce the differences in health outcomes. SDG 6 describes the importance of

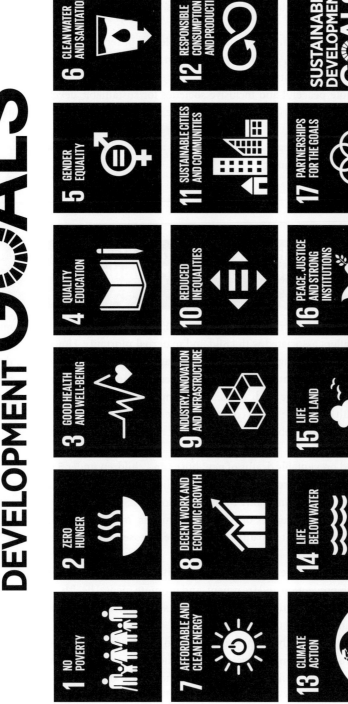

Figure 7.1 The Sustainable Development Goals (SDGs)

United Nations. (n.d.-b). Sustainable development goals: Communications materials [online]. Copyright © WHO. Available at: <https://www.un.org/sustainabledevelopment/news/communications-material/>

Case Box 7.7 The Sustainable Development Goals (SDGs) *(continued)*

Goal 14. Conserve and sustainably use the oceans, seas, and marine resources for sustainable development

Goal 15. Protect, restore, and promote sustainable use of terrestrial ecosystems, sustainably manage forests, combat desertification, and halt and reverse land degradation and halt biodiversity loss

Goal 16. Promote peaceful and inclusive societies for sustainable development, provide access to justice for all and build effective, accountable, and inclusive institutions at all levels

Goal 17. Strengthen the means of implementation and revitalize the global partnership for sustainable development

---

Case Box 7.8 Health Targets of Sustainable Development Goal 3: Ensuring Healthy Lives and Promoting Well-Being for All at All Ages

Significant strides have been made in increasing life expectancy and reducing some of the common killers associated with child and maternal mortality. However, ensuring healthy lives and promoting the well-being at all ages is essential to sustainable development in the future. Continuous efforts are needed to manage the persistence and emergency of a wide range of diseases. According to Goal 3 of SDGs, the following targets for health should be achieved by 2030. These include:

3.1 By 2030, reduce the global maternal mortality ratio to less than 70 per 100,000 live births.

3.2 By 2030, end preventable deaths of new-borns and children under 5 years old, with all countries aiming to reduce neonatal mortality to at least as low as 12 per 1,000 live births and under-5 mortality to at least as low as 25 per 1,000 live births.

3.3 By 2030, end the epidemics of AIDS, tuberculosis, malaria, and neglected tropical diseases and combat hepatitis, water-borne diseases, and other communicable diseases.

3.4 By 2030, reduce by one-third premature mortality from non-communicable diseases through prevention and treatment, and promote mental health and well-being.

3.5 Strengthen the prevention and treatment of substance abuse, including narcotic drug abuse and harmful use of alcohol.

3.6 By 2020, halve the number of global deaths and injuries from road traffic accidents.

3.7 By 2030, ensure universal access to sexual and reproductive healthcare services, including for family planning, information, and education, and the integration of reproductive health into national strategies and programmes.

Case Box 7.8 Health Targets of Sustainable Development Goal 3: Ensuring Healthy Lives and Promoting Well-Being for All at All Ages (*continued*)

3.8 Achieve universal health coverage, including financial risk protection, access to quality essential health-care services, and access to safe, effective, quality, and affordable essential medicines and vaccines for all.

3.9 By 2030, substantially reduce the number of deaths and illnesses from hazardous chemicals and air, water, and soil pollution and contamination.

3. A Strengthen the implementation of the World Health Organization Framework Convention on Tobacco Control in all countries, as appropriate.

3. B Support the research and development of vaccines and medicines for the communicable and non-communicable diseases that primarily affect developing countries, provide access to affordable essential medicines and vaccines, in accordance with the Doha Declaration on the TRIPS Agreement and Public Health, which affirms the right of developing countries to use to the full the provisions in the Agreement on Trade Related Aspects of Intellectual Property Rights regarding flexibilities to protect public health, and, in particular, provide access to medicines for all.

3. C Substantially increase health financing and the recruitment, development, training, and retention of the health workforce in developing countries, especially in the least developed countries and small island developing states.

3. D Strengthen the capacity of all countries, in particular developing countries, for early warning, risk reduction, and management of national and global health risks.

Notably, most of these health-related targets have been monitored since 2000 for tracking the status of the Millennium Development Goals (2000–2015).

Source: United Nations (n.d.-a).

availability of access to water and sanitation. As illustrated in Chapter 6 and throughout this book, clean drinking water and sanitation are key environmental determinants of health. Lack of access to safe and adequate water can heighten a population's health risk and their vulnerability in a crisis.

SDG 7 concerns energy access while SDG 8 links economic growth and development and these issues have important implications on health outcomes (see Chapter 8 on energy and economic transitions). SDG 9 and SDG 11 describe the importance of having resilient infrastructure and making cities and human settlements inclusive, safe, resilient, and sustainable. Resilient infrastructure and cities will reduce loss of human life in crises and emergencies (see Chapter 4 on Natech). SDG 12 describes the importance of balancing of consumption and production patterns in sustainable development. Coordinated management in natural resources, food waste, hazardous waste, and recycle efforts are critical to the maintenance of health and well-being of people and the environment.

SDG 13 focuses on climate change, one of the major drivers of the increase in the frequency and intensity of hazards such as temperature extremes, possible rainfall variability (leading to increased flooding or droughts), sea-level rise, extreme weather events (e.g. typhoons and storms), and climate-sensitive diseases (e.g. dengue and malaria). Health risks and health protection intervention strategies in the overlapping spheres of development, climate change, and disasters should be considered and assessed holistically. SDGs 14 and 15 concern land and marine resources that affect global ecology, human environment, diseases risks, and food access.

Conflicts, wars, violence, and terrorism are direct threats to life and large-scale violence and conflict leads to population displacement when people fear for their lives, and survival becomes the principal goal of existence (WHO, 2000). The ability and capacity to protect health and maintain human security decline in conflict-riven communities and fragile states as basic services and provisions for basic needs such as food and water are reduced. Furthermore, conflicts have not only acute effects on violence-related mortality and injuries but also broader and lingering effects on the level of communicable diseases, malnourishment, non-communicable disease treatments and mental health. SDG 16 promotes peaceful and inclusive societies for sustainable development. It also advocates access to justice for all, and builds effective, accountable, and inclusive institutions at all levels. SDG 10 highlights the importance of the equalities within and among nations while SDG 17 stresses the importance of strengthening the means of implementation and revitalization of the global partnership for sustainable development.

Planetary health is also associated with sustainable development goals. Lo, Lyne, Chan, and Capon (2018) highlighted the need to expand current academic focus and encourage knowledge developing in related areas. This involves strengthening health governance in the commitment to the SDGs, universal health coverage, and health policies and engage in multidisciplinary health protection actions. Case Box 7.9 describes the 'triple billion goals' advocated by the WHO (2019) in an attempt to achieve universal health coverage, protect the community from emergencies, and enable more people to enjoy better health and well-being.

Current gaps in global policies

In a globalized world, the reduction of health risks and environmental hazards is a collective/public good and requires multinational and transitional efforts. In addition to the environmental policies described in Chapter 6, global agreements in sustainable development are important to health protection at the global level. Throughout several landmark UN agreements adopted in 2015–2016, including the Sendai Framework for Disaster Risk Reduction 2015–2030, the 2030 Sustainable Development Goals (SDGs), the Paris climate agreement, and the New Urban Agenda (Habitat III), 'health' is recognized as an inevitable outcome. Health emergency and disaster risk management, as a joint venture of this cross-over health discipline has emerged as an umbrella field that encompasses public health, emergency and disaster medicine, disaster risk reduction, humanitarian response, development studies, community health resilience, and health system resilience (Chan and Shaw, 2019; see also Chapter 4 on Health-EDRM). The evolution of the interdisciplinary discussions regarding it will no doubt benefit future global health protection

Case Box 7.9 'Triple Billion Goals': Achieving Universal Health Coverage and Health Protection 2019–2023

Ryoma Kayano

Significant global health progress was made after the Millennium. People have longer life expectancy, the population experiences fewer child mortality, essential vaccination reaches a larger number of people than ever, and access to HIV treatment has improved. Nevertheless, globally, people are facing increasingly complex mix of health risks and threats such as poor access to health services, financial hardship as a result of medical expenses, increasing burden of non-communicable diseases, and emergence of antimicrobial resistance and high-impact health emergencies (e.g. epidemics, pandemics, conflicts, and natural and technological disasters). To respond to those new challenges building on past achievements, the WHO developed its thirteenth general programme of work 2019–2023 (GPW 13) in the context of achieving the Sustainable Development Goals (SDGs) (WHO, 2018).

GPW 13 sets '*triple billion goals*' that aim to enable 1 billion further people benefitting from universal health coverage, 1 billion more people better protected from health emergencies, and 1 billion more people enjoying better health and well-being. These strategic priorities are not mutually exclusive. As it is frequently highlighted that 'global health security and universal health coverage are two sides of the same coin', the achievement of these strategic priorities requires implementation that is mutually reinforcing (Wenham, Katz, Birungi, Boden, Eccleston-Turner, et al., 2019). For example, strengthening health systems (e.g. towards better universal health coverage) will make a system more resilient to emergencies and disasters. In communicable disease outbreaks, more capacity to detect and control outbreaks before such health risks are disseminated or spread (better health protection) in a world with fewer strict national borders. In order to ensure such goals are achieved, collaboration and joint efforts of Member States, the WHO, and other partners with all level (local, national, regional, global) are required.

efforts (Collaborating Centre for Oxford University and CUHK for Disaster and Medical Humanitarian Response [CCOUC], 2018; Kayano, Chan, Murray, Abrahams, and Barber, 2019).

Conclusion

Globally, the pressures and resources demands of human living, socio-economic development, technology innovations, and policy decisions have all contributed to the dynamic changes in planetary health and intergenerational sustainability of human's living ecosystem. One of the major concerns for future health protection is if our planet has the capacity to sustain the health, well-being, and current consumption patterns of its population. Adverse health and environmental consequences such as transboundary pollution, deforestation, climate change, loss of biodiversity have all changed the dynamics of health risks.

For health protection in the coming decades, an expanded conceptual framework is needed for health protection to encompass the complex dynamics surrounding its robustness. This chapter discusses a number of concepts that might facilitate further conceptual, research, and policy development that impacts on the overall well-being of humans, animals. and the planet. For example, One Health and the development of planetary health as fields of academic and research have expanded traditional public health approaches to incorporate examination of the interdependencies of human, animals, culture, and natural systems on health protection. These concepts argue that the protection of human health requires the analysis and strategic solution formulation that encompasses human choices and activities, the well-being of animals and the ecosystem, as well as intergenerational justice in decisions taken about the environment and related practices.

References

Atlas, R. M. and Maloy, S. (2014). The future of One Health. *Microbiol Spectr 2*(1) doi:10.1128/microbiolspec.OH-0018-2012.

Baker, J. L. (2012). *Climate Change, Disaster Risk, and the Urban Poor: Cities Building Resilience for a Changing World*. Washington DC: World Bank Publications.

Bonnefoy, X. (2007). Inadequate housing and health: An overview. *Int J Environ Pollut 30*(3/4) 411–29.

Chan, E. Y. Y. and Shaw, R. (eds). (2019). *Public Health and Disasters: Health Emergency and Disaster Risk Management in Asia*. Singapore: Springer.

Collaborating Centre for Oxford University and CUHK for Disaster and Medical Humanitarian Response (2018). *Planetary health for Health-EDRM*. Paper presented at Research Summit on Health-related Emergency and Disaster Risk Management (H-EDRM), 9–10 July 2018, Hong Kong.

Dorfman, M. and Rosselot, K. S. (2011). Testing the waters: A guide to water quality at vacation beaches: Twenty-first annual report. Available at: https://www.nrdc.org/sites/default/files/ttw2011.pdf.

Frankson, R., Hueston, W., Christian, K., Olson, D., Lee, M., et al. (2016). One Health core competency domains. *Front Public Health 13*(4) 192.

Goodland, R. (1995). The concept of environmental sustainability. *Ann Rev Ecol, Evol S 26* 1–24.

Horton, R., Beaglehole, R., Bonita, R., Raeburn, J., McKee, M., et al. (2014). From public to planetary health: A manifesto. *The Lancet 383*(9920) 847.

Kayano, R., Chan, E. Y. Y., Murray, V., Abrahams, J., and Barber, S. L. (2019). WHO Thematic Platform for Health Emergency and Disaster Risk Management Research Network (TPRN): Report of the Kobe expert meeting. *Int J Environ Res Public Health 16*(7) 1232. doi:10.3390/ijerph16071232.

Lener, H. and Berg, C. (2017). A comparison of three holistic approaches to health: One Health, EcoHealth, and planetary health. *Front Vet Sci 4*(163). doi:10.3389/fvets.2017.00163.

Inter-Agency Standing Committee (2017). The gender handbook for humanitarian action. Available at: https://interagencystandingcommittee.org/system/files/2018-iasc_gender_handbook_for_humanitarian_action_eng_0.pdf.

Lo, S., Lyne, K., Chan, E. Y. Y., and Capon, A. (2018). Planetary health and resilience in Asia. In H. Legido-Quigley and N. Asagari-Jirhandeh (eds), *Resilient and People-Centred Health*

Systems: Progress, Challenges and Future Directions in Asia. (pp. 56–93). Available at: https://apps.who.int/iris/bitstream/handle/10665/276045/9789290226932-eng.PDF?sequence=5&isAllowed=y.

Marcolino, M. S., Oliveira, J., D'Agostino, M., Ribeiro, A. L., Alkmim, M., et al. (2018). The impact of mHealth interventions: Systematic review of systematic reviews. *JMIR mHealth and uHealth, 6*(1), e23. doi:10.2196/mhealth.8873

McMichael, T. (2005). Global environmental changes, climate change and human health. In K. Lee and J. Collin (eds), *Global Change and Health.* Maidenhead: Open University Press. pp. 126–45.

United Nations (n.d.-a). Goal 3: Ensure healthy lives and promote well-being for all at all ages. Available at: https://www.un.org/sustainabledevelopment/health/.

United Nations (n.d.-b). Sustainable development goals: Communications materials. Available at: https://www.un.org/sustainabledevelopment/news/communications-material/.

United Nations (1992). Convention on biological diversity. Available at: https://www.cbd.int/doc/legal/cbd-en.pdf.

United Nations (2016). New Urban Agenda. Available at: http://habitat3.org/wp-content/uploads/NUA-English.pdf.

United Nations Department of Economics and Social Affairs (2018). World urbanization prospects: The 2018 revision. Available at: https://esa.un.org/unpd/wup/Publications/Files/WUP2018-KeyFacts.pdf.

United Nations General Assembly (2015). Transforming our world: the 2030 Agenda for Sustainable Development (A/RES/70/1). Available at: https://www.un.org/en/development/desa/population/migration/generalassembly/docs/globalcompact/A_RES_70_1_E.pdf.

United States Centers for Disease Control and Prevention (2017). Saving lives by taking a One Health approach: Connecting human, animal, and environmental health. Available at: https://www.cdc.gov/onehealth/pdfs/OneHealth-FactSheet-FINAL.pdf.

United States Centers for Disease Control and Prevention. (2018). One Health. Available at: https://www.cdc.gov/onehealth/basics/index.html.

Wenham, C., Katz, R., Birungi, C., Boden, L., Eccleston-Turner, M., et al. (2019). Global health security and universal health coverage: From a marriage of convenience to a strategic, effective partnership. *BMJ Glob Health 4* e001145.

World Commission on Environment and Development (1987). Report of the World Commission on Environment and Development: Our common future. Available at: https://www.are.admin.ch/dam/are/en/dokumente/nachhaltige_entwicklung/dokumente/bericht/our_common_futurebrundtlandreport1987.pdf.download.pdf/our_common_futurebrundtlandreport1987.pdf.

World Health Organization (2000). Conflict and health. Available at: https://www.who.int/hac/techguidance/hbp/Conflict.pdf.

World Health Organization (2002). Health and sustainable development: Key health trends. Available at: https://www.who.int/mediacentre/events/HSD_Plaq_02.2_Gb_def1.pdf.

World Health Organization. (2011). *mHealth: New Horizons for Health Through Mobile Technologies: Based on the Findings of the Second Global Survey on ehealth* (Global Observatory for eHealth Series, Volume 3). Geneva: WHO.

World Health Organization (2018). Thirteenth general programme of work, 2019–2023. Available at: http://apps.who.int/gb/ebwha/pdf_files/WHA71/A71_4-en.pdf?ua=1.

World Health Organization (2019). WHO unveils sweeping reforms in drive towards 'triple billion' targets. Available at: https://www.who.int/news-room/detail/06-03-2019-who-unveils-sweeping-reforms-in-drive-towards-triple-billion-targets.

World Health Organization, and Secretariat of the Convention on Biological Diversity (2015). Connecting global priorities: Biodiversity and human health: A state of knowledge review. Available at: https://apps.who.int/iris/bitstream/handle/10665/174012/9789241508537_eng.pdf?sequence=1.

Zinsstag, J., Schelling, E., Waltner-Toews, D., and Tanner, M. (2011). From 'one medicine' to 'one health' and systematic approaches to health and well-being. *Prevent Vet Med 101*(3-4), 148–56. doi:10.1016/j.prevetmed.2010.07.003.

Chapter 8

Challenges and Opportunities of Health Protection in the Twenty-First Century

Globally, changes of macro-determinants of health occur as consequences of population movement, urbanization, globalization, technology advancement, and globalized living environments in the twenty-first century. Regardless of development status, population are experiencing a range of health transitions that result in changes of the health determinants (Caldwell et al., 1990). One of the latest frontiers in public health is the examination of how large-scale transitions might affect health risks and outcomes. Human activities associated with these changes alter human health, disease risks, and the ecosystems that support and sustain living creatures. Rayner and Lang (2012) argue that a number of transitions have changed the dynamics of health, actions, and the ecosystems that humans interact with. This chapter discusses a number of these transitions including globalisation, demographic, epidemiological, economic, ecological, energy, technological, nutrition, and urban transitions.

Humans' health and well-being are intimately linked to their immediate environment, circumstances, and behavioural changes associated with their living context. Changes in environment will lead to **environmental risk transitions**, which alter the types of health risk exposure and subsequently health outcomes of human population (Hutchinson and Kovats, 2016). Case Box 8.1 discusses how air pollution might have multiple implications on human physiological changes (see Chapter 6 on pollution).

Health transition describes how health status and outcomes of a population evolve alongside with changes in behavioural, social, and cultural determinants that may influence health (Caldwell, Findley, Caldwell. Santow, Crawford, et al., 1990; see also Chapter 2 on health transition). Health determinants evolve and often change with socioeconomic development and alter health outcomes in a community and how stakeholders might protect and plan for relevant needs of the population (Lo, Lyne, Chan, and Capon, 2018). In this chapter, major changes in macro health determinants, globalization, and demographic, epidemiological, economic, ecological, energy, technological, nutrition, and urban transitions will be discussed.

Essentials for Health Protection. Emily Ying Yang Chan, Oxford University Press (2020).
© Oxford University Press
DOI: 10.1093/oso/9780198835479.001.0001

Case Box 8.1 Case Study on Air Pollution: Air Pollution Is Destroying Our Health

Xiang Qian Lao

Ambient air pollution is the leading contributor to the global disease burden. World Health Organization (WHO) estimated that fine particulate matter (PM2.5) alone contributed to 4.2 million deaths (7.5% of all-cause deaths) worldwide in 2016 (World Health Organization [WHO], 2018a). Some 91% of those premature deaths occurred in low- and middle-income countries, and the greatest number in the WHO South-East Asia and Western Pacific regions (WHO, 2018a).

Previous research on the link between air pollution and health mostly focuses on short-term effects such as mortality, mainly for sensitive individuals or vulnerable populations. Scientists recently found that long-term exposure to air pollution may cause physiopathological changes in all individuals, resulting in a much more serious disease burden. For example, studies show that long-term exposure to PM2.5 air pollution may increase the level of inflammation and coagulation (Zhang, Chang, Lau, Chan, Chuang, et al., 2017; Zhang, Chan, Guo, Chang, Lin, et al., 2018) and the risk of hypertension and chronic kidney disease (Chan, Zhang, Lin, Lin, Deng, et al., 2018; Zhang, Guo, Lau, Chan, Chuang, et al., 2018), which ultimately cause cardiovascular morbidity and mortality. Long-term exposure to air pollution can also reduce pulmonary function and result in chronic obstructive pulmonary disease (Guo, Zhang, Lau, Lin, Chuang, et al., 2018) and mortality.

Besides, of global health protection concern, more than 90% of the world's population currently lives in a place where the air quality does not reach the standards recommended by the WHO. From 30 October to 1 November 2018, the First WHO Global Conference on Air Pollution and Health took place in Geneva and an aspirational goal was proposed to reduce the number of deaths from air pollution by two-thirds by 2030 (WHO, 2018a).

Globalization transition

In the twenty-first century, one of the most significant changes to human experience and living context is associated with **globalization**. These globalized changes can be categorized into three main dimensions, namely **spatial, temporal**, and **cognitive** (Hanefeld and Lee, 2015). Major **spatial changes** occur with travelling in long physical distances. Technology advancement in transportation and better infrastructure (e.g. roads) development have increased speed and the possibility of mobility and movement. Compared with historical patterns of human movement, travel options and migration patterns have altered drastically across the globe. Populations have better access to water, food, job opportunities, and healthcare services, which were not available for previous generations. **Temporal** changes occur with the increased efficiency and frequency of human interactions. Information acquisition and more intense communication exchange occurs over much shorter timescales and over longer geographic distances. For medical and health protection, better communication enables the easy exchange of medical expertise and scientific advances in technology that facilitate better health protection. Global inter-connectedness allows for the possibility of information exchange and better global disease surveillances, alerts about extreme events, and emergency response facilitation, which supports health protection. In addition, multinational collaboration maximizes clinical capacity in the organization of medical services and care options (e.g. remote consult-ation; refer also to the discussion about **technological transition** following), research collaboration, and education opportunities.

Globalized living contexts expand ideas and influence perceptions, leading to **cognitive** changes in human ideas and thinking. Personal preference, norms, cultural values, ideologies, and knowledge change with the alternation in living context. In a globalized, interconnected world, exposure to international media and communication platforms (e.g. Internet) brings about consensus and convergence of values, approaches, and solutions that require transnational collaborations (e.g. pollution control and banning use of plastics) to be addressed effectively. Case Box 8.2 discusses the challenges of Gavi, a global public–private partnership programme, and the approaches it undertakes to address a changing global health landscape.

Along with positive changes, globalization and a globalized living context may also bring negative consequences to human health and challenges effectiveness of trad-itional health protection approaches. Historically, health protection attempts have been driven and managed by discrete national or territory policies and programmes. With the disappearing of physical boundaries between nation states, management of health de-terminants, promotion of well-being, and engagement of disease control have become a transnational or global affair. Health protection is thus likely to become less effective if attempted only by a single nation or geographic area. Preferences, interests, and prac-tices from distant and foreign context are increasingly more likely to affect local patterns if the community is closely interlinked to the globalized lifestyle. Nevertheless, the im-pact of globalization on health-affecting habits and mental health is yet to be quantified. Rapidly evolving patterns of population movement, trade of goods, diseases, and infor-mation change risk profile and disease outcomes. For example, infectious disease control and food and product safety often illustrate how globalization might change the nature of health protection. Adverse health-related incidents (e.g. food-safety incidents) with adverse health outcomes are no longer able to be controlled entirely by local rules and regulations, or single country-based behavioural interventions or policies. Changing em-ployment patterns and working hours in a globalized community (e.g. the 24-hour multi-national office context) may also lead to specific occupational hazards and environmental impacts on a community.

Fundamentally, one of the major challenges in health protection for the global-ized world is the lack of clear leadership in governance, resources, and financial and infrastructural support for the health protection efforts in the increasingly complex

Case Box 8.2 Gavi's Evolving Strategy in Response to Changing Global Health Landscape

Caroline Dubois

Childhood vaccination remains one of the most cost-effective health investments with proven strategies that make it accessible to even the most vulnerable populations (WHO, 2018b). Founded in partnership between WHO, UNICEF, and the Bill and Melinda Gates Foundation, Gavi the Vaccine Alliance is a global public–private partnership that brings countries, international agencies, industry, and civil society together to improve equal access to new and underused vaccines for children in low-income countries (Gavi, 2019).

While immunization programmes worldwide continue to face long-standing barriers, the global landscape is changing fundamentally and Gavi's strategy adapts to meet challenges of the future. It becomes increasing challenging to maintain its core focus on accelerating access to vaccines and increasing equitable coverage. One example is the need to expansion Gavi's vaccine investment strategy to build new life-course delivery platforms in countries, which will strengthen primary healthcare as a whole by providing more opportunities where children, adolescents, or adults are in contact with health workers (Tissandier, 2018). This approach will be in line with achieving universal health coverage under SDG 3. In 2013, Gavi introduced its human papillomavirus vaccine programme, whose success requires wider counselling and adolescent health education beyond vaccine delivery (Sussman, Helitzer, Bennett, Solares, Lanoue, et al., 2015).

In addition, Gavi aims to introduce six additional vaccines to its portfolio by 2021. Among these vaccines, some will require the integration of immunization with other health services above and beyond the scope of traditional infant-centric programmes. These include hepatitis B birth dose, a challenge in contexts where the number of births in health facilities or attended by skilled personnel is low and vaccine delivery will require coordination with wider maternal health programmes (Wang, Smith, Peng, Xu, and Wang, 2016). Another is human rabies post-exposure prophylaxis, whose programme faces unique challenges in predictability, diagnosis, and response logistics, and must be supported with broader health education and system strengthening (Kessels, Recuenco, Navarro-Vela, Deray, Vigilato, et al., 2017).

---

transnational context. With multinational stakeholders and actors that range from nation states and commercial entities to non-governmental agencies and individuals in the civil society, there is an urgent need for the establishment and strengthening of global systems for monitoring, implementing, as well as enforcing various essential health protection commitments. For example, the surge of incidences of food-borne or related disease patterns have shown how globalized food production and distribution changes might affect health risks and potential disease manifestations. The promotion of international food safety standards and guidelines is likely to promote health and trade in both developed and developing countries. Ensuring effective health protection regulations and policies in a globalized world remains a major challenge for current diverse, global, nation-state systems.

Demographic transition

Birth, death, and population movement are the three main components that affect **demographic structure** of a society or community. These dynamics alter health risk profile, health outcomes, and types of approaches harnessed to address health protection needs in a community (McCracken and Philips, 2017). Population growth (by birth and emigration), ageing, and movement (death or immigration) affect population structure and the dynamics of health risks, needs, and medical outcomes. **Mortality transition** is a demographic description of how mortality rates of each age groups across a lifespan decrease as longevity increase and as a result, life expectancies increase. **Fertility transition** describes the decrease of the birth rate and the delay of the child-bearing age of a female population in their reproductive span. **Ageing transition** (or ageing of population) describes the number of older individuals which is increasing at a faster rate than that of the number

---

Case Box 8.3 Palliative/End-of-Life Care

End-of-life care refers to care and support received during the last stage of life. People with terminal diseases (e.g. cancer, HIV/AIDs, and chronic respiratory diseases) might require multidisciplinary support. In addition to physical medical needs (e.g. palliative treatment for pain relief), these patients might benefit from psycho-social and spiritual support. **Palliative care** refers to care and services that improve quality of life of patients and their family who are facing problems associated with life-threatening illness through the prevention and relief of suffering (World Health Assembly, 2014). However, while end-of-life care often involves palliative treatment support, palliative care might be offered to patients in an early stage of their treatments or therapy that intends to extend life expectancy. So palliative care might not always equivalent to end-of-life care.

Pain management usually constitutes the main component of palliative care, and support also ranges from social to logistic to counselling of patients and family. Although end-of-life care should be an integral part of the pathway of care, WHO has estimated that only 14% of those who need end-of-life and palliative care are receiving such support and services globally (WHO, 2018d). Most of the current service availability is concentrated in developed, high-income countries. The unmet needs are likely to remain huge and will expand in volume with global ageing of population and the increase of non-communicable diseases (e.g. cancer).

Case Box 8.4 Migration and Health in the Twenty-First Century

Historically, migration and health have a complex relationship. Migration might be internal (within) and external (beyond) a country. People migrate for various reasons. Voluntary movement include for job and education opportunities, travel for leisure as well as for a better quality of life or retirement purpose. Reasons for involuntary or forced movement include war, conflict, and to escape discrimination. There is currently a limited amount of publicly available data on levels of active migration.

For health protection, migration presents both opportunities and threats to a community. The term 'healthy migrants' usually refers people who are of working age with good health status who can contribute to the economy (formal or informal) of the recipient community. These migrants contribute to the economy and work force and help relieve the pressure of in communities who are experiencing a decreasing working population due to ageing. However, for any community, an emigration of well-educated, young professionals (e.g. doctors, nurses, and engineers), also known as the 'brain drain' of the origin community, might have important implications for health system capacity and for education resources planning. With a global shortage of 2.4 million medical and health staff, this has important implications on the ethics of international recruitment of health workers (WHO, 2014).

Migrants may also be displaced people (or refugees if migration is beyond country of origin) who have endured hardship during major crises (e.g. war, conflict, and economic hardship) and emergencies (e.g. natural disasters and accidents). Given their migration context, displaced persons tend to have significant health needs and are in vulnerable status (see Chapter 4).In addition to the increased regular global travel individuals undertake for leisure and business reasons, events that involve large number of people gathering, such as religious (annual Hajj migration to Mecca) or sporting events (Olympics), present challenges to health protection across a number of risks associated with communicable disease control, injury, and disaster prevention. Overall, it is important to highlight the potential health threats presented by transient migrants or travellers.

of children being born in a population. Specifically, ageing transition typically occurs when mortality transition and fertility transition occur in a society. In the 21st century, population ageing is becoming one of the more prominent demographic features of both developed and developing countries (see Chapter 2). Globally, the percentage of population aged over 60 will double between 2000 and 2050 from 10% to 21% and significant increases will occur for those over 80 years (United Nations Department of Economic and

Social Affairs [UN DESA], 2017). If the demographic pattern continues to evolve with its dynamics, authorities and stakeholders will need to re-orientate their medical, health, and social services, facilities, and economic capacity to support a more ageing-friendly context for the health protection of these greying communities. Although life expectancy is likely to lengthened with the changes of risks and socio-economic transitions, with physical decline in older age and the complexity of health problems in the later stage of physiological age, maintaining the quality of life of older age might present a new range of health protection needs. For example, physical environments will need to be changed to accommodate physical limitations associated with old age (see also Case Box 8.3 on palliative and end-of-life care).

Migration patterns affect the demographic structure of a community. Large-scale population movement, voluntarily or involuntarily, affects community demographic profile and its health protection needs (see Case Box 8.4). Disease patterns and population health needs also follow population movement.

Demographic transition occurs when the proportion of the working population of the whole region/geographic area has reached its peak and then subsequently it is expected to decline in size and the proportion of older persons in these countries will increase. In many developed countries, the tipping point of the maximum size of the working-age population (the specific time point when working population as % of total population starts to decline) might have passed decades ago. These communities are now facing major population ageing and an increased economic and social burden has been imposed on a declining proportion of working population in the community. In general, global population growth in many regions has demonstrated a slowdown for the past few decades.

With demographic transition, health protection efforts will need to assess how the evolving demographic structure may affect community. For example, a community with a predominantly aged population will likely to have different health risks and medical needs from a migrant-based healthy young population. An aged population will thus need specific services adaptation and protection policies (e.g. access barrier-free facilities and timing adjusted for traffic lights to avoid injury), while a migrant-based young community might require updated occupational protection guidelines and access to social hygiene clinics for health and well-being protection purposes. **Sex-ratio imbalance** might identified by examining demographic structure when planning health protection strategies in communities. Although females tend to have longer life expectancy when compared with males globally, such a female biological advantage might be lost due to the systematic discrimination and disadvantages experienced by the female gender throughout their life course. The sex-ratio imbalance phenomenon may also have important social and healthcare implications in developing context and countries that are facing such demographic patterns (refer to Case Box 8.5).

Case Box 8.5 Sex-Ratio Imbalance: Implication of Health Protection

Sex-ratio imbalance is a specific phenomenon when communities report an unnatural balance of sex/gender ratio. Migration is one of the key demographic drivers for such patterns. Specific migration worker profile (e.g. male-dominated industries such as mining, and female-dominated industries such as services and the hospitality industry) might tip the sex-ratio balance of a community. Cultural and social preferences for sons or boys may be another fundamental demographic determinant for community gender imbalance. With female infanticide and abandonment still occurring in some developing countries such as China and India, Asia is particular hard hit by such patterns. With the increasing availability and accessibility of technology (e.g. ultrasound prenatal diagnosis), gender selection through abortion might occurs more easily during prenatal period. Even if gender-identification tests are outlawed, social and cultural influences cannot be ignored. In 2017, an estimated 160 million girls went missing globally (McCracken and Philips, 2017). In countries with a specific demographic policy, such as China's 'one-child policy' that was in place from the 1970s to mid-2010s, such phenomena are more prominent. China reported a ratio of 116 boys to 100 girls in 2014, compared to the global average ratio of 105 boys to 100 girls. The China pattern demonstrates a number of indirect long-term social consequences.

One of the main concerns for males, especially those in the low socio-economic subgroup, in this context might be the challenge of finding partners for marriage. In less-developed countries, the trafficking of women, demand for commercial sex workers, and social instability due to sexual violence against women leads to major health implications for women at risk. Moreover, females often assume the role as caregiver in the family, looking after vulnerable and older people within the household. The absence of women and daughters have led to concern of how social and care support might be organized, especially in these situations.

Although education, campaigns, and changes in policy (e.g. outlawing foetal sex selection, changes of the one-child policy in China in 2015, etc.) may help reduce inequality, it takes generations to redress these phenomena. Notably, similar patterns are observed even if population policies in the context are not as strictly observed. For example, Vietnam has also reported an gender ratio of 120 boys to 100 girls. The consequences of sex-ratio imbalance will remain an important concern for health and social protection as well as the organization of medical and social services for decades to come.

Epidemiological transition

Disease patterns that affect a community is inextricably linked to demographic profile and various health determinants such as genetic predisposition, lifestyles, social (income disparity), environmental, and policy factors. **Epidemiological transition** marks a shift from the disease pattern of predominantly infectious diseases to that of chronic non-communicable diseases. With changes in modern living, activities, and consumption patterns, disease risks have shifted from unsafe food, undernutrition, and preventable childhood diseases to lifestyle-related risks of addiction (e.g. smoking and alcohol), obesity, physical inactivity, and pollution. As changes of community health determinants would affect disease patterns, **disease risk transitions** will alter disease patterns. For example, while the loss of healthy life (in terms of disability-adjusted life years, DALYs) from communicable diseases and new-born, nutritional, and maternal causes have all been on the decline, the losses from non-communicable diseases such as cancer, cardiovascular and respiratory conditions, and mental health diseases are on rising trends. For health protection in the decades to come, new programme approaches and policy initiatives need to be developed to address disease risks and profile that are relevant to the specific disease risk transition a country or a community may be experiencing. Case Box 8.6 discusses the current gap in breast cancer screening in Hong Kong and Case Box 8.7 describes the current lack of a comprehensive approach to manage dementia patients in China.

Case Box 8.6 Community-Based Activities Needed in Response to the Threat of Breast Cancer Among Women

May Hang-mei Lee

Breast cancer is the most common female cancer worldwide, affecting more than 2 million women all over the world (Bray, Ferlay, Soerjomataram, Siegel, Torre, et al., 2018). Secondary preventive measures (i.e. breast cancer screening) have been adopted worldwide for early cancer diagnosis and treatment. Eleven countries or regions had already reported significant clinical stage shifting and achieved mortality reduction in certain age groups after the implementation of population-wide screening programmes. However, in many developed contexts, despite the emphasis on prevention and screening, population-wide screening programmes for breast cancer are not available.

In Hong Kong, an urban Asian city, while the age-standardized incidence rates for the more commonly known cancers (lung, colorectal, cervical) did not show a significant increase, an average of 2.5% annual increase had been observed in breast cancer over the period 2007–16 (Hong Kong Cancer Registry, Hospital Authority, 2018). On average, over half of all breast cancer cases in Hong Kong were diagnosed at more advanced clinical stages (stage II or above diseases requiring more invasive treatment such as mastectomy and chemotherapy). Moreover, the five-year survival rate for breast cancer is high when detected early (97.5% for stage I), but it greatly reduces to 19.3% at stage IV (Kwong, Mang, Wong, Chau, and Law, 2011).

Currently, Hong Kong women rely largely on self-awareness and will seek medical consultation if any changes in their breasts are suspected. As reported in studies, women's awareness of breast cancer here is suboptimal. One-quarter of breast cancer patients sought medical advice only after the symptoms persisted for three months or more (Hong Kong Breast Cancer Foundation, 2018). Under these circumstances, probably the most direct and effective approach for protecting women from breast cancer would be to raise their awareness by organizing more community-based activities about breast cancer and to promote mammography screening for women at the community level.

Case Box 8.7 Call for National Strategies to Deal with China's Surging Dementia Population

Hermione Hin-man Lo and Janice Ying-en Ho

China has one of the fastest growing older populations in the world. The estimated number of national dementia cases is projected to increase from 9.48 million in 2017 (Wu, Ali, Guerchet, Prina, Chan, et al., 2018) to 32 million (Alzheimer's Disease International [ADI], 2014) in 2050. Economic reforms have eroded the Chinese traditional way of older people care taking (Chen, Boyle, Conwell, Xiao, and Chiu, 2014). Decreased family size and increased job mobility have led to the segregation and isolation of older people in rural areas. A difference in dementia prevalence, with 6.05% in rural area and 4.4% in urban in 2008 to 2009, was result (Jia, Wang, Wei, Zhou, Jia, et al., 2014). The estimated total annual costs of dementia in China increased from US$0.9 billion in 1990 to US$47.2 billion in 2010, and are predicted to reach US$114.2 billion by 2030 (ADI, 2014).

Despite the elevating demand in dementia care, China has not introduced any national policies to address the problem directly (ADI, 2014; Chen, et al., 2014). Dementia was included as a sub-part of national policies to tackle the ageing population in the National Mental Health Plan 2000–10 and 2011–20 and the Five-year plan (2016–20) on older people's care issued by the State Council (ADI, 2014; Jia et al., 2014). Although the Government mounted an effort to expand primary care services to support dementia care, specialized and outreach services to address the needs of dementia patients and their carers are still limited by public resources and lack of public awareness (Wu, Gao, Chen, and Dong, 2016). The escalating dementia population may lead to psychological burdens and social and financial distress, if the problem is not promptly managed (Dua, Seeher, Sivananthan, Chowdhary, Pot, et al., 2017).

Some disease patterns evolve with environmental and climate changes. For example, malaria and dengue infection risks change with urbanization as well as changes in temperature and rainfall patterns. Attitudes, knowledge, and behavioural patterns of citizens might affect environmental and disease risks. Case Box 8.8 discusses how an urban community may perceive the risks of dengue infection and control.

In addition, disease risks and pattern transitions might occur at a different pace for different demographic subgroups due to variation of socio-economic status and other social determinants. Thus, it should be emphasized that epidemiological changes do not occur in linear patterns and changes in risks are associated with changes of health status, disease occurrence, and their resulting outcomes. For example, despite better socio-economic and infrastructure support (e.g. water and sanitation), which changes communicable disease-based disease profiles to non-communicable disease profiles, the emerging infectious diseases (EIDs) and re-emerging of communicable diseases and antibiotic-resistant infections will make communicable disease remains as a main health protection and disease control focus in communities (see Case Box 5.5 on antimicrobial drug-resistant infections and global surveillance mechanisms).

Case Box 8.8 Knowledge and Protective Behaviours of Dengue Fever in a Subtropical City: The Case of Hong Kong

Holly Ching-yu Lam

Dengue fever is an increasing global health risk that associated with climate changes (World Health Organization Western Pacific Regional Office, 2017). Unlike malaria, another major climate change-related vector-borne disease, vectors of dengue infection are present in many cities and urban populations. Community's awareness, knowledge, risk patterns (mosquito bites), and protective behavioural practices are essential to effective disease prevention. With no effective treatment, the most efficient control measures currently available to reduce the disease burden are through risk factor management and diseases prevention.

A population-based randomized telephone survey (n = 590) has been conducted among adults ($\geq$ 18 years old) three weeks after the Government announcement of a local dengue outbreak in Hong Kong, a subtropical urban city in Southern China in August 2018, to examine the awareness, knowledge, risk patterns and protective behaviour practices as well as the sociodemographic-associated factors of increased knowledge and preventive practices (Lam, Chan, Lo, Tsang, Man, et al., 2019).

Overall, about 40% of respondents claimed to have been bitten by mosquitoes during the study period, a high season for mosquito bites in Hong Kong. Although study results showed high levels of community awareness of the local outbreak (96.1%), symptom identification (84.0%), and adoption rate of at least one mosquito preventive measure (nearly 80%), there are community disparities in knowledge and health protection practices. The older people ($\geq$ 65 years old) and those with primary level education or below were less likely to identify dengue's symptoms. Females and those who were educated to secondary level or higher were more likely to adopt more protective measures against mosquito bites. As a high-risk community, current protective measures against mosquito bites practised by the community were shown not to be effective. Relevant knowledge and anti-mosquito bites practices should be reinforced among the older people, males, and especially for those with lower education level in order to reduce risk.

When comparing two communities, differences in demographic characteristics and access to resources may present a different health profile and needs for health protection consideration. Thus, for health protection efforts in health risk management, although understanding of general trends of epidemiological transitions may facilitate programme and policy planning, the diversity of epidemiological patterns may present challenges to the adequate addressing of health risks and concerns.

Moreover, disease pattern and health needs might alter as a result of successful health protection and promotion measures such as control of harmful substances (tobacco) and provision of enabling environment (e.g. better road- and transport-related policies to protect from traffic accidents, and barrier-free access and stress-free contexts). Case Box 8.9 discusses how behavioural risk patterns might change with policies interventions.

Case Box 8.9 How Policies Change and Shift Alcohol Drinking Patterns

Jean H. Kim

Two serial cross-sectional telephone surveys were conducted in adult Chinese women prior to the 2007–08 beer and wine tax eliminations in 2006 ($n = 4946$) and in 2011. Over the study period, only women in the 36–45-year-old stratum reported significant increases in all three drinking patterns: past-year drinking (38.1–45.2%); past-month binge drinking (2.3–5.2%); and weekly drinking (4.0–7.3%) ($P\ 0.05$). Results indicated middle-aged women, unemployed or retired women, and those ascribing to alcohol's health benefits emerged as new binge-drinking risk groups. In 2011, 3.5% of all drinking-aged women (8.8% of past-year drinkers, 20.7% of binge drinkers, and 23.1% of weekly drinkers) re-ported an increased drinking frequency after the tax policy changes. The main contexts of increased drinking included social events and with restaurant meals. Beliefs regarding alcohol's health benefits were common to all contexts of increased drinking. Among women who increased their drinking frequency, the largest proportion attributed it to peer effects/social environment conducive to drinking, and brand marketing/advertising influences.

The authors hypothesized that the increased drinking among certain subgroups of Hong Kong Chinese women, a traditionally low-alcohol consumption group, are likely to be arising from the combined influences of increased societal acceptance of social drinking, aggressive marketing promotions, and personal beliefs in the health benefits of drinking that have recently emerged in the region. Hence, multi-prong strategies are required to combat potential drinking harms among these women.

Source: Wong, Kim, Goggins, Lau, Wong, et al. (2018).

Economic transition

Economic transition refers to the change of employment profile from traditional eco-nomic industry (e.g. agriculture and fishing) to manufacturing-based and service- and knowledge-based economy. Globally, increased economic growth has also broadened inequalities within and between countries. Whilst economic wealth might increase in a society or country, development and rapid expansion usually leads to various access disparities and in the process of development, potentially leads to massive environmental degradation. The increase in poverty, the widening of socio-economic inequalities, and job insecurity in changes to economic structure will affect individuals' well-being and health outcomes. Reduced material access, and precarious living and working conditions can predispose vulnerable population to major risks of injury and occupational hazards that lead to poor health outcomes (see Case Box 8.10).

To ensure sustained economic performance, active attempts should also be made to reduce inequality and to minimize adverse environmental consequences (see Case Box 8.10 on child labour). Governments and stakeholders should create favourable economic conditions and opportunities to address vulnerabilities, increase resilience, inclusiveness, and sustainability to withstand the potential economic downward trend that may arise from an ageing popula-tion, slower capital accumulation, and modest productivity growth. Case Box 8.11 discusses

Case Box 8.10 Child Labour

In many developing context, child labour remains a reality in both formal and informal sectors. Although children in the workforce might potentially bring economic benefit to their families, especially those who are in poverty, children are more prone to injury and lose education opportunities, which might hamper later occupational possibilities in life. In addition to the physical and psychological damage, children are also more vulnerable to abuses in all forms (e.g. physical and sexual abuse and trafficking).

Case Box 8.11 Read-Across Implications of Self-Management by Diabetes Mellitus Patients Among the Working Population: Public Health, Social Welfare and Labour Policies

Heidi H. Y. Hung

   Diabetes mellitus (DM) is a chronic disease characterized by increased concentrations of blood glucose, with type 2 DM accounting for over 90% of all DM cases. DM is a significant risk factor for cardiovascular diseases and is associated with a range of complications. DM is one of the main cause of death related to chronic diseases worldwide, with the global prevalence rising from 4.7% in 1980 to 8.8% in 2017 (International Diabetes Federation, 2017). The age-standardized DALY rate stood at 1887.6 per 100,000 for DM in 2016, higher than that for ischaemic stroke and haemorrhagic stroke combined (Hay, Abajobir, Abate, Abbafati, Abbas, et al., 2017). The primary objective of type 2 DM management is to prevent complications. Self-management is a cornerstone for the DM regimen as patients have to perform complex care activities every day, including adherence to recommended diets, physical activities, and medications, self-monitoring of blood glucose, and attend preventive screenings.

   Meanwhile, self-management by DM patients among the working population receives limited support and merits special attention from the health protection angle. With the early or young onset of type 2 DM, the ageing workforce and potential disease implication on economic productivity on the total workforce both add to urgency to the issue. Specifically, if DM patients among the working population are unable to manage their conditions, not only does it imply extra burden on the health system but also loss of productivity at the social level and disruption to livelihood at individual and family levels that may lead to reliance on social welfare.

   In addition to better health education and service support, labour policies are critical in supporting the self-management by DM patients at work, in particularly regulations of sick leave and standard working hours. With a recent study illustrating that DM patients had a higher increased risk of acute myocardial infarction admissions than non-DM patients during extreme temperatures (Lam, Chan, Luk, Chan, and Goggins, 2018), working conditions and the emergency preparedness of outdoor workers call for further research.

the challenges of managing diabetes mellitus, an important non-communicable disease experiencing a rising trend throughout the world, for the working population.

For the health sector, there is an increased emphasis on increasing financial resources (e.g. privatization of healthcare services) to alleviate the public resources burden of healthcare cost and to improve access, options, and service quality. Although such changes might improve certain aspects of healthcare systems, reforms in developing countries have also resulted in budget cuts in public health systems and programmes that have sought to engage in health protection activities. The burden of protecting communities may shift to the non-governmental and private voluntary organization service providers. Access to care and health support that aims to protect health, especially for the vulnerable such as older people and women, might be profoundly affected if policy initiatives are not considered carefully.

In addition, with the increased involvement of the commercial sector in health, governance of health protection efforts might experience new challenges. While self-regulation, corporate social responsibility, and professional code of conduct are typical approaches used to monitor, regulate, and examine specialized technology-based industries, the lack of competition on a similar scale of economic activities, the ability to monitor and regulate a monopolized health-related industry (e.g. drug research and production) will become increasingly challenging (Lee, 2005).

Ecological transition

Ecological transition is a complex phenomenon that involves transitions in population, mobility, natural resources, social structures, humans and other species, the Earth/physical environment, and human settlements. Not only have global environmental changes (see Chapter 7) put pressure on the ecological transition to the living environment, but such a transition also has social and technological dimensions (Lindfield and Steinberg, 2012). **Loss of biodiversity** (see Case Box 7.3), habitat loss (e.g. alteration and fragmentation), overexploitation of wild species populations, pollution, climate change, and invasive species—most of these stem from human demand for food, water, energy, and land. The **ecological footprint** is an accounting framework (Global Footprint Network [GFN], 2018) that is used to measure the amount of biologically productive land and sea area that humanity needs to produce the resources it consumes, provide for its infrastructure, and absorb waste. It has been reported that if the ecological footprint exceeds the bio-capacity of a country, it will deplete its natural environment to meet human needs or import from other countries, which might be unsustainable (GFN, 2018).

Socially, rapid population growth and urbanization are key drivers of environmental degradation. Human migration driven by displacement, population growth, economic development, inequality, and climate change/extreme events has environmental consequences such as changing patterns of consumption/energy use, pressures on ecosystem services, and agricultural expansion (United Nations Development Programme [UNDP], 2016). Other drivers are unsustainable consumption patterns and waste production. In urban areas, needs for transport and therefore air pollution related to fossil fuel consumption, the increase of the middle class, the reduction in fertility and mortality rates, and an ageing population also drive environmental degradation. Water stress will present major health protection risks of ecological transition in the decades ahead. Ineffective protection of existing water sources, climate change (lack of precipitation and unsustainable melting of the glacier ice that supports water access for some populations), and the resource stress of supporting mega-cities are factors that pose ecology challenges for human sustainability as well as barriers for health protection for communities. Availability, accessibility, and cost of accessing safe drinking water may hamper health maintenance and potentially lead to crises and conflicts. For example, although water efficiency has been improved by 90% in developing countries in the region, overall water use per US dollar of GDP still fared far worse than the world average in 2015 (UNDP, 2016). Moreover, the poor and vulnerable will be most affected by climate change and environmental risks (Watts, Amann, Arnell, Ayeb-Karlsson, Belesova, et al., 2018) (refer to Case Box 8.12).

Case Box 8.12 Vulnerability and Climate Change-Related Floods

Zhe Wang and Emily Ying Yang Chan

Flooding has been the most frequently occurred disaster with the highest economic losses and a reported increase in incidents globally. In addition to the massive damage on infrastructure and society, it also brings about severe negative impact on human health. With its effect of land use, global climate change has increased the frequency and intensity of extreme weather events (e.g. heavy precipitation and flooding). Approaches to reduce the health risks associated with floods has become a major concern for disaster health response and risk management in China.

The Sichuan province is situated in the south-west of the China. It is one of the most disaster-prone provinces frequently affected by natural hazards, including earthquake, floods, and landslides (e.g. the Wenchuan earthquake in 2008 which killed more than 80,000 people and was one of the most catastrophic natural disasters in human history). Meanwhile, despite not being seen as devastating, flooding also poses a major health protection threat due to its highly recurrent nature and its relationship to climate change. Flooding hazard potentially causes severe economic losses and more severe negative health effects to local communities in the long run.

Using routinely collected provincial data, a study attempts to quantify and describe the spatial distribution of vulnerability to the health impacts at prefectural levels of flooding disaster which occurred in Sichuan in 2016. Based on the result of this assessment, community adaptive capacity is associated with the sensitivity or the extent of human health effect of a prefecture. In this study, adaptive capacity refers to the ability to adapt to the threat and reduce potential losses or cope with the health consequences of natural disasters. Regular health vulnerability assessment is strongly recommended to identify the potential gaps and to support evidence-based policy-making in disaster risk reduction and preparedness. Resources can be better allocated to provide early warning and intervention efforts to those communities vulnerable to natural disasters.

Source: Wang, Yang, Sun, Jinghuan, Li, and Chan (2019).

Energy transition

Moving away from reliance on human and animal energy towards fossil fuel energy has shaped a new form of society in the twentieth century. Achieving a modern, globalized, energy-intense standard of living has become almost universally a norm, particularly in countries with an active middle class. The **energy transition** is described as a series of steps from traditional energies (usually renewable) towards fossil fuels such as coal, gas, and oil, and then to nuclear and various renewable energy sources. While access to energy and energy source transitions have benefits to society, transportation, communications, and public health, the current widespread reliance on fossil fuels brings direct risks to human health from toxic pollution (i.e. cardiac, respiratory, and neurological effects).

Moreover, energy distribution is unequal. For example, many countries in South East Asia face shortfalls in meeting energy demands. A total of 95% of people do not have access to adequate modern clean energy in Indonesia, Cambodia, Myanmar, and the Philippines. Reliance on traditional use of burning biomass, rapid urbanization, and increasing energy demands cause substantial air quality issues. Most of the PM emissions from households are from the use of fuel wood and charcoal for cooking and heating, with 40% of the population reliant on solid biomass for cooking (International Energy Agency [IEA], 2017) (see also Chapter 6).

With the rapid socio-economic development in developing countries, large expansion in a region's power system will be required (coal and renewables accounting for almost 70% of new capacity). Coal-based power source will remain as 40% of the global total energy requirement mix by 2040 (IEA, 2017). Despite the uncertainty of clean energy use, the declining energy cost also means more energy access in remote areas. Energy transition offers an opportunity for new, affordable policy and technology options, which offer energy security and environmental benefits, but this requires substantial investment (IEA, 2017) (see Case Box 8.13).

Case Box 8.13 New Energies and Crises

Various forms of renewable, non-combustible, and supposedly clean new energy like solar, wind, tidal, hydropower, and geothermal energy can reduce carbon emission to benefit both the environment and human health. However, many of these new energies have meteorological, temporal, or geographical limitations. Nuclear energy, while free of these limitations, brings its own problems and poses huge environmental risks. In 2016, nuclear power and hydropower accounted for 10.4% and 16.6% of global electricity production, while wind, solar, tidal and other non-combustible energies combined constituted 5.6% (International Energy Agency, n.d.). In early 2019, there were 450 nuclear power reactors in operation and 55 under construction worldwide, with the highest concentration in East Asia, North America, and Western Europe, and the lowest in Latin America and Africa. The nuclear accidents in Chernobyl in 1986 and in Fukushima in 2011 reminded people of the environmental health risks involved (Chan, 2017). Dams built for the generation of hydropower destroy the landscape and result in deforestation and soil erosion. Facilities for solar and wind power also occupy precious land resources.

Technological transition

The impact of technology on human lives might be transformation in well-being mainten-ance. Not only will **technology transition** enhance efficiencies in transport, information exchange, and agriculture and industrial production, It should also simplify and reduce the cost of travel. Communication and information technology advances (e.g. the avail-ability of smartphone and the Internet) in particular has facilitated access to education and learning, expertise exchange, and service efficiencies (e.g. medical record keeping and design). Notably, more global travel might lead to unforeseeable environmental costs (e.g. air and noise pollution, and transport-related accidents) and challenges in disease control associated with people, animal, and product movement within and across na-tional boundaries. In addition, although technology advances enhance food and agricul-tural production efficiencies (more food with less resources/time input), the long-term health implications of consuming these food products (e.g. genetically modified food) are yet to be proven. Information access via technology is adopted by different segments of society differently and total reliance on new technology in health protection (e.g. risk communication) might bring unintended effect of creating 'left-behind' populations (see Case Box 8.14 on risk communication in extreme weather events).

Case Box 8.14 Community Capacity Building Through More Effective Risk Communication: Evidence-Based Recommendations for an Urban Chinese City

Gloria Kwong-wai Chan, Heidi H. Y. Hung, and Zhe Huang

Risk communication plays a role in every aspect of community capacity building, from disseminating risk information, building risk literary, developing public know-ledge about relevant disaster risk, shaping public practices including personal hygiene, uptake of vaccination, and improving individual and household level preparedness. Effective communication about health risks and related self-help approaches in ex-treme events and disaster may be a critical factor in community capacity building for better resilience. Tools and approaches should be developed to target community com-munication patterns and information needs. Research has indicated that effectiveness of risk communication may be associated with various community determinants, such as social demographic characteristics, previous disaster experiences, as well as health governance and systems.

The Collaborating Centre for Oxford University and CUHK for Disaster and Medical Humanitarian Response (CCOUC) conducted a series of studies in Hong Kong, fo-cusing in particular on individual and household preparedness and significance of warning dissemination channels. Given its location as a developed coastal metrop-olis in the Pacific Rim region and its subtropical climate, the topography and built environment of high skyscraper-based Hong Kong is vulnerable to the impact of ty-phoons, floods, and fires. Its high-density living context, heavy reliance of infrastruc-ture lifeline support, and active population movement (e.g. travellers) have rendered the

Case Box 8.14 Community Capacity Building Through More Effective Risk Communication: Evidence-Based Recommendations for an Urban Chinese City *(continued)*

Hong Kong population at high risk of infectious diseases such as avian influenza A (H5N1) in 1997 and 2003, the SARS epidemic in 2003, and swine influenza H1N1 in 2009.

Research in recent years has, however, found that general public perception of disaster remained low, with only 12.8% of the respondents considering Hong Kong susceptible to disasters. The level of household preparedness, as quantified by preparedness measures (equipped with a first aid kit, basic aids supplies, emergency food and drinking water, basic medication, and a fire extinguisher), was also low, with only 28.3% of the respondents equipped with all items. Such findings indicated that disaster risk communication in Hong Kong needs to start from basic risk literacy and aims to encourage a more active role at individual and household levels (Chan, Yue, Lee, and Wang, 2016). The limited knowledge, awareness, and action of the public echoed the findings of previous studies conducted specifically on the A/H7N9 influenza epidemic in mainland China, coinciding with a period of high levels of seasonal flu in Hong Kong. Studies found that in spite of the previous experience of having SARS cases brought into Hong Kong from mainland China, the Hong Kong public had a poor understanding of H7N9 influenza and were practising protective measures sufficiently. It was hypothesized that prolonged health risk warnings might have caused public fatigue towards outbreaks, and hence indicated the need to pay special attention to risk communication in the context of repeated outbreaks (Chan, Cheng, Tam, Huang, and Lee, 2015a). Another study conducted in the context of A/H7N9 on community capacity building was concerned with the public attitude towards vaccine uptake, which is one of the most important public health measures for disease outbreak prevention. It was found that more than 60% of respondents confused seasonal influenza and A/H7N9 influenza and willingness to get vaccinated was affected by anxiety level and vaccine history, independent of socio-demographic factors (Chan, Cheng, Tam, Huang, and Lee, 2015b). This finding contradicted sharply with the factors found to be associated with other protective behaviours, including personal hygiene, being female, older age, living in the city centre, and being a white-collar worker (Chan et al., 2015a). Such findings supported the need to develop specific communication and education strategies for community vaccine uptake promotion, as opposed to other forms of protective behaviours.

Apart from a general understanding about the risk knowledge and preparedness level of the public, it is of utmost importance to identify the effective communication channels for the community. Following advances in mobile communications, communication channels, or warning/risk information dissemination channels are being developed rapidly, in particular smartphone and related mobile applications. CCOUC studies conducted in 2014 and 2016 revealed an extremely interesting finding in terms of risk information dissemination channels. A study conducted in 2014 on infectious disease outbreak preparedness indicated that the preferred channels to obtain

Case Box 8.14 Community Capacity Building Through More Effective Risk Communication: Evidence-Based Recommendations for an Urban Chinese City *(continued)*

infectious disease information were television (56%) and the Internet (16%), while smartphone/apps were one of the least popular options (Chan, Huang, Mark, and Guo, 2017). Another study with similar methodology, a population-based, cross-sectional, random digit-dialling telephone survey, conducted in 2016 on communication channels for weather information acquisition found that TV and smartphone apps were reported to be the two most widely used channels, and among those who were not using a preferred channel, 61.3% would like to switch to a smartphone app (Chan, Huang, Mark, and Guo, 2017) (See Figure 8.1). While noting the differences in the research questions and other variations between the two studies, the dramatic rise in the popularity of smartphone apps warrants much attention: this could be because of more widespread use of smartphone app over the two years, or the difference in the qualities of smartphone app for infectious disease information dissemination (by health authorities) and weather information dissemination (by the observatory), or other factors that might prove to be critical in improving risk information communication. Further study for a better understanding on the risk information communication channels is therefore required.

For healthcare and health protection, technology can improve access to care and services, and enhance the capacity of a system to provide services to its target community. Better diagnosis technology might enhance screening and treatment capacity for disease throughout life course. Improved capacity to protect preventable disease manifestation and improve survival rates might be available from pre-natal diagnosis to early cancer screening. Information and communication technology (ICTs) for medicine and healthcare management lead to major developments in eHealth (the use of mobile devices for health purposes) and mobile health (mHealth). These advances allow better communications, data collection, trends and pattern prediction, and continuous health and medical education. It might also improve information sharing across the continuum of care and service providers (e.g. by sharing patient history-related information for better care management).

Scientific advances also allow new drug and vaccine development for disease prevention and health protection. New drugs and medicines might have fewer side-effects, longer storage times, and less storage specification (e.g. temperature requirement) to enable transportation of and access to relevant medications despite logistic challenges. Better treatment options might be available with improved biomaterials (to avoid tissue and immune rejection) that have better bio-compatibility. 3D-printing technology might provide body part replacement and support better recovery. Nanotechnology can increase a range of treatment possibilities from drug delivery to gene therapy. Genetic engineering enables better cancer treatment (e.g. gene therapy) and vector-borne disease control with genetically modified mosquitoes.

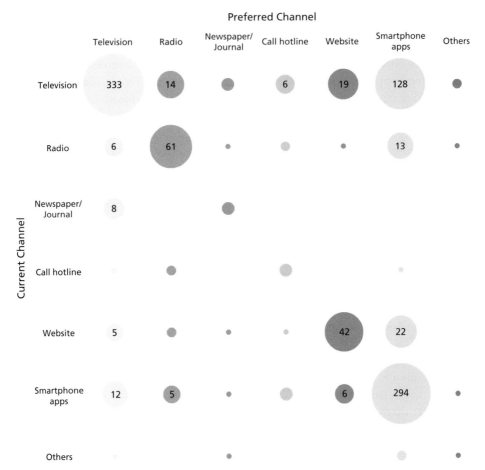

Figure 8.1 Comparison between current and preferred channels of weather information acquisition in Hong Kong, January/February 2016

Note: The number of each circle is the actual frequency. Numbers less than 5 were not shown in the figure.

Source: data from Chan, E. Y. Y. and Murray, V. (2017). What are the health research needs for the Sendai Framework? The Lancet, 390(10106), e35-e36. Copyright © 2017 Elsevier.

Nevertheless, even with all the advances in improving longevity and enhancing treatment options, technology brings with it uncertainty about the potential unintended environmental consequences (e.g. genetically modified mosquitoes might change natural ecological systems and subsequently threaten human health). As highlighted earlier, the range of technology options that improve health and well-being might not be accessible equally across the general population. In addition to the concern over equality, quality (biosecurity risks), services, and the ethics dimension of the utilization of these technologies should also be considered (see Case Box 8.5 on the potential use of technology and the issue of sex-ratio imbalance).

Nutrition transition

Nutrition transition describes the change of dietary pattern and the nutritional status of a community. It refers to the evolution of a low-variety, cereal-predominant diet to fat and sugary processed-food-based diet. Major health implications are observed with such dietary changes. Diet-related risk and disease profile of the community will change from risks of food insecurity (famine) and the development of nutritional deficiency associated diseases (e.g. stunting, wasting) to the risks of over-consumption of certain nutritional products (e.g. fat and refined sugar) and the development of non-communicable degenerative diseases such as obesity, diabetes, and cardiovascular and hypertension disease. Nutrition transition had been observed in a change in diet and physical activity witnessed in the twentieth century around the world as people had access to more resources. Modern societies tend to converge towards a 'Western' diet high in saturated fats, sugar, salt, and refined food (Popkin, 2002; Lo, Lyne, Chan, and Capon, 2018). Moreover, some important health determinant shifts that occur alongside with or preceding the nutrition transition are demographic (e.g. family planning leading to fewer children and less pressure on food, ageing, etc.) and epidemiological transitions (e.g. better infectious disease control and less susceptibility to nutrition deficiency as worm infestation may cause iron deficiency in children). Case Box 8.15 describes the phenomenon of the 'triple burden of malnutrition'.

Urban transition

Urban populations in the world continue to grow. While 55% of population in the world lived in urban areas in 2018, this proportion is anticipated to rise to 68% by 2050. Asia was home to 54% of the world's urban population in 2018. By 2050, India and China together with Nigeria in Africa will account for 35% of the projected growth of the global urban population (UN DESA, 2018). The growth in urban population also tend to be

---

Case Box 8.15 Triple Burden of Malnutrition in Asia

Rising incomes and food availability not only resulted in malnutrition rate reduction but also increased the burdens of obesity and associated non-communicable diseases potentially. In the twenty-first century, many countries are actually experiencing thee 'triple burden' of malnutrition (i.e. some segments of the population are experiencing wasting and stunting while others may suffer from overweight and obesity). Global stunting prevalence in 2016 was 22.9%. Prevalence of stunting in Asia among children below 5 years declined by 37% between 2000 and 2016 but remained high in many sub-regions. Nearly half of the 41 million children under 5 worldwide who were overweight or obese in 2016 lived in Asia.

Sources: Lo, Lyne, Chan, and Capon. (2018), WHO (2018c).

in countries that are prone to natural hazards. It was estimated that by 2050, the urban population exposed to cyclones will increase from 310 million to 680 million, while exposure to major earthquakes will increase from 370 million to 870 million (World Bank, 2009).

Urban transition describes the changes in population living context or lifestyle from being rural- to urban-based. This change might be related to population movement from rural to urban settlement (accounting for about 20–30% of urban population growth in Asia-Pacific region). It may also result from the change of material and service access of a population which lives in a context evolving from a rural into an urbanized context. People who are originally living in rural areas might be reclassified as 'living in urban areas' (i.e. '*in-situ* urbanization') (Zhu, 2000) and adopt an 'urbanized lifestyle'. Such change will subject the residents to both the positive and negative health risks that are associated with this lifestyle. Environmental changes will also follow an increasingly urbanized community. Air pollution, poor waste management, water safety and sanitation, and suboptimal housing of high-density living will render the population susceptible to infectious diseases outbreak, prompting challenges to health security (see Case Box 8.16).

The accepted notion of growing 'urban ill health' has been well described (Lang and Rayner, 2012). Natural population growth occurs when births outnumber deaths and this

Case Box 8.16 Transitional Community in China

Zhe Huang and Emily Ying Yang Chan

A transitional community may be defined as a traditional rural village in the process of urbanization, representing an important living context with respect to villagers in rural China nowadays (Chan 2010; Chan, Ho, Huang, Kim, Lam, et al., 2018). Socio-economic development in these communities might often be related to the national policy of regional development as well the migration of workers who work in urban settings in cities. Theses migrant workers bring incomes, new ideas, and urban lifestyles when they return home (Chan, 2010). Although economic development improves material access and living standard of the village, villagers may lack the knowledge of health risks, and health-enhancing habits and practices due to the new way of life. Some undesirable and unhealthy lifestyles (e.g. a fatty diet) may become prevalent, and such risks might increase the prevalence of chronic diseases. Thus, many of the residents in transitional communities face the threat of chronic diseases in conjunction with the risks of pre-existing health problems (e.g. infectious diseases) in the high-speed of social transformation. This double burden has formed a special background for rural health problems during this period. Health needs in transitional communities are complex, and health education should be tailored and evaluated to raise awareness, promote habit-changing behaviour, and minimize unfavourable health outcomes.

phenomenon accounts for about 60% of urban growth worldwide. Intense living density and urban poverty results in increasing vulnerability to disaster events in developing countries. Unless proactive disaster risk reduction efforts can be invested in these communities, people in Asia, the global region with the fastest growing megacities in low-lying areas like Bangkok, Dhaka, Ho Chi Minh City, Jakarta, and Kolkata, will be vulnerable to extreme event risks.

Growing inequality and urban consumption patterns pose challenge to health protection. Demands in housing, education, health services, and transportation will all subject to pressure of urban population growth. The ageing populations in many areas and changing gender roles due to the improved education and employment of women and falling fertility rates will pose special challenges for future Asian cities. Various pollutions (e.g. air, noise, and light) have specific health, environmental/climate, and economic consequences as people move away to less polluted areas (Landrigan, 2017). Despite the challenges of urban transition, cities. The opportunity to build a healthy and sustainable environment rests on planning, implementation, and determination of authorities and institutions.

Other challenges in health protection: health systems and regulation of the diversity of health services and systems

Traditional medicine and complementary medicine

Although Western medical systems have been the predominant international scientific cornstone for how medical and health services are structured, complementary or alternative medical systems also significantly contribute to health and medical service provision globally. Traditional medicine and complementary medicine (T&CM) provides important resources to bridge health service gaps in many health systems throughout the world. However, medical pluralism, the co-existence and the use of more than one type of medical approach, is not a common system or policy practice across the globe. Regulations and policies towards T&CM practitioners and formal access to related treatment and products vary. To effectively protect community health, T&CM presents a number of challenges in communities health protection management in communities. In some countries, especially in Asia and Africa, 80% of the population may depend on traditional medicine (TM) for their primary healthcare. Nevertheless, the lack of relevant scientific evidence, capacity to establish good quality control, application of safety standards, and priority setting based on effectiveness of treatment approaches are some major gaps hampering health protection efforts. Unqualified practitioners, misdiagnosis or delayed of treatment of conventional treatments, poor quality, adulterated, or counterfeit products, exposure to misleading information, and direct adverse health effects (e.g. poisoning incidents) are some health risks associated with potential services and use of traditional and complementary drugs and health products (WHO, 2013a) (see Case Box 8.17 on adverse health events of over-the-counter drugs).

Case Box 8.17 Adverse Events of Over-the-Counter Chinese Herbal Medicine

Jean H. Kim

Limited published literature is available to understand prevalence and factors associated with adverse events of over-the-counter traditional Chinese herbal medicine (COTC) despite its common use in the treatment of everyday illness in many parts of the world. A cross-sectional telephone survey was conducted among Hong Kong Chinese adults in 2011 ($n = 1100$) with informed verbal consent. Stepwise logistic regression of demographic, attitudinal, and behavioural variables was used to determine factors associated with past-year adverse events. Of study respondents, 71.7% reported past-year COTC use and 2.3% reported at least one COTC-related adverse event in the past year. Of the 27 adverse events cases reported among COTC users, the most common were allergic reactions, dizziness, and gastrointestinal problems. Pills/capsules were the dosage form that caused the highest proportion of adverse events, followed by plasters, creams/ointments, and ingestible powders. A large proportion of COTC users demonstrated low levels of COTC-related knowledge, while the main impediment to greater information-seeking was the belief that reliable COTC information is not obtainable from Western health professionals. Although COTC users reporting adverse events were more likely to report adopting more practices to avoid adverse events (OR = 6.47; 95% CI: 1.38–30.3), they were also more likely to come from lower education levels (OR = 9.64, 95% CI: 2.20–42.3) and to have received COTC information from non-reliable, mass-media information sources such as magazines (OR = 3.32; 95% CI: 1.01–8.50) or TV (OR = 2.93; 95% CI: 1.03–10.7). Around 42.9% of COTC users found information on package labels unclear.

Source: Kim, Kwong, Chung, Lee, Wong, et al (2013).

With the increased access to and distribution of health and medical products internationally, protecting the health and well-being of users will be an important aspect in health protection. Traditional approaches adopted by national drug/poison regulation mechanisms might not be able to monitor the use of products beyond national boundaries and with international access. In addition, despite global movements toward more stringent complementary medicine regulation, the unequal global distribution of reliable information and widespread misperceptions among consumers present major challenges to the safe use of complementary medicine (Kim, Kwong, Chung, Lee, Wong, et al., 2013). Whilst better integration of T&CM services into the formal healthcare systems might enhance monitoring and coordination, inertia from formal medical establishments, business communities (e.g. insurance services provider), as well as scientific community will remain important obstacles. To ensure health protection, approaches might be needed to facilitate cross-training (western medicine and T&CM), regulations, and monitoring of potential health consequences of T&CM services.

Research methodology

In the face of the challenges and issues in environmental and health risks that require cross-national and multi-disciplinary solutions, new methodologies (see Case Boxes 8.18 and 8.19) and corresponding awareness toward related ethical issues are urgently needed (Chan, Wright, and Parker, 2019).

Although 'health-protection effectiveness' is often measured by a lack of incidents/emergencies, with all the health threats and challenges of the twenty-first century, not all significant incidents might be anticipated or preventable. For example, the impact of disasters on cities with a greater concentration of people can be devastating. Poorer segments of population are particularly vulnerable in disasters, especially when a significant proportion live in more hazardous settlements and lack the necessary safety nets to recover from economic or environmental shocks (World Bank, 2018a). It is estimated that 10% of the world's population (i.e. 735.9 million people) lived on less than US$1.90 a day in 2015 despite a noted progress in poverty reduction from 2013. The poverty rate was 12.4% in South Asia, 2.3% in East Asia, and 1.5% in Central Asia, compared to 41.1% in Sub-Saharan Africa (World Bank, 2018b).

In order to offer health protection to a community, a robust system, relevant decision-making supporting scientific evidence, clear communication and education capacity, and strong multi-disciplinary partnership (Commonwealth, 2016; Ghebrehewet, Stewart, Baxer, Shears, Conrad, et al., 2016) are required.

Case Box 8.18 The Health Vulnerability Index

Zhe Huang and Emily Ying Yang Chan

The ability to measure vulnerability is a crucial step to strengthen action to protect health. Conducting vulnerability assessment helps identify people at high risks of health effect as well as specify solutions to respond (WHO, 2013b). However, there are major technical gaps to describe vulnerability since existing vulnerability indicators/indexes mostly focus on economic and social vulnerability. Even though some vulnerability indicators/indexes include health elements, they neglect an important health-affecting factor, chronic disease, which has been cited as the most important cause of mortality and morbidity (WHO, 2009). In addition, vulnerability assessment is subject to the country's own method and capacity in data collection, raising difficulties for multi-country comparisons.

A Health Vulnerability Index (Chan, Huang, Lam, Wong, and Zou, 2019) is proposed using open-access data. The indicators identified are publicly available in most countries, making country comparison possible. Suggested indicators include proportion of population below 15 years and above 65 years, under-5 mortality ratio, maternal mortality ratio, prevalence of tuberculosis, the age-standardized raised blood pressure, physician ratio, hospital bed ratio, and coverage of the MCV1 and DTP3 vaccines. Findings could provide evidence to support health risk reduction, and serve as a basis for the development of a population-based risk assessment tool.

Case Box 8.19 Future of Environmental Epidemiology

Peter Ka-hung Chan

In the twenty-first century, environmental epidemiology is set to face major challenges from global climate change, urbanization, and demographic transition. Substantially more people are exposed to emerging environmental risk factors such as ambient air pollution, extreme temperature events, and loss of green space, especially in low- and middle-income countries (Nieuwenhuijsen, 2016; Intergovernmental Panel on Climate Change [IPCC], 2018). While challenges from infectious diseases remain, the global disease burden will continue to be dominated by chronic non-communicable diseases, which are already the leading causes of premature mortality globally. These changing exposure and disease patterns pose new challenges for understanding how the ever-changing environmental risks are interrelated, linked to social and behavioural risk exposures (e.g. reduced physical activity due to air pollution), and impact population health.

Nonetheless, the emerging challenges come with new opportunities. There have been rapid advances in exposure assessment technologies, particularly wearable sensors and OMICs assays (Tonne, Basagana, Chaix, Huynen, Hystad, et al., 2017). As the costs of sensor and OMICs technologies continue to decline and more large-scale biobanks are established, comprehensive and accurate assessment of personalized, multi-dimensional environmental exposures will be increasingly feasible. This will lead to an explosion of data across the internal and external 'exposome', the totality of human environmental exposures during a lifetime. While this brings enormous opportunities for holistic and in-depth quantification of the dose–response relationships of a range of environmental exposures with adverse health outcomes, more advanced statistical methods are urgently needed to integrate data from vastly different sources and to account for the complex inter-exposure correlation. There is also a pressing need to establish systematic protocols to evaluate the reliability, validity, and practicality of wearable sensors, both in laboratory and field-based settings, in order to distinguish the robust scientific instruments from less reliable consumer products, as the commercial market grows rapidly. More importantly, one must strike a balance between conventional hypothesis-driven investigations and data-driven exploration in order to find the right path in the woods.

Preparing cities for disaster risks and strengthening resilience is fundamental to ensuring sustainable development and poverty reduction. The concept of disaster resilience has gained wide interest, especially after the adoption of the Hyogo Framework for Action 2005–2015: Building the Resilience of Nations and Communities to Disasters (hereafter 'Hyogo Framework'), with the main goal of hazard planning, and disaster prevention, preparedness, and mitigation shifting to focus more on building community resilience rather than reducing vulnerability. The Sendai Framework for Disaster Risk Reduction 2015–2030 (hereafter 'Sendai Framework') succeeding the Hyogo Framework focuses on disaster risk management, with reduction of disaster risk as an expected outcome, and health resilience promoted throughout the framework.

The concept of 'resilience' is frequently discussed alongside with health protection. **Resilience** is the ability of a system, community, or society that is exposed to hazards to resist, absorb, accommodate, and recover from the effects of a hazard in a timely and efficient manner (United Nations International Strategy for Disaster Reduction [UNISDR], 2009; Chan, 2017). **Disaster preparedness** refers to specific 'activities', often intentional, that seek to reduce disaster risk, while resilience is a parameter that describes a **condition** of an individual, a community, or a country, which can improve survival and capacity to absorb shock and stress. Raising preparedness would increase resilience, but other circumstances that may not constitute preparedness activities, such as previous exposures to incidents/ disasters or having a stable healthcare workforce, are also factors that enhance resilience.

Resilience building to ensure health protection is a common feature shared across disciplines which seek to protect community well-being (Castleden, McKee, Murray, and Leonardi, 2011). Communication, learning (education, knowledge), adaptation, risk awareness, social capital (trust, social cohesion), good governance, planning/preparedness, redundancy, economic capacity and diversification, well-being (physical, mental) are some key characteristics discussed in their thinking. Case Box 8.20 describes efforts to build bottom-up Health-EDRM for community resilience in rural communities (Chan, 2018).

Case Box 8.20 The Ethnic Minority Health Project in Rural China for Bottom-up Health Emergency and Disaster Risk Management (Health-EDRM) for Community Resilience

Gloria Kwong-wai Chan, Heidi H. Y. Hung, Carol Ka-po Wong, and Emily Ying Yang Chan

Across the world, ethnic minority communities are often associated with higher disaster risk due to poverty, social segregation, residence in unsafe settlement, etc. (Chan, 2018). Health protection in these communities is challenging as underlying socio-demographic-social vulnerabilities mean higher health risks. Physical, psychological, and social impacts of extreme events and disasters in ethnic minorities are often more severe, and they tend to have less resilience or capacity to bounce back. In order to develop bottom-up health risk reduction efforts in emergency and disaster risk management among ethnic minorities in China, the Collaborating Centre for Oxford University and CUHK for CCOUC initiated the multi-site-based Ethnic Minority Health Project (EMHP) in 2009 in remote, poor, and disaster-prone ethnic minority villages in China with the following objectives (CCOUC, 2018):

1. To empower vulnerable communities in rural and remote settings to prepare and mitigate the adverse impact of natural disasters;

2. To bring science to the people by adapting technical 'know-how' developed in academic settings to concrete practice in the field;

3. To develop human resources to work in rural and remote communities by offering practice and field-based trainings;

Case Box 8.20 The Ethnic Minority Health Project in Rural China for Bottom-up Health Emergency and Disaster Risk Management (Health-EDRM) for Community Resilience *(continued)*

4. To raise global awareness of issues related to disaster impact and preparedness among remote communities in developing countries; and

5. To document empirical findings to support future development of related intervention for other rural, community-based health projects.

Field-based interventions and social study laboratories were conducted to develop, implement, and evaluate public health interventions targeting health emergency and disaster risk management (Chan and Murray, 2017; Lo, Chan, Chan, Murray, Ardalan., 2017) appropriate for the specific settings of individual sites and research findings were generated. An early mixed-method study from the EMHP conducted in a predominately Hui minority-based village in Gansu Province indicated that while previous disaster exposure was significantly associated with a higher disaster risk perception, the perception did not translate into preparedness effort, as only 10.7% of households possessed a disaster emergency kit, and only 9.6% of households with chronic disease patients stockpiled medications (Chan, Kim, Lin, Cheung, and Lee, 2014). The study findings indicated the need to understand the barriers behind carrying out basic preparedness action in spite of the knowledge and perceptions about the disaster risk. Communication and education efforts demonstrating the benefits of preparedness efforts and removing the barriers would suit the needs of such vulnerable communities.

With increasing knowledge about the disaster risk perceptions and practices of different ethnic minority communities in China and the general level of preparedness, public health interventions practicable for resource-deficient settings were then developed and tested under the EMHP. CCOUC developed the disaster preparedness kit with reference to the principles under the Sphere Standards, public health principles, and the specific needs of the ethnic minority-based community and its individuals. The experience of developing a disaster preparedness kit as a disaster risk reduction intervention at community level under the EMHP was shared and reviewed in a recent international study on 'grab bags', which found that these had now been widely recognized as a major disaster risk reduction strategy, but more evidence was called for on the effectiveness of such measure in order to justify the necessary investment (Chan, Guo, Lee, Liu, and Mark, 2017; Pickering, O'Sullivan, Morris, Mark, McQuirk, et al., 2018) (see Figure 8.2).

Two major public health interventions that have been studied to build bottom-up community resilience in the ethnic minority regions are the preparation of homemade oral rehydration solutions (ORS) and the possession of a disaster preparedness kit. The experience of an ethnic Yi community in Sichuan Province, which had experienced recurrent floods, was analysed and documented. Villagers were educated on the preparation of ORS and allocated disaster a preparedness kit, and a 12-month follow-up study found that project participants retained the knowledge on both ORS and disaster preparedness kit intervention (Chan et al., 2017). Another study also found intervention resulted in temporal stability (Chan, Ho et al., 2018).

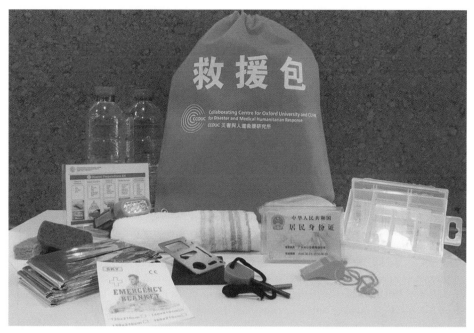

Figure 8.2 Disaster preparedness kit/'grab bag' distributed under the EMHP by the CCOUC

As highlighted with the various transitions of macro-determinants of health, health sectors, regardless of development status, are facing pressure to evolve, adapt, and cope with changes and the risks of health protections. Legido-Quigley and Asagari-Jirhandeh (2018) argued that a resilient health system had to be people-centred, which included planning people's experiences as they moved through the journey to health. Such a system should also be resilient in order to absorb, respond to, and recover from various challenges from natural disasters and infectious disease outbreaks to the growing burden of non-communicable diseases to challenges posed by the population ageing. Moreover, the quality of care in such systems should be monitored and safeguarded by regulatory mechanisms. Universal health coverage (UHC) offers an important platform for reducing inequality and increase resilience to pressures such as climate change.

Conclusion

Macro health determinants that influence well-being and health outcomes are discussed in this chapter. In addition to understanding the dynamics of transitions in health risks and new choices in ecosystems described here, public health workers, researchers, and policy-makers should be aware of the need to confront what constitutes 'normality' and revisit the 'necessary' health harm of an action or a policy (Rayner and Lang, 2012). Public health is a field of study that offers a conceptual framework regarding how health and public health implications affect the transformational relationships between people, behavioural, environmental, social, and cultural circumstances. In the coming decades, new conceptual frameworks will be developed in public health and these new ideas are likely to be interdisciplinary and multidisciplinary to facilitate the formulation of approaches required to address the range of health risks that confront, and the best methods to protect, the community.

References

Alzheimer's Disease International (2014). Dementia in the Asia Pacific region: Alzheimer's Disease International report 2014. Available at: https://www.alz.co.uk/adi/pdf/Dementia-Asia-Pacific-2014.pdf.

Bray, F., Ferlay, J., Soerjomataram, I., Siegel, R. L., Torre, L. A., et al. (2018). Global cancer statistics 2018: GLOBOCAN estimates of incidence and mortality worldwide for 36 cancers in 185 countries. *CA: Cancer 68*(6) 394–424. doi: 10.3322/caac.21492.

Caldwell, J., Findley, S., Caldwell. P., Santow, G., Crawford, W., et al. (1990). *What We Know About Health Transition: The Cultural, Social and Behavioral Determinants of Health.* Canberra: Australia National University Printing Services.

Castleden, M., McKee, M., Murray, V., and Leonardi, G. (2011). Resilience thinking in health protection. *J Public Health 33*(3) 369–77. doi:10.1093/pubmed/fdr027.

Chan, E. Y. Y. (2017). *Public Health Humanitarian Responses to Natural Disasters.* London: Routledge.

Chan, E. Y. Y. (2018). *Building Bottom-up Health and Disaster Risk Reduction Programmes.* Oxford: Oxford University Press.

Chan, E. Y. Y., Cheng, C. K., Tam, G., Huang, Z., and Lee, P. (2015a). Knowledge, attitudes, and practices of Hong Kong population towards human A/H7N9 influenza pandemic preparedness, China, 2014. *BMC Public Health 15*(1) 943. doi:10.1186/s12889-015-2245-9.

Chan, E. Y. Y., Cheng, C. K. Y., Tam, G., Huang, Z., and Lee, P. Y. (2015b). Willingness of future A/H7N9 influenza vaccine uptake: A cross-sectional study of Hong Kong community. *Vaccine 33*(38) 4737–40. doi:10.1016/j.vaccine.2015.07.046.

Chan, E. Y. Y., Guo, C., Lee, P., Liu, S., and Mark, C. K. M. (2017). Health Emergency and Disaster Risk Management (Health-EDRM) in remote ethnic minority areas of rural China: The case of a flood-prone village in Sichuan. *Int J Disast Risk Sc 8*(2) 156–63. doi:10.1007/s13753-017-0121-1.

Chan, E. Y. Y., Ho, J. Y., Huang, Z., Kim, J. H., Lam, H. C., et al. (2018). Long-term and immediate impacts of Health Emergency and Disaster Risk Management (Health-EDRM) education interventions in a rural Chinese earthquake-prone transitional village. *Int J Disast Risk Sc 9*(3) 319–30.

Chan, E. Y. Y., Huang, Z., Lam, H. C. Y., Wong, C. K. P., et al. (2019). Health Vulnerability Index for disaster risk reduction: Application in Belt and Road Initiative (BRI) region. *Int J Environ Res Public Health 16*(3) 380.

Chan, E. Y. Y., Huang, Z., Mark, C. K. M., and Guo, C. (2017). Weather information acquisition and health significance during extreme cold weather in a subtropical city: A cross-sectional survey in Hong Kong. *Int J Disast Risk Sc 8*(2) 134–44. doi:10.1007/s13753-017-0127-8

Chan, E. Y. Y., Kim, J. H., Lin, C., Cheung, E. Y. L., and Lee, P. P. Y. (2014). Is previous disaster experience a good predictor for disaster preparedness in extreme poverty households in remote Muslim minority based community in China? *J Immigr Minor Health 16*(3) 466–72. doi:10.1007/s10903-012-9761-9.

Chan, E. Y. Y. and Murray, V. (2017). What are the health research needs for the Sendai Framework? *The Lancet 390*(10106) e35–e36.

Chan, E. Y. Y., Wright, K., and Parker, M. (2019). Health-emergency disaster risk management and research ethics. *The Lancet, 393* 112–13.

Chan, E. Y. Y., Yue, J., Lee, P., and Wang, S. S. (2016). Socio-demographic predictors for urban community disaster health risk perception and household based preparedness in a Chinese urban city. *PLoS Currents*. doi:10.1371/currents.dis.287fb7fee6f9f4521af441a236c2d519.

Chan, K. W. (2010). The global financial crisis and migrant workers in China: 'There is no future as a labourer; Returning to the village has no meaning'. *Int J Urban Reg Res 34*(3) 659–77.

Chan, T. C., Zhang, Z., Lin, B. C., Lin, C., Deng, H. B., et al. (2018). Long-term exposure to ambient fine particulate matter and chronic kidney disease: A cohort study. *Environ Health Perspect 126*(10) 107002.

Chen, S., Boyle, L. L., Conwell, Y., Xiao, S., and Chiu, H. F. K. (2014). The challenges of dementia care in rural China. *Int Psychogeriatr 26*(07) 1059–64. doi:10.1017/s1041610214000854.

Collaborating Centre for Oxford University and CUHK for Disaster and Medical Humanitarian Response (2018). Ethnic Minority Health Project. Available at: http://www.ccouc.ox.ac.uk/home-5.

The Commonwealth (2016). Commonwealth health ministers meeting 2016: Ministerial statement. Available at: http://thecommonwealth.org/sites/default/files/events/documents/Ministerial%20Statement%20-%20Commonwealth%20Health%20Ministers%20Meeting%202016.pdf.

Dua, T., Seeher, K. M., Sivananthan, S., Chowdhary, N., Pot, A. M., et al. (2017). World Health Organization's global action plan on the public health response to dementia 2017-2025. *Alzheimers Dement 13*(7, Suppl) P1450–Pl1451. doi:10.1016/j.jalz.2017.07.758.

Gavi (2019). About Gavi. Available at: https://www.gavi.org/about/.

Ghebrehewet, S., Stewart, A. G., Baxer, D., Shears, P., Conrad, D., et al. (2016). *Health Protection Principles and Practice*. Oxford: Oxford University Press.

Global Footprint Network (2018). Ecological footprint. Available at: https://www.footprintnetwork.org/our-work/ecological-footprint/.

Guo, C., Zhang, Z., Lau, A. K. H., Lin, C. Q., Chuang, Y. C., et al. (2018). Effect of long-term exposure to fine particulate matter on lung function decline and risk of chronic obstructive pulmonary disease in Taiwan: A longitudinal, cohort study. *Lancet Planetary Health 2* e114–e125.

Hanefeld, J. and Lee, K. (2015). Introduction to globalization and health. In J. Hanefeld (Ed.), *Globalization and health* (Understanding Public Health Series; 2nd ed.; pp. 1–13). Maidenhead, England: Open University Press.

Hay, S. I., Abajobir, A. A., Abate, K. H., Abbafati, C., Abbas, K. M., et al. (2017). Global, regional, and national disability-adjusted life-years (DALYs) for 333 diseases and injuries and healthy life expectancy (HALE) for 195 countries and territories, 1990-2016: A systematic analysis for the Global Burden of Disease Study 2016. *Lancet 390*(10100) 1260–344.

Hong Kong Breast Cancer Foundation (2018). Hong Kong Breast Cancer Registry report No. 10. Available at: http://www.hkbcf.org/document/BCR10_Fullview_01.pdf.

Hong Kong Cancer Registry, Hospital Authority (2018). Hong Kong cancer statistics 2016: Cancer registration in Hong Kong. Available at: http://www3.ha.org.hk/cancereg/pdf/overview/Summary%20of%20CanStat%202016.pdf.

Hutchinson, E. and Kovats, S. (2016). *Environment, Health and Sustainable Development* (2nd edn). London: Open University Press.

International Diabetes Federation (2017). IDF diabetes atlas eighth edition. Available at: https://diabetesatlas.org/resources/2017-atlas.html.

Intergovernmental Panel on Climate Change (2018). Global warming of 1.5°C. Available at: https://www.ipcc.ch/sr15/.

International Energy Agency (n.d.). Electricity statistics. Available at: https://www.iea.org/statistics/electricity/.

International Energy Agency (2017). Southeast Asia energy outlook 2007. Available at: https://www.iea.org/southeastasia/.

International Atomic Energy Agency (2019). Power reactor information system (PRIS). Available at: https://pris.iaea.org/PRIS/home.aspx.

Jia, J., Wang, F., Wei, C., Zhou, A., Jia, X., et al. (2014). The prevalence of dementia in urban and rural areas of China. *Alzheimers Demen 10*(1) 1–9. doi:10.1016/j.jalz.2013.01.012.

Kessels, J. A., Recuenco, S., Navarro-Vela, A. M., Deray, R., Vigilato, M., et al. (2017). Pre-exposure rabies prophylaxis: A systematic review. *Bull WHO 95*(3) 210–19C. doi:10.2471/BLT.16.173039.

Kim, J. H., Kwong, E. M. S., Chung, V. C. H., Lee, J. C. O., Wong, T., et al. (2013). Acute adverse events from over-the-counter Chinese herbal medicines: A population-based survey of Hong Kong Chinese. *BMC Complement Altern Med 13* 336. doi:10.1186/1472-6882-13-336.

Kwong, A., Mang, O. W. K., Wong, C. H. N., Chau, W. W., and Law, S. C. (2011). Breast cancer in Hong Kong, Southern China: The first population-based analysis of epidemiological characteristics, stage-specific, cancer-specific, and disease-free survival in breast cancer patients: 1997–2001. *Ann Surg Oncol 18*(11) 3072–8. doi:10.1245/s10434-011-1960-4.

Lam, H. C. Y., Chan, E. Y. Y., Lo, E. S. K., Tsang, S. N. S., Man, A. Y. T., et al. (2019). *Sociodemographic predictors of knowledge, risk patterns and protective behaviours of dengue fever in subtropical city: The case of Hong Kong.* Paper presented at Annual Meeting of the International Society of Environmental Epidemiology, Netherlands.

Lam, H. C. Y., Chan, J. C. N., Luk, A. O. Y., Chan, E. Y. Y., and Goggins, W. B. (2018). Short-term association between ambient temperature and acute myocardial infarction hospitalizations for diabetes mellitus patients: A time series study. *PLoS Medicine 15*(7) e1002612. doi:10.1371/journal.pmed.1002612.

Lang, T. and Rayner, G. (2012). Ecological public health: The 21st century's big idea? *Br Med J 345* e5466. doi:10.1136/bmj.e5466.

Landrigan, P. L. (2017). Air pollution and health. *Lancet Public Health 2*(1) Pe4–e5. doi:10.1016/S2468-2667(16)30023-8.

Lee, K. (2005). Introduction to the global economy. In K. Lee and J. Collin (eds), *Global Change and Health*. Maidenhead: Open University Press, pp. 63–82.

Legido-Quigley, H. and Asagari-Jirhandeh, N. (2018). *Resilient and people-centred health systems: Progress, challenges and future directions in Asia*. Available at: https://apps.who.int/iris/bitstream/handle/10665/276045/9789290226932-eng.PDF?sequence=5&isAllowed=y.

Lindfield, M. and Steinberg, F. (2012). *Green Cities*. Manila: Asian Development Bank.

Lo, S., Lyne, K., Chan, E. Y. Y., and Capon, A. (2018). Planetary health and resilience in Asia. In H. Legido-Quigley and N. Asagari-Jirhandeh (eds), *Resilient and People-Centred Health Systems: Progress, Challenges and Future Directions in Asia* (pp. 56–93). Available at: https://apps.who.int/iris/bitstream/handle/10665/276045/9789290226932-eng.PDF?sequence=5&isAllowed=y.

Lo, S. T. T., Chan, E. Y. Y., Chan, G. K. W., Murray, V., Ardalan, A., et al. (2017). Health Emergency and Disaster Management (H-EDRM): Developing the research field within the Sendai Framework paradigm. *Int J Disast Risk Sc 8*(2) 145–9.

McCracken, K. and Philips, D. R. (2017). *Global Health: An Introduction to Current and Future Trends* (2nd edn). London: Routledge.

Nieuwenhuijsen, M. J. (2016). Urban and transport planning, environmental exposures and health—New concepts, methods and tools to improve health in cities. *Environ Health 15*(Suppl 1) S38.

Pickering, C. J., O'Sullivan, T. L., Morris, A., Mark, C., McQuirk, D., et al. (2018). The promotion of 'grab bags' as a disaster risk reduction strategy. *PLoS Currents 10*. doi:10.1371/currents.dis.223ac4322834aa0bb0d6824ee424e7f8.

Popkin, B. (2002). An overview on the nutrition transition and its health implications: The Bellagio meeting. *Public Health Nutr 5*(1A) 93–103.

Rayner, G. and Lang, T. (2012). *Ecological Public Health: Reshaping the Conditions for Good Health.* Abingdon: Routledge.

Sussman, A. L., Helitzer, D., Bennett, A., Solares, A., Lanoue, M., et al. (2015). Catching up with the HPV vaccine: Challenges and opportunities in primary care. *Ann Fam Med 13*(4) 354–60. doi:10.1370/afm.1821.

Tissandier, F. (2018). Gavi board starts framing alliance's approach to 2021–2025 period. Available at: https://www.gavi.org/library/news/press-releases/2018/gavi-board-starts-framing-alliance-s-approach-to-2021-2025-period/.

Tonne, C., Basagana, X., Chaix, B., Huynen, M., Hystad, P., et al. (2017). New frontiers for environmental epidemiology in a changing world. *Environ International 104* 155–62.

Wong, E. C., Kim, J. H., Goggins, W. B., Lau, J., Wong, S. Y. S., et al. (2018). Chinese women's drinking patterns before and after the Hong Kong alcohol policy changes. *Alcohol Alcohol 53*(4) 477–86. doi:10.1093/alcalc/agy010.

World Bank (2018a). City resilience program. Available at: https://www.worldbank.org/en/topic/disasterriskmanagement/brief/city-resilience-program.

World Bank (2018b). Poverty. Available at: https://data.worldbank.org/topic/poverty.

World Bank (2009). *Density and disasters: Economics of urban hazard risk* (Policy Research Working Paper No. 5161). Available at: http://documents.worldbank.org/curated/en/456301468148146720/pdf/WPS5161.pdf.

United Nations Department of Economic and Social Affairs (UN DESA) (2017) World population prospects: The 2017 revision. Available at: https://esa.un.org/unpd/wpp/publications/Files/WPP2017_KeyFindings.pdf.

United Nations Department of Economic and Social Affairs (UN DESA) (2018). 2018 revision of world urbanization prospects. Available at: https://population.un.org/wup/.

United Nations Development Programme (2016). Human development report 2016: Human development for everyone. Available at: http://hdr.undp.org/sites/default/files/2016_human_development_report.pdf.

United Nations International Strategy for Disaster Reduction (2009). 2009 UNISDR terminology on disaster risk reduction. Available at: https://www.unisdr.org/files/7817_UNISDRTerminologyEnglish.pdf.

Wang, S., Smith, H., Peng, Z., Xu, B., and Wang, W. (2016). Increasing coverage of hepatitis B vaccination in China: A systematic review of interventions and implementation experiences. *Medicine (Baltimore) 95*(19) e3693. doi:10.1097/MD.0000000000003693.

Wang, Z., Yang, Z., Sun, H., Jinghuan, R., Li, Q., and Chan, E. Y. Y. (2019). *The Spatial Distribution of Vulnerability to the Health Impacts of Flooding in Three Counties, Sichuan Province.* Beijing: Public Health Emergency Center & Branch for Health Hazards and Disaster Response. Chinese Center for Disease Control and Prevention.

Watts, N., Amann, M., Arnell, N., Ayeb-Karlsson, S., Belesova, K., et al. (2018). The 2018 report of the Lancet Countdown on health and climate change: Shaping the health of nations for centuries to come. *The Lancet 32*(10163) 2479–514.

World Health Assembly (2014). Strengthening of palliative care as a component of comprehensive care throughout the life course: Report by the Secretariat. Available at:: https://apps.who.int/iris/bitstream/handle/10665/158962/A67_31-en.pdf?sequence=1&isAllowed=y.

World Health Organization (2009). Global health risks: Mortality and burden of disease attributable to selected major risks. Available at: https://www.who.int/healthinfo/global_burden_disease/GlobalHealthRisks_report_full.pdf

World Health Organization (2013a). WHO traditional medicine strategy 2014–2023. Available at: http://www.searo.who.int/entity/health_situation_trends/who_trm_strategy_2014-2023. pdf?ua=1.

World Health Organization (2013b) . Protecting health from climate change: Vulnerability and adaptation assessment. Available at: http://www.who.int/iris/handle/10665/104200.

World Health Organization (2014). *Migration of Health Workers: The WHO Code of Practice and the Global Economic Crisis*. Geneva: WHO Document Production Services.

World Health Organization (2018a). Ambient (outdoor) air quality and health. Available at: http://www.who.int/en/news-room/fact-sheets/detail/ambient-(outdoor)-air-quality-and-health.

World Health Organization (2018b). Immunization. Available at: https://www.who.int/topics/immunization/en/.

World Health Organization (2018c). Obesity and overweight. Available at: https://www.who.int/news-room/fact-sheets/detail/obesity-and-overweight.

World Health Organization (2018d). Palliative care. Available at: https://www.who.int/en/news-room/fact-sheets/detail/palliative-care.

World Health Organization Western Pacific Regional Office (2017). Dengue fever and malaria: Global and regional situation summary. Available at: http://www.wpro.who.int/southpacific/programmes/communicable_diseases/malaria/page/en/index2.html.

Wu, C., Gao, L., Chen, S., and Dong, H. (2016). Care services for elderly people with dementia in rural China: A case study. *Bull WHO* 94(3) 167–73. doi:10.2471/blt.15.160929.

Wu, Y. T., Ali, G. C., Guerchet, M., Prina, A. M., Chan, K. Y., et al. (2018). Prevalence studies of dementia in mainland China, Hong Kong and Taiwan: An updated systematic review and meta-analysis. *Intern J Epidemiol* 47(3) 709–19. doi:10.1093/ije/dyy007.

Zhang, Z., Chan, T. C., Guo, C., Chang, L. Y., Lin, C., et al. (2018). Long-term exposure to ambient particulate matter ($PM_{2.5}$) is associated with platelet counts in adults. *Environ Pollut* 240 432–9.

Zhang, Z., Guo, C., Lau, A. K. H., Chan, T. C., Chuang, Y. C., et al. (2018). Long-term exposure to fine particulate matter, blood pressure, and incident hypertension in Taiwanese adults. *Environ Health Perspect* 126(1) 017008.

Zhang, Z. L., Chang, L. Y., Lau, A. K. H., Chan, T. C., Chuang, Y. C., et al. (2017). Satellite-based estimates of long-term exposure to fine particulate matter are associated with C-reactive protein in 30034 Taiwanese adults. *Int J Epidemiol* 46 1126–36.

Zhu, Y. (2000). *In situ* urbanization in rural China: Case studies from Fujian Province. *Dev Change* 31(2) 413–34.

Chapter 9

Health Protection and Health Risks in a Changing World

Protecting the health of the population has always been the main objectives of public health policies and actions. As illustrated throughout this book, human beings today face major challenges to manage a rapidly expanding repertoire of health risks as well as experience major transitions during their life courses. In an increasingly globalized, urbanized world, carelessness and suboptimal attempts in health protection in a densely populated, interconnected living context can easily transform a relatively minor localized health risk to catastrophic health outcomes that transcend national boundaries.

Due to the dynamic changes that influence modern living, the scope and nature of health protection will only become more complex. The decisions and choices human beings make influence future health trends and the well-being of our global population. In addition to the major health protection themes of emergency and disaster preparedness (including Health Emergency and Disaster Risk Management (Health-EDRM)), climate change, infectious disease control, environmental risks, and issues of sustainability and planetary health discussed earlier, various dynamics and transitions that may contribute to major changes in health profile and risks deserve careful monitoring and policy reconsideration. With longer life expectancies, changing disease patterns, and diversity of human habitat and consumption patterns, research and academic communities are presented with the enormous responsibility to catch up, propel knowledge advancement, and understand the health implications of these changes. Whilst some of the potential outcomes of health-shaping trends and risks may be predicted and extrapolated from previous patterns, health implication of many of the new phenomena (e.g. Natech events mentioned in Chapter 3) are yet to be mapped out.

Successful attempts in the protection of health and well-being of individuals are often invisible in a community. In a community that is supported by effective health-protection measures, the probability of escalating a known health risk to a catastrophic health-affecting event may be minimized. Moreover, policies and programmes that address the complex interaction of human, living and natural environments, socio-economic development, and technology advances may alter health risks as well as potentially create opportunities to improve and advance the welfare and well-being of the entire living ecosystems.

In the coming decades, the capacity to coordinate and participate in a multidisciplinary team and to work with interdisciplinary actors will be crucial in health protection.

Essentials for Health Protection. Emily Ying Yang Chan, Oxford University Press (2020).
© Oxford University Press
DOI: 10.1093/oso/9780198835479.001.0001

To protect health effectively, practitioners and workers in health protection, whether health- or non-health-based, must learn terminology, acquire knowledge and skills, and broach the frontiers of other relevant disciplines associated with health. The principles and concepts of public health introduced in this book serve as the basic knowledge building blocks to facilitate the conceptualization, analysis, identification, and evaluation of issues and potential solutions associated with human health and well-being in an increasingly complex world. Mutual learning and collaboration across disciplines and sectors will be essential to enable the formulation of effective cross-disciplinary policies and actions to protect health and well-being.

Nevertheless, the dynamic and complex interaction among human behaviour, living and natural environments, and technology advances are incessantly creating unknown health risks and threats. Human well-being depends on an environment that promotes health-enhancing opportunities and effectiveness in health protection attempts to control health risks. Policy-makers and public health practitioners must remain vigilant and resourceful to manage these ever-increasing emerging health risks. Ultimately, our collective intelligence, actions, and determination will dictate our capacity for protecting, maintaining, and improving the health and well-being of humanity in the twenty-first century.

Index

Tables, figures and boxes are indicated by *t, f* and *b* following the page number
For the benefit of digital users, indexed terms that span two pages (e.g., 52–53) may, on occasion, appear on only one of those pages.